Handbook of
Sports Medicine
and Science

Football (Soccer)

EDITED BY

Björn Ekblom MD
Karolinska Institute, Stockholm

OXFORD

Blackwell Scientific Publications

LONDON EDINBURGH BOSTON

MELBOURNE PARIS BERLIN VIENNA

© 1994 International Olympic Committee

Published by
Blackwell Scientific Publications
Editorial Offices:
Osney Mead, Oxford OX2 0EL
25 John Street, London WC1N 2BL
23 Ainslie Place, Edinburgh EH3 6AJ
238 Main Street, Cambridge
    Massachusetts 02142, USA
54 University Street, Carlton
    Victoria 3053, Australia

Other Editorial Offices:
Librairie Arnette SA
1, rue de Lille
75007 Paris
France

Blackwell Wissenschafts-Verlag GmbH
Düsseldorfer Str. 38
D-10707 Berlin
Germany

Blackwell MZV
Feldgasse 13
A-1238 Wien
Austria

First published 1994

Set by Setrite Typesetters, Hong Kong
Printed and bound by Bell and Bain Ltd., Glasgow

DISTRIBUTORS

Marston Book Services Ltd
PO Box 87
Oxford OX2 0DT
(*Orders*: Tel: 0865 791155
        Fax: 0865 791927
        Telex: 837515)

USA
    Blackwell Scientific Publications Inc.
    238 Main Street
    Cambridge, MA 02142
    (*Orders*: Tel: 800 759-6102
            617 876-7000)

Canada
    Times Mirror Professional Publishing Ltd
    130 Flaska Drive
    Markham, Ontario L6G 1B8
    (*Orders*: Tel: 800 268-4178
            416 470-6739)

Australia
    Blackwell Scientific Publications Pty Ltd
    54 University Street
    Carlton, Victoria 3053
    (*Orders*: Tel: 03 347-5552)

A catalogue record for this title
is available from the British Library

ISBN 0-632-03328-2

Library of Congress
Cataloging-in-Publication Data

Football (Soccer)/edited by Björn Ekblom.
        p.   cm.
    (Handbook of sports medicine and science)
    Includes bibliographical references
    and index.
    ISBN 0-632-03328-2
    1. Soccer.   2. Sports medicine.
    I. Ekblom, Björn.   II. Series.
    [DNLM: 1. Soccer — injuries.
    2. Soccer — physiology.
    3. Sports medicine.   QT 260 S6775 1994]
RC1220.S57S64   1994
617.1'027 — dc20
DNLM/DLC
for Library of Congress

Contents

List of contributors

Paul Balsom *Karolinska Institute, Stockholm, Sweden*

Jens Bangsbo *August Krogh Institute, Copenhagen, Denmark*

Carlos Bestit Carcasona *Barcelona, Spain* (died September 1993)

Björn Bolling *University of Sports, Stockholm, Sweden*

John Brewer *Lilleshall National Sports Centre, Lilleshall, UK*

Jackie Davis *Lilleshall National Sports Centre, Lilleshall, UK*

Jan Deneve *AZ St Jan, Brugge, Belgium*

Michel D'Hooghe *AZ St Jan, Brugge, Belgium*

Eric Dunning *University of Leicester, Leicester, UK*

Hans-Joerg Eissmann *DFB Football Training Centre, Leipzig, Germany*

Jan Ekstrand *University of Linköping, Linköping, Sweden*

Heinz Liesen *Sports Medicine Institute, Paderborn, Germany*

Pekka Luhtanen *University of Jyväskylä, Jyväskylä, Finland*

J. Michael Lynch *Pennsylvania State University, University Park, Pennsylvania, USA*

Stefan Muecke *Sports Medicine Institute, Paderborn, Germany*

Lars Peterson *Gothenburg Medical Center, Gothenburg, Nebraska, USA*

Thomas Reilly *John Moores University, Liverpool, UK*

Per Renström *University of Vermont College of Medicine, Burlington, Vermont, USA*

Roland Watteyne *AZ St Jan, Brugge, Belgium*

Clyde Williams *University of Loughborough, Loughborough, UK*

Forewords

On behalf of the International Olympic Committee I should like to welcome the new volume in our Handbook of Sports Medicine and Science series: *Football.*

My sincere appreciation goes to the IOC Medical Commission. This book will prove a valuable publication and will contribute in many ways to team coaches, athletic trainers, club physiotherapists and other health related professionals working with football players.

Juan Antonio Samaranch
Marqués de Samaranch

The International Olympic Committee's Medical Commission takes this opportunity to present the new volume in the Handbook of Sports Medicine and Science series: *Football.*

Our thanks go to the IOC Medical Commission's Publications Advisory Sub-Committee, with a special mention for the efforts of Professor Björn Ekblom and the contributing authors.

Prince Alexandre de Merode
Chairman, IOC Medical Commission

Acknowledgements

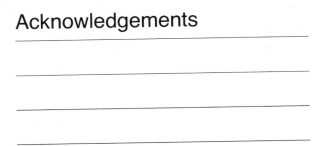

I wish to thank the Medical Commission of the International Olympic Committee and, in particular, Prince Alexandre de Merode for valuable support in the production of this handbook.

I also wish to acknowledge Howard G. Knuttgen for all his help and patience. His friendship and never-failing support throughout the years have ensured that this project could be finished.

Finally, to Blackwell Scientific Publications, Peter Saugman, Helen Harvey and Jane Andrew, I am most grateful for unfailing help and professional work.

Bjorn Ekblom
Stockholm, March 1994

Chapter 1

The history of football (soccer)

The first issue that has to be addressed in discussing the history of football is the origin and meaning of the terms "football" and "soccer." This is because, in virtually every country in the world, it is usual to refer to the game simply as "football" or by the translation of that English word into the native tongue, e.g. *Fussball* in German, *voetbal* in Dutch, *futebol* in Portuguese, *futbol* in Spanish, and *fotboll* in Swedish. The only exception in Europe is in Italy where use of the term *calcio* reflects the claim of that country to having been the birthplace of the modern game, though this claim is probably false. Although not so widely used as the term "football," in England the term "soccer" is widely understood. It is not so widely understood in continental Europe or Central and South America. In fact, the principal countries where the term "soccer" is used are those of North America where its use is made necessary by the fact that Americans and Canadians use "football" to refer to their native, "gridiron" games.

This discussion may seem needlessly pedantic; however, it is essential, if only because it is commonly believed outside Canada and the USA that "football" implies a solely or mainly kicking game, i.e. "soccer." Such a belief is erroneous. "Football" is a generic term which refers to a whole class of ball games, central among them being Association football (soccer), Rugby football, American football, Canadian football, Australian football, and Gaelic football. "Soccer" is a corruption of the term, "association", and thus refers to the highly specific Association way of playing. The term is said to have originated in the late nineteenth century at Oxford University when a student named Charles Wreford-Brown was asked one day by a friend at breakfast: "I say, Charles, are you playing rugger [Rugby] today?" "No," he replied, "I'm playing soccer" (Glanville 1969, p. 29). The practice of adding "-er" to

abbreviations was apparently fashionable among the English upper and middle classes at that time. Nevertheless, such a story is probably apocryphal. If it is not, it represents one of the few instances in the history of sport where the introduction of a specific practice can be authentically traced to a named individual. The key word in the last sentence is "authentically" for there are numerous mythical accounts which trace the origins of sports to the innovative actions of specific individuals and do not see the need to locate these individuals in a social context.

There are two broad kinds of mythical accounts of the origins of sports: those which trace them to the actions of an individual and those which trace them to a collection of individuals. An example of an individual origin myth in this field is the one which traces Rugby to the alleged deviant act in 1823 of William Webb Ellis, a Rugby schoolboy. Another example traces baseball to the alleged act of General Abner Doubleday in Cooperstown, New York, in 1839 (Gardner 1974, pp. 60–61; Dunning & Sheard 1979, p. 66). Both are highly implausible.

Most attempts to explain the origins of football are myths of the collective rather than the individual kind. Again, they take different forms. For example, it used to be believed in Kingston upon Thames, Surrey, that the local game traditionally played there each Shrove Tuesday originated from a Saxon defeat of Danish invaders in the early Middle Ages. The head of the defeated Danish chieftain, it was said, was kicked in celebration around the streets, and the game grew out of that. A similarly implausible belief used to be held in Derby, only this time the game is said to have originated from a defeat of Roman troops by native Britons in the third century AD (Marples 1954, pp. 6–7). Such beliefs are mythical because there is simply no evidence to support them from the time when the supposed originating events are said to have taken place.

Origin myths of an anthropologically more plausible kind trace the origins of football to a pagan fertility rite. Writing in 1929, for example, W.B. Johnson noted that it is common in primitive rituals for a globular object to symbolize the sun. In other words, the football is a symbolic representation of the bringer and supporter of life, a hypothesis which receives indirect support from the fact that *la soule*, the French name for a form of football which traditionally flourished in

Normandy and Brittany, appears to be cognate with *sol*, the Latin word for "sun" (Marples 1954, pp. 12–13). What is not explained in this origin myth, however, is why the symbolic sun should have been kicked and thrown around in what is generally agreed to have been a rough and physically dangerous game.

An earlier variant of this hypothesis was proposed by E.K. Chambers who argued that the football symbolically represents, not the sun, but the head of a sacrificial beast (Marples 1954, pp. 14–15). The object of the game, he conjectured, was for the players to get hold of the symbolic head and bury it on their lands in the hope of ensuring abundant crops. Indirect support for such a hypothesis was said to be provided by the fact that the object of some forms of folk football, for example that played at Scone in Scotland, was to place the ball in a hole (Marples 1954, p. 12). Further indirect support was said to come from "the Haxey Hood game," a folk ritual which still survives in Haxey, Lincolnshire. The "hood" in this game is a roll of sacking or leather and the aim of the players is to fight for possession of the roll and convey it to their respective village inns. That the roll or "hood" is the symbolic representation of an animal is said to be indicated by a speech traditionally made by "the Fool," an official in the ceremony, which takes place the day before the game. The relevant part of the Fool's speech goes as follows:

> We've killed two bullocks and a half but the other half we had to leave running field: we can fetch it if it's wanted. Remember it's
> *Hoose agin hoose, toon agin toon,*
> *And if you meet a man, knock him doon.**
> (Marples 1954, pp. 14–15)

It is deduced from this that the "hood" represents half a bullock, i.e. part of a sacrificial beast. The point about hypotheses of this kind is that it is impossible to support them by reference to evidence of a substantive kind. They are thus bound to remain more or less plausible speculations and there is no way of determining whether the idea of playing with a football originated from a fertility rite in which the ball symbolically represented the sun, the head of a sacrificial beast, both of these things or, for that matter, anything else. Indeed, there is no way of determining conclus-

ively whether football had a ritual origin or not. However, the traditional speech of the Fool in the Haxey Hood ceremony does point in a sociologically more plausible direction. More particularly, while it may not allow one to determine what the origins of football were, it does permit one to establish with some certainty its function as a violent and enjoyable means for expressing conflict between rival groups which enabled them to confirm one dimension of their superiority or inferiority relative to one another.

Yet another form of collective origin myth holds that football is a more or less direct derivative of one of the following: the ancient Chinese game of *tsu chu* (kick ball); Japanese *kemari*; Roman *harpastum*; Greek *episkyros*; or the Italian *gioco del calcio* (game of kicking) (Green 1953, pp. 5–6; Young 1966, p. 2). In none of these cases, with the partial exception of *calcio*, is there evidence which allows one to trace a line of descent. A somewhat more plausible explanation was proposed by Jusserand in 1901 and accepted by Magoun in 1938 (Magoun 1938, pp. 134–137; Marples 1954; Gardner 1974). Noting the existence of several parallels between the folk football of England and France, Jusserand suggested they must have had a common origin. And since the extant records go further back in France than England, he concluded that football must have originated in France and been brought to England in the eleventh century by the Normans. If Jusserand is correct, it is more than a little ironic for he will have proved the French origins of what is widely regarded as having been an originally English sport! The author's view is that Jusserand's desire to prove the superiority of the French over the English probably helped to tilt him towards this conclusion. This is because — apart from the name which is obviously English — all the evidence suggests that, while football *per se* may not have originated in England, soccer and Rugby, the game forms which developed in the nineteenth century, most certainly did. As will be shown, such a view is not mere speculation but can be supported by reference to reliable data.

Marples accepts the plausibility of the Jusserand hypothesis but speculates, equally plausibly, that the existence of football-like games such as "hurling" and "knappan" in Cornwall, Ireland and Wales, the Celtic regions of Britain, is consistent with what he calls "the Celtic hypothesis," namely that football and football-

---

* *House against house, town against town,*
And if you meet a man, knock him down.

like games underwent an independent but parallel evolution among the Franks and Anglo-Saxons on the one hand and among the Celts on the other. Although it is impossible to support it by direct evidence, this line of reasoning is convincing. However, it can be taken further. Since the Chinese, the Japanese, the Greeks, the Italians, the Romans, the English, the French, and the Celts all, at some stage in their histories, played forms of ball game which have been proposed with varying degrees of plausibility as the ancestral form of football, it seems plausible to hypothesize that football-like games most probably had multiple origins, being played in different forms in all or most societies with the technological ability to construct appropriate types of ball and the freedom from material and military necessity to engage in forms of play. It is possible that, the lower the division of labour in such societies, the more closely they approximated structurally to the pattern of social organization called "mechanical solidarity" by Durkheim, the more their game forms would have had a ritual and religious character (Durkheim 1964, p. 70 ff.). That is because, in societies of that type, the ritual and the sacred are all-pervasive, an observation which is consistent with Carl Diem's assertion that: "All physical exercises were originally cultic" (Diem 1971, pp. 1, 3).

In short, although it is necessary to maintain a critical distance from the particular anthropological explanations of the origins of football proposed by Johnson and Chambers, there are sociological reasons for believing that such hypotheses may not be totally wide of the mark. However, these reasons necessarily remain speculative. They may be more or less plausible but it is impossible to support them by reference to concrete data. However, there is evidence about the history of football and, if properly interpreted, such evidence begins to allow one to distinguish fact from myth.

Folk football in medieval and early modern Britain

Reliable evidence for the existence in Britain of a game called "football" does not begin to accumulate until the fourteenth century. However, between 1314 and 1660, orders prohibiting football and other popular games were issued by the central and local authorities of Britain on more than 30 occasions. The list in Table 1.1 gives an idea of the frequency with which it was felt necessary to re-enact such prohibitions, together with an indication of how widely in a geographical sense the folk antecedents of modern football were played.

The 1496 statute of Henry VII was re-enacted several times during the reign of Henry VIII (1509–1547), the last English monarch to re-enact such legislation. However, it remained on the statute book until 1845 under the title "The bill for maintaining artillery and the debarring of unlawful games" (Marples 1954, p. 43).

The prohibition of 1314 and that issued by Edward III in 1365 show the two main reasons why the state authorities wished to ban football and similar games. The order of 1314 was issued in the name of Edward II by the Lord Mayor of London and referred to "great uproar in the City, through certain tumult arising from great footballs in the fields of the public, from which many evils perchance may arise..." It aimed "on the King's behalf" to forbid the game "upon pain of imprisonment" (Marples 1954, pp. 439–441). Edward III's prohibition was connected with the belief that playing games like football was having adverse effects on military preparedness. It is significant that this was the time of the Hundred Years War with the French which had broken out in 1338. The prohibition of 1365 reads as follows:

> To the Sherriffes of London. Order to cause proclamation to be made that every able bodied man of the said city on feast days when he has leisure shall in his sports use bows and arrows or pellets and bolts...forbidding them under pain of imprisonment to meddle in the hurling of stones, loggats and quoits, handball, football...or other vain games of no value; as the people of the realme... used heretofore to practise the said art in their sports when by God's help came forth honour to the kingdom and advantage to the King in his actions of war; and now the said art is almost wholly disused and the people engage in the games aforesaid and in other dishonest, unthrifty or idle games, whereby the realm is likely to be without archers. (Marples 1954, pp. 181, 182)

It is clear, then, that the state authorities in medieval Britain tried to suppress football and other traditional games because they regarded them both as a waste of time and as a threat to public order. As a result, they

Table 1.1 Selected list of prohibitions by state and local authorities of the folk antecedents of modern football (Magoun 1938; Marples 1954; Young 1966)

Year	Monarch	Place	Year	Monarch	Place
1314	Edward II	London	1478		London
1331	Edward III	London	1488		Leicester
1349	Edward III	London	1491	James IV of Scotland	
1365	Edward III	London	1496	Henry VII	London
1388	Richard II	London	1533		London
1401	Henry IV	London	1570		Chester
1409	Henry IV	London	1572		Peebles
1410	Henry IV	London	1581		London
1414	Henry V	London	1594		London
1424	James I of Scotland	Perth			Shrewsbury
1450		Halifax	1608		Manchester
1454		Halifax	1609		Manchester
1457	James II of Scotland	Perth	1615		London
1467		Leicester	1655		Manchester
1471	James III of Scotland	Perth	1656		Manchester
1474	Edward IV	London	1657		Manchester
1477	Edward IV	London	1660		Bristol

Local rather than state authorities were responsible for those prohibitions where the name of the reigning monarch is not included.

tried to direct the energies of the people into what they (the authorities) regarded as more useful channels such as military training.

Official prohibitions may tell us about how the authorities in medieval and early modern Britain viewed folk football and similar games but they provide comparatively little information about the character of such games. A discussion of an early seventeenth century account by Sir Richard Carew of a Cornish game called "hurling" will show that these folk antecedents of modern football and related modern sports were forms of inter-group combat games that were closer to "real" fighting than is the case with their twentieth century offspring.

According to Carew, hurling matches were usually organized by "gentlemen." The "goals" were either these gentlemen's houses or two towns or villages some 5 or 6.5 km (3 or 4 miles) apart.* There was, he said, "neither comparing of numbers nor matching of

---

* Carew also provides an account of a more regulated and orderly type of hurling which he calls "hurling to goales" (see Dunning & Sheard 1979, p. 35 ff.).

men." The game was played with a silver ball and the object was to carry it "by force or trickery" to the goal of one's own side. Carew described the game in the following terms:

Whoever gains possession of this ball generally finds himself pursued by the other side and they will not leave him alone until he is laid flat on God's dear earth. Once he has fallen, he is not allowed to retain the ball and therefore throws it to the most distant of his team-mates who then tries, for his part, to make an escape.

The hurlers play over hills, dales, hedges, ditches; yes, and through bushes, briars, bogs, pools and rivers so that you will sometimes see 20 or 30 lie tugging in the water, scrambling and scratching for the ball. A game that is, indeed, rude and rough, yet one that is not entirely lacking in stratagems in some ways resembling those of war. Thus there are horsemen placed on either side ready to ride away with the ball if they can catch it. But, however fast they gallop, they are certain to be met at some hedge corner, crossroads, bridge or stretch of deep water which their opponents know they must pass. And if luck is not with them, the horsemen are likely to pay the price of their theft with their own and their horses' overthrow to the ground.

The ball in this game may be compared to an infernal spirit. Whoever catches it behaves immediately like a madman, struggling and fighting with those who try to hold him...I cannot decide whether I should more commend this game for its manliness and exercise, or condemn it for its boisterousness and the harms it causes. For, while it makes their bodies strong, hard and nimble, and puts courage into their hearts to meet an enemy face to face, it is also accompanied by many dangers. For proof of this, when the hurling is ended you will see them returning home as if from a pitched battle, with bloody heads, bones broken and out of joint, and such bruises as will shorten their lives. Yet it is a good game and never causes trouble for attorneys or the coroner. (Carew 1602; author's translation into modern English)

Carew's account gives a good idea of the loose overall structure of this type of game. There was, for example, no limitation on numbers of participants, no stipulation of numerical equality between the sides and no restriction on the size of the playing area. Hurlers did not play on a specifically demarcated pitch but on the territory surrounding what were agreed on as the goals of the two sides, i.e. the places to which they had respectively to transport the ball in order to win. Cornish hurling was a rough but by no means totally unregulated game. One of the customary rules emerges clearly from Carew's account: when tackled, a player was obliged to pass the ball to a team-mate. There was also a rudimentary division of labour within each team into what Carew, using a then-contemporary military analogy, called a "fore-ward," a "rere-ward," and two "wings." This shows that use of the terms, "forward" and "wing" to denote particular playing positions (a practice which survives in present-day football and Rugby) has a long ancestry. Carew also mentioned a division between players on horseback and players on foot. This is interesting because it suggests that, in these folk games, elements of what were later to become separate games — in this instance, hurling and polo — were rolled together into a single undifferentiated whole.

The roughness described by Carew is what one would expect of games played by such large numbers

according to loosely defined oral rules. There was no referee to arbitrate and keep control, and no outside body to appeal to in cases of dispute. That games of this type continued to be played until the nineteenth century emerges from an account of a kind of football that was played each Christmas Day in the early 1800s in South Cardiganshire, Wales:

At Llanwennog, an extensive parish below Lampeter, the inhabitants for football purposes were divided into the Bros and Blaenaus...The Bros... occupied the high ground of the parish. They were nick-named "Paddy Bros" from a tradition that they were descendants from Irish people. The Blaenaus occupied the lowlands and, it may be presumed, were purebred Brythons...the match did not begin until about mid-day...Then the whole of the Bros and Blaenaus, rich and poor, male and female, assembled on the turnpike road which divided the highlands from the lowlands. The ball...was thrown high in the air by a strong man, and when it fell Bros and Blaenaus scrambled for its possession, and a quarter of an hour frequently elapsed before the ball was got out from the struggling heap...Then if the Bros could succeed in taking the ball up the mountain to Rhyddlan they won the day; while the Blaenaus were successful if they got the ball to their end of the parish...The whole parish was the field of operations, and sometimes it would be dark before either party secured a victory. In the meantime, many kicks would be given and taken, so that on the following day the competitors would be unable to walk, and sometimes a kick on the shins would lead the two men concerned to abandon the game until they had decided who was the better pugilist...the art of football playing in the olden time seems to have been to reach the goal. When once the goal was reached, the victory was celebrated by loud hurrahs and the firing of guns, and was not disturbed until the following Christmas Day. (Dunning & Sheard 1979, pp. 29–30)

In fact, ball games of this type continue to be played in parts of Britain. Hallaton "bottle-kicking" and Ashbourne and Atherstone football are perhaps the best-known examples.

Some authorities have been reluctant to use accounts of "bottle-kicking," "hurling," "knappan," and similar games such as East Anglian "camp ball" as evidence regarding the folk antecedents of modern football. That is understandable but arguably based on a failure fully to appreciate the nature of this type of game. They were based on local custom, not on common national rules; hence the chances of variation between communities were great because there were neither written rules nor central organizations to unify the manner of playing. Given that, references to "football" in medieval or early modern sources do not imply a game played according to a single set of rules. Identity of names is therefore no guarantee of identity of the games to which these names refer. By the same token, the differences between folk games that were given different names were rarely as great as those between modern sports. That is, as far as one can tell, the differences between hurling, knappan, camp ball, bottle-kicking, and, as referred to in the medieval and early modern sources, football, were neither so great nor so clear-cut as are those between Rugby, soccer, hockey, and polo today.

These similar games may have different names because they were played with different implements. The "knappan," for example, was a wooden disc. The "bottle" in the Hallaton game was (is) a wooden keg. Similarly, references to football in some early accounts seem to refer more to a type of ball than to a type of game. For example, the prohibition of football in Manchester in 1608 referred to playing "*with* the ffotebale" rather than to "playing ffotebale" (Dunning & Sheard 1979, p. 22). As far as can be ascertained, the type of ball to which this name was given was an inflated animal bladder, usually, but not always, encased in leather.

Balls of this type probably lent themselves better than smaller, solid balls to kicking. This could explain the name "football." Alternatively, the term could have signified a game that was played *on* foot as opposed to horseback. Nevertheless, it would still be wrong to assume that, in folk games called "football," the ball was only propelled by foot or, conversely, that in games called "hurling" or "handball" it was only propelled by hand. That is because prohibitions in these folk games were less clearly defined and less rigidly enforceable than is the case in modern sports.

Such games were traditionally associated with religious festivals such as Shrovetide, Easter, and Christmas. However, they could also be played on an *ad hoc* basis at any time in the autumn, winter, or spring. They were played across country and through the streets of towns and often by females as well as males. One played as the member of a specific group — e.g. for Hallaton vs. Medbourne, the "Bros" vs. the "Blaenaus," the shoemakers vs. the drapers, the bachelors vs. the married men, the spinsters vs. the married women — rather than as the member of a club one had joined voluntarily and where the primary reason for associating was in order to play football. In these folk games, communal identity took precedence over individual identity, the pressure to take part was intense, and the degree of individual choice that players had was relatively small.

Whatever their names and whether associated with a specific festival or not, the folk antecedents of modern football were openly emotional affairs characterized by physical struggle. Such restraints as they contained were loosely defined and imposed by custom as opposed to elaborate formal regulations which are written down, requiring players to exercise a high degree of self-control and involving the intervention of external officials when this self-control breaks down. As a result, the basic game-pattern — the character of these folk games as struggles between groups, the open enjoyment in them of excitement akin to that aroused in battle, the riotousness, and the relatively high level of socially tolerated physical violence — was always and everywhere the same. In short, these games were cast in a common mould which transcended differences of names and locally specific traditions of playing.

Folk football in Europe

Ball games similar to the British folk antecedents of modern football were played, as has been shown, in France. Just as in Britain, these folk games were prohibited by royal edict, for example by Philippe V in 1319 and Charles V in 1369 (Marples 1954, p. 25). In fact, such attempts were made right up until the Revolution which suggests that the French authorities were just as unsuccessful at suppressing these games as their counterparts in Britain. Similar edicts were also enacted in colonial America showing that the earliest English settlers must have played such games as well (Gardner 1974, p. 96).

Although there were a few signs of similar developments simultaneously in England (Dunning & Sheard 1979, p. 35), in Italy, a somewhat more restrained and regulated game, the *gioco del calcio*, had developed by the sixteenth and seventeenth centuries. The participants were "young Cavaliers of good purse," we are told, and two teams of 27 members per side played every evening in the Piazza di Santa Croce in Florence from Epiphany to Lent (Marples 1954, p. 67). It remained a rough game. Indeed, it continues to be rough to the present day. Its roughness is brought out well in an English translation of a description by Boccalini which was published in London in 1656. The beginning reads as follows:

> The Noble Florentines plaid the last Tuesday at the Calcio in the Phebean field...and though some, to whom it was a new sight to see many of these Florentine Gentlemen fall down to right cuffs, said, that that manner of proceeding in that which was but play and sport, was too harsh, and not severe enough in real combat...the Commonwealth of Florence had done very well in introducing the Calcio among the Citizens, to the end that having the satisfaction of giving four or five good round buffets in the face to those to whom they bear ill will, by way of sport, they might the better appease their anger (than by the use of daggers). (Young 1966, pp. 88–90)

The presence of pike-carrying soldiers in pictorial representations of the game, however, (Marples 1954, facing p. 21), suggests that the social control function attributed to *calcio* by Boccalini may not always have been performed. It is reasonable to suppose that pikemen were necessary in case the excitement of the struggle led either the young noble players or members of the crowd to get carried away and lose their self-restraint (Guttman 1986, p. 51).

Development of modern football

Although *calcio* was known to a handful of English writers and their readers for around 100 years, they were members of a small élite and it is doubtful whether their knowledge had any direct effects on the British folk antecedents of modern football. With or without gentry support, these continued to be widely played by the common people in the traditional manner until the nineteenth century, while, as far as one can tell, Florentine *calcio* froze at the developmental level reached in the sixteenth and seventeenth centuries. In short, the development of modern football appears to have been a process which occurred autonomously in England. Two processes that occurred more or less

simultaneously in the eighteenth and nineteenth centuries are of relevance in this connection: (a) the cultural marginalization of folk football, a process that began in the middle of the eighteenth century and gathered pace as the nineteenth wore on; and (b) the development of newer forms of football in the public schools and universities from about the 1840s onwards.

Cultural marginalization of folk football

The cultural marginalization of folk football need not detain us long. It is sufficient just to note that, these forms of playing seem to have fallen foul of the "civilizing" and "state-formation" processes as they were experienced in eighteenth and nineteenth century Britain (Elias 1939). That is, increasing numbers of people came to regard the roughness of folk football with repugnance. At the same time, the formation of the new police force in the 1820s and 1830s placed in the hands of the authorities a more efficient instrument of social control than any previously available. The prohibitions that had begun in 1314 ould thus be made to stick and "the bill for maintaining artillery and the debarring of unlawful games" could be removed from the statute book. Another influence may have been at work as well. It is possible that the survival of folk football in the face of centuries of opposition had been predicated in part on support from sections of the aristocracy and gentry. If that is, indeed, a reasonable supposition, then a further reason for the cultural marginalization of these antecedents of modern football may have been connected with the way in which industrialization involved an augmentation of the power of rising bourgeois groups. As a result, status competition between members of the bourgeoisie and the landed ruling classes grew more intense, leading the latter to grow more status-exclusive in their behavior and withdraw their support from traditional sports and games. Possible support for such an hypothesis is provided by an anonymous Old Etonian* who wrote contemptuously in 1831 that:

> I cannot consider the game of football as being at

* The term "Old Etonian" refers to a former Eton pupil. It remains common usage in the UK to refer to former pupils of a school as "old boys" and is not confined simply to public schools.

completely oblivious to what was happening at the other public schools. However, they are unlikely to have been such "cultural dopes." They considered their school to be the leading public school in all respects. It was, after all, the second oldest, only Winchester being able to take pride in a longer pedigree. Having been founded by Henry VI in 1440, Eton was also able to boast about being a royal foundation. Moreover, being located next to Windsor, it continued to have connections with the royal court. One can easily imagine how the Eton boys would have reacted to the development of a distinctive way of playing football at Rugby, in their eyes an obscure Midlands establishment that catered primarily for parvenues.

Under Thomas Arnold, the fame of Rugby had begun to spread and with it, the fame of their way of playing football. The Rugby boys, it seems reasonable to suppose, were hoping to draw attention to themselves by developing a distinctive game. However, it would seem similarly not unlikely that, by developing a form of football that was equally distinctive but in key respects diametrically opposite to the game at Rugby, the Etonians were deliberately attempting to put the "upstart" Rugbeians in their place and to "see off" this challenge to the Etonians' status as *the* leading public school.

Emergence of Association football as a national game

Starting in the 1850s, the embryonic Association football and Rugby games spread into the wider society. Two wider social developments underpinned this process: (a) an expansion of the middle classes that occurred correlatively with continuing industrialization and urbanization; and (b) an educational transformation usually referred to as the "public school games cult" (Marples 1954, pp. 119 ff.). There is no need to analyze these wider developments here. It is enough simply to note that the games cult helped to establish social conditions that were conducive to the spread of football in its embryonic modern forms, above all playing a part in transforming what were destined to become Association football and Rugby into status-enhancing activities for adult "gentlemen."

This process of diffusion led to pressure for unified rules. An attempt was made to form a single national game but there was no basis for consensus among the participating groups. Or more precisely, there were

two: support polarized around the embryo Association football and Rugby models but neither camp was able to establish unequivocal dominance. Consequently, the bifurcation of Association football and Rugby which appears to have been set in motion by Eton–Rugby rivalry in the 1840s, was perpetuated on a national level, leading to the formation of separate ruling bodies, the Football Association (FA) in 1863 and the Rugby Football Union (RFU) in 1871. Only the formation of the FA need concern us here. Two partly independent developments are of relevance in this connection: (a) the formation of the earliest clubs; and (b) the growth in the importance of football as a leisure activity at the Universities of Oxford and Cambridge.

The first reliable record of a football club comes from Sheffield, Yorkshire, where occasional matches were recorded as early as 1855 and where Sheffield FC issued a constitution and a set of rules in 1857 (Young 1966, pp. 76–78). Another club is recorded in the Sheffield suburb of Hallam in the same year and, by 1862, there were 15 clubs in the district. Numbers 5 and 8 of the rules formulated by the Sheffield Committee in 1857 show that Sheffield football was modelled on one or more of the embryo Association football games. These rules were:

> **5** Pushing with the hands is allowed but no hacking or tripping up is fair under any circumstances whatever.
> **8** The ball may be pushed or hit with the hand, but holding the ball except in the case of a free kick is altogether disallowed.
> (Young 1966, p. 77)

The extant data suggest, however, that most early clubs were founded in the south of England, particularly in and around London. For example, Forest FC, a club which played at Snaresbrook, Essex, was founded in 1859 by a group of Old Harrovians, prominent among them C.W. and J.F. Alcock, the sons of a Sunderland Justice of the Peace who were shortly to figure prominently in the formation of the FA. Forest changed its name of Wanderers in 1864 but maintained the Harrow connection. Another club with Harrow associations was N.N. (No Names), Kilburn, but the date of its foundation remains unknown. Other clubs known to have been in existence by 1863 include Blackheath (1858), Richmond (1859), and Harlequins (1859), all three of them playing variants of the Rugby game. Also founded by that time were the following embryo Association football clubs: Crystal Palace (1860), vided by Table 1.3. Table 1.4 provides data on participants in and attendances at World Cup Finals and sheds further light on the global spread of Association football.

During the twentieth century, Association football emerged as the world's most popular team sport. The

Table 1.3 The growth of FIFA (1904–1994)

Year	Number of Associations
1904	7
1914	24
1920	20
1923	31
1930	41
1938	51
1950	73
1954	85
1959	95
1984	150
1991	165
1994	178*

* This will probably increase to 190 in June 1994.

Table 1.4 The World Cup Finals: venues, participants, and attendances (1930–1990)

Date	Venue	Winner	Attendances	Number of matches
1930	Uruguay	Uruguay	434 500	18
1934	Italy	Italy	395 000	17
1938	France	Italy	483 000	18
1950	Brazil	Uruguay	1337 000	22
1954	Switzerland	West Germany	943 000	26
1958	Sweden	Brazil	86 000	35
1962	Chile	Brazil	776 000	32
1966	England	England	1614 677	32
1970	Mexico	Brazil	1673 975	32
1974	West Germany	West Germany	1774 022	38
1978	Argentina	Argentina	1610 215	38
1982	Spain	Italy	1766 277	52
1986	Mexico	Argentina	2199 941	52
1990	Italy	West Germany	2510 686	52

reasons for its comparative success are not difficult to find. It does not require much equipment and is comparatively cheap to play. Its rules — apart perhaps from the offside law — are relatively easy to understand. Above all the rules of Association football regularly make for fast, open, and fluid play and for a game that is finely balanced among a number of interdependent polarities such as force and skill, individual and team play, and attack and defense (Elias & Dunning 1986, pp. 191–204; Murphy et al. 1990, pp. 1–19). As such, its structure permits the recurrent generation of levels of tension and excitement that are enjoyable for players and spectators alike. At the heart of this is the fact that matches are physical struggles between two groups governed by rules which allow the passions to rise yet keep them — most of the time — in check. To the extent that they are enforced and/or voluntarily obeyed, the rules of Association football also limit the risk of serious injury to players. That is another respect in which it can be said to be a "civilized" game.

Given such a structure, at a football match one is able to experience in a socially acceptable manner and a concentrated period of time a whole gamut of strong feelings: hope when one's team looks close to scoring and elation when they do; fear when the opponents threaten to score and disappointment when they succeed. During a closely fought match, the spectators flit constantly from one emotion to another until the issue is resolved. Then, the supporters of the winning team experience triumph and jubilation, those of the losers dejection and despair. If the match has ended in a draw, the supporters of both sides are liable to experience a mixture of emotions. But to experience excitement at a soccer match, one has to care. For the "gears" of one's passions to "engage," one has to be committed, to be identified with one or other of the teams, and to want to see that team win.

Of course, other sports involve some of the characteristics listed here but only Association football involves them all. That, it is reasonable to believe, is why it has become the world's most popular sport. In turn, its worldwide popularity and the degree to which fans identify with their teams help to explain why it is the sport most frequently associated with "hooliganism" and spectator disorders (Dunning et al. 1988, Williams et al. 1989, Murphy et al. 1990). Limitations of space mean that football hooliganism can only be dealt with briefly here.

A plausible reason for the frequency of Association football-related spectator disorders might appear to be the fact that, given its relative lack of overt violence compared with Rugby and American football, the game of Association football provides fewer opportunities for spectators to experience violence vicariously, hence allowing them less chance cathartically to release aggressive feelings. Among the many weaknesses in this hypothesis, however, is the fact that spectator violence is a regular accompaniment of Rugby in the South of France (Holt 1981, pp. 135–136) and is increasing in English Rugby at the moment. Nor is spectator violence by any means entirely unknown in conjunction with gridiron football in the USA. In that country, a pattern of "celebratory rioting" is well established at most major sports, not infrequently involving the use of guns and sometimes leading to deaths (Murphy *et al.* 1990, pp. 194–212).

In fact, the relative frequency of hooliganism at Association football matches is easy to explain without reference to catharsis. It can be said to be primarily a function of the social composition of crowds, of the fact that, worldwide, the majority of football spectators tend to be drawn from the lower reaches of their societies, a fact which leads to behavior in terms of norms which permit the relatively open expression of excitement and aggression. Such a pattern is spiced by the fact that, in most societies, groups lower down the social scale, are more likely to form intense "we-group" bonds that involve an equally intense hostility towards "they-groups" or "outsiders." At a football match, of course, the "outsiders" are provided by the opposing team and its supporters.

The greater relative frequency of crowd disorderliness at Association football matches is also partly a function of the greater media exposure the game receives. This serves to contribute both to a popular conception of football hooliganism as more frequent and of spectator violence at other sports as less frequent than is actually the case. In short, the greater relative frequency of hooligan behavior at football matches is partly a question of fact and partly one of media-generated myth. For example, in the period up to and including the mid-1960s, the occurrence of football hooliganism in Central and South America, continental Europe and Britain's "Celtic fringe" was regularly reported in the British press, together with statements to the effect that such behavior "never happened in England." However, that was a myth because spectator violence had been rife at English Association football matches before the First World War and never died out completely. Similarly, following the Heysel tragedy in 1985, it came to be widely believed in continental Europe, indeed the world at large, that football hooliganism is a uniquely English "disease." That is another myth for at least two reasons. The first is the fact that the worst *reported* hooligan-related football tragedy in modern times occurred at the match between Peru and Argentina in Lima in 1964 when no fewer than 318 people are reported to have died. The second is the fact that, although its incidence varies between countries and within countries over time, football hooliganism has never been restricted to a single country. What was unique about the English until the mid-1980s was the readiness of a minority of fans to engage in hooligan behavior abroad. Now, in the early 1990s, football hooliganism is reported more regularly in Germany, Italy, and the Netherlands than in England. It would, though, be premature to conclude that football hooliganism in England has died out. All that can be said with certainty is that this threat to the world's number one team sport will not be seriously diminished in any country until it has been tackled at its social roots.

Appendix: some significant dates in the history of football

1314   First recorded reference to "football."
1845   First written rules of football produced at Rugby School.
1849   First written rules of a non-handling form of football produced at Eton.
1863   Formation of the Football Association.
1871   Formation of the Rugby Football Union.
1885   Professionalism ratified by the Football Association.
1888   Formation of the Football League.
1906   Formation of FIFA.
1930   Inauguration of the World Cup.
1964   At the match between Peru and Argentina in Lima 318 people die.
1985   The Heysel tragedy at the European Cup Final in Brussels between Liverpool and Juventus; 39 people die, most of them Italians.

References

Arlott J. (1977) *The Oxford Companion to Sports and Games.* Paladin, London.

Carew R. (1602) *The Survey of Cornwall.* London.

Diem C. (1971) *Weltgeschichte des Sports*, 3rd edn. Cotta, Frankfurt.

Dunning E. (1961) *Early stages in the development of football as an organised game.* MA thesis, University of Leicester.

Dunning E., Murphy P. & Williams J. (1988) *The Roots of Football Hooliganism.* Routledge, London.

Dunning E. & Sheard K. (1979) *Barbarians, Gentlemen and Players.* Martin Robertson, Oxford.

Durkheim E. (1964) *The Division of Labour in Society.* Free Press, Glencoe, Illinois.

Elias N. (1939) *Über den Prozess der Zivilisation.* Haus zum Falken, Basle.

Elias N. & Dunning E. (1986) *Quest for Excitement.* Basil Blackwell, Oxford.

Gardner P. (1974) *Nice Guys Finish Last.* Allen Lane, London.

Glanville B. (1969) *Soccer Panorama.* Eyre & Spottiswoode, London.

Green G. (1953) *The History of the Football Association.* Naldrett, London.

Guttmann A. (1986) *Sports Spectators.* Columbia University Press, New York.

Holt R. (1981) *Sport and Society in France.* Macmillan, London.

Macrory J. (1991) *Running with the Ball: the Birth of Rugby Football.* Collins-Willow, London.

Magoun F.P. (1938) *A History of Football from the Beginnings to 1871.* Kolner Anglistische Arbeite, Cologne.

Marples M. (1954) *History of Football.* Secker & Warburg, London.

Murphy P. Williams J. & Dunning E. (1990) *Football on Trial.* Routledge, London.

Williams J., Dunning E. & Murphy P. (1989) *Hooligans Abroad*, 2nd edn. Routledge, London.

Young, P.F. (1966) *A History of British Football.* Stanley Paul, London.

Further reading

Dunning E. (1971) *The Sociology of Sport: A Selection of Readings.* Frank Cass, London.

Elias N. (1978) *What is Sociology?* Hutchinson, London.

Elias N. (1978) *The Civilizing Process*, Vol. 1. *The History of Manners.* Basil Blackwell, Oxford.

Elias N. (1982) *The Civilizing Process*, Vol. 2. *State Formation and Civilization.* Basil Blackwell, Oxford.

Fishwick N. (1987) *English Football and Society, 1910–1950.* Manchester University Press, Manchester.

Guttmann A. (1978) *From Ritual to Record.* Columbia University Press, New York.

Holt R. (1989) *Sport and the British.* Clarendon Press, Oxford.

Johnson W.B. (1929) Football: a survival of magic, *Contemporary Review*, cxxv (quoted in Marples 1954).

Jusserand J.J. (1901) *Les Sports et les Jeux d'Exercise dans l'ancienne France* (quoted in Marples 1954).

Kitchin L. (1966) The contenders, *The Listener*, 27 October.

Mason T. (1980) *Association Football and English Society, 1863–1915.* Harvester, Brighton.

Tomlinson A. & Whannel G. (1986) *Off the Ball: the Football World Cup.* Pluto, London.

Chapter 2

The evolution of

football tactics

It is almost impossible to compare great football teams of the past and to determine "the best team ever", but successful teams have often added new tactics or ideas to the game. This is one of the reasons for their success. But without skilful players there can be no success and, therefore, one of the most important reasons for the improvement of the game over time is due to the development of the players' technical and physical standards. This chapter describes the tactical development of the game in five countries. In order to lead the development of a new strategy, the country represented by its national team must of course be successful. The results in the World Cup and Olympic Game finals can be used as a measure of success. Thus Germany, Italy, Brazil, and Hungary are selected. For obvious reasons England — the native country of football — must also be included.

Football tactics and rules

In the nineteenth century, names were given to the players according to their tasks and positions. The roles of the different players are traditionally connected with the numbers on their backs, which were introduced in the 1930s. The following numbers will be used for future reference.

1 Goalkeeper.
2 Right fullback.
3 Left fullback.
4 Right halfback.
5 Center halfback.
6 Left halfback.
7 Outside right forward.
8 Inside right forward.
9 Center forward.
10 Inside left forward.
11 Outside left forward.

The practical application of the rules of the game is also worth mentioning. In order for a game to develop, the participants must be challenged, for example in football it must not be too easy or too difficult to score. This is determined by the rules that limit or extend playing possibilities. One example of this is the offside rule. Around 1860, football was mainly played in England. The British Football Association was founded in 1863, and at that time adopted the following offside rule: "When a player has kicked the ball anyone in the same team is regarded as offside if he is nearer to the opponent's goal-line than the kicker."

The consequence of this rule was obvious. The only way to score was to dribble, which made the games unorganized, chaotic, and very unpredictable. This style of play was named "the dribbling game." However, although almost all the players were attackers it was still very difficult to score. Therefore, in 1868 the offside rule was altered so that a player could not be offside if three opponents were nearer to their own goal-line when the ball was last played forward.

The pioneers

Queen's Park AFC in Glasgow was one of the first clubs to discover the tactical possibilities of the new rule. They were a well-organized team which consisted of two fullbacks, two halfbacks, and six forwards. This style of play was incredibly successful, from 9 July 1867, when the club was founded, until 16 January 1875, the team did not have a goal scored against them!

Attacking play improved among the British football teams. The six forwards were grouped forming three pairs of which one forward supported the others from behind. This was the birth of the inside forwards and the center halfback. The center halfback was consequently an attacking supporting midfield player, the strategist, and often the dominant player of the team. Gradually, this position became more withdrawn but some of the offensive tasks remained. This formation was given many names including "the pyramid formation," "the classical formation," "the offensive formation," and "the two back formation" and became the starting point for all tactical developments.

The teams soon became better organized and as a consequence specialized players emerged, for example

1 Combi
2 Monzeglio
3 Allemandi
4 Ferraris IV
5 Monti
6 Bertolini
7 Guaita
8 Meazza
9 Schiavio
10 Ferrari
11 Orsi
Coach: Pozzo

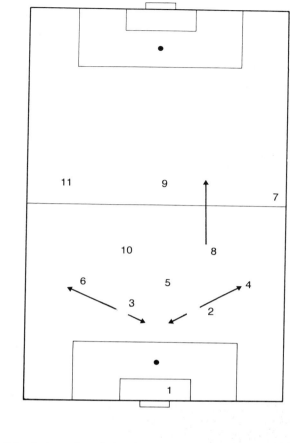

Fig. 2.4 Italy in the 1934 World Cup Final in Rome against Czechoslovakia (2−1 in extra time).

the 1912 Olympic Games in Stockholm; a position he maintained for 36 years until 1948. During these years he maintained the principle of the two back formation, but he had to adapt his team's style to the new offside rule. The two fullbacks covered deep back while the wing halfbacks and the center half marked the three forwards. The characteristics of Italy included:
1 Formation: two back formation with five midfield players (three halfbacks and two inside forwards), one center forward, and two wingers.
2 Defensive playing style: a combination of zone-marking and zone-covering. A withdrawn center half-back and deep inside forwards. The two fullbacks were zone-covering.
3 Offensive playing style: counter-attacks with long passes to the forwards.
4 Results: in 49 games against other national teams between 1930 and 1936, Italy won 33 games, tied 10, and lost 6.

It is obvious that the Italians accepted the defensive role of the center-half but kept the two fullbacks as extra cover. This defensive type of play became tough and sometimes brutal. One can see signs of this even today in Italian football.

Gradually Germany and Hungary adopted the three back formation while Italy remained with the two back concept, as did their Latin cousins in Brazil.

The revolutionary Hungarian style

Up to the beginning of the 1950s football was fairly "static" with restricted working areas for the players. However, new winds blew in from the Hungarian Steppe. The Hungarian team played with two inside forwards in the front line and the center forward withdrawn as a play-maker. The offense involved quick changing of positions which caused the previously stable three back defensive system to break up. An illustration of that is the well-known game at Wembley in London 1953, when Hungary defeated England 6−3; England's first ever home defeat by a continental side (Fig. 2.5).

The Hungarians had adopted the British three back formation in the 1940s. However, in Hungary they were used to playing against two top forwards in their league games. Because of this, they had to withdraw one of the two wing halfbacks as an extra defender. This was the beginning of the four back formation:

1 Formation: a strengthened three back formation with two center forwards and the wingers somewhat withdrawn.

2 Defensive playing style: a combination of zone-marking and zone-covering.

3 Offensive playing style: frequent changing of positions and a very high standard in passing and ball control.

4 Results: in 51 games against other national teams between 1950 and 1955, Hungary won 43 games, tied 7, and lost only 1.

The four back line

Brazil played against Hungary in the 1954 World Cup and lost. It is possible that this caused the South Americans to change their style of play. In the 1958 World Cup in Stockholm, Brazil had adopted the Hungarian style of play with two top inside forwards and a center forward behind them, which gave great mobility and a stable four back defense line. This copy of the Hungarian style was as good as the original (Fig. 2.6). Brazil won the World Cup by beating Sweden 5−2 in the final. Brazil's characteristics included:

1 Formation: a strengthened three back formation with two center forwards and one offensive winger.

2 Defensive playing style: a combination of zone-marking and zone-covering.

1 Grosics
2 Buzánszky
3 Lantos
4 Bozsik
5 Lóránt
6 Zakariás
7 Budai
8 Kocsis
9 Hidegkúti
10 Puskás
11 Czibor
Coach: Sebes

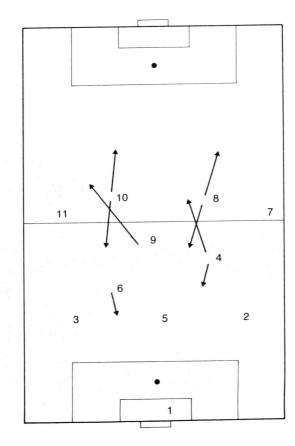

Fig. 2.5 Hungary in London (1953) against England (6−3).

1 Gylmar
2 D. Santos
3 N. Santos
4 Zito
5 Bellini
6 Orlando
7 Garrincha
8 Vava
9 Didi
10 Pelé
11 Zagallo
Coach: Feola

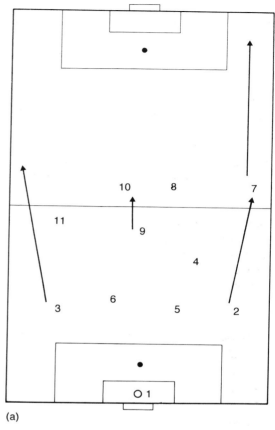

(a)

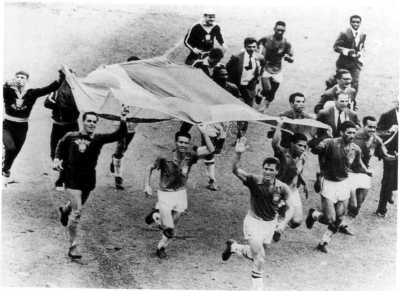

(b)

Fig. 2.6 (a) Brazil in the 1958 World Cup Final against Sweden (5−2). (b) A lap of honor by the Brazilian team. © Popperfoto, UK.

1 Banks
2 Cohen
3 Wilson
4 Stiles
5 J. Charlton
6 Moore
7 Ball
8 Hurst
9 R. Charlton
10 Hunt
11 Peters
Coach: Ramsey

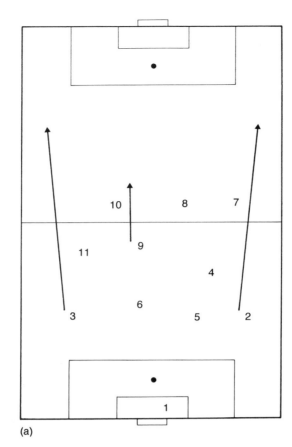

(a)

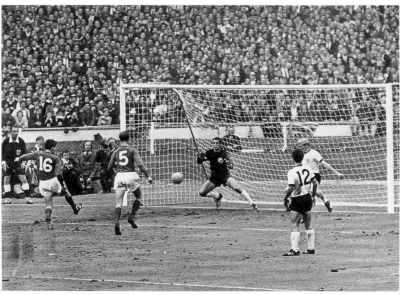

(b)

Fig. 2.7 (a) England in the 1966 World Cup Final in London against West Germany (4−2 in extra time). (b) England's second goal. © Popperfoto, UK.

1 Sarti
2 Picchi
3 Guarneri
4 Burgnich
5 Bedin
6 Fachetti
7 Jair
8 Peiró
9 Mazzola
10 Suarez
11 Corso
Coach: Herrera

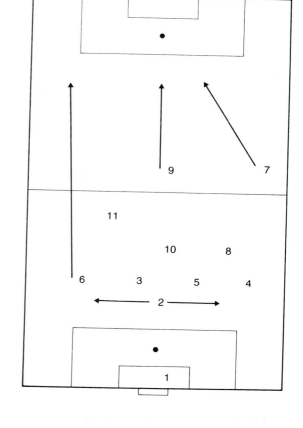

Fig. 2.8 The playing style of the Italian club team Internazionale in the 1965 European Cup Final in Milan against the Portuguese club team Benefica (1−0).

3 Offensive playing style: very quick short passing combined with individual actions on a very high technical level.

4 Results: in 22 games against other national teams between 1957 and 1958, Brazil won 17 games, tied 3, and lost 2.

At the beginning of the 1960s the traditional three back formation had lost its role. Skillful and quick forwards who were always changing positions had demonstrated the disadvantage of this system and new defensive solutions became necessary. The solutions to this problem were varied, though the English way was identical to the Brazilian one. At the 1966 World Cup in London, England demonstrated that this recipe was still effective by winning the competition (Fig. 2.7).

Although, the formation was not new, the style of play was. The team worked as a unit with a very compact appearance. The players worked over large areas and supported each other in all situations. England's characteristics included:

1 Formation: a strengthened three back formation with three midfielders, two center forwards, and a withdrawn outside left.

2 Defensive playing style: zone-marking. Both wing halves had defensive roles.

3 Offensive playing style: no traditional wingers. The two fullbacks attacked along the sidelines.

4 Results: in 26 games against other national teams in 1965 and 1966, England won 19 games, tied 6, and lost only 1.

The libero

In Italy the solution to the problem with the two center forwards was that one of the fullbacks moved up to mark one of the center forwards while the center half-back took care of the other. The second fullback had no marking duties, therefore acquired the name "libero" (sweeper). The inside forwards had assistance from the left winger, who in turn had a supporting role in the midfield. The center forward and the right winger were in front. The successful Italian club team FC Internazionale (Fig. 2.8) were a typical exponent of that system:

1 Formation: a developed two back formation with two center forwards and one winger. The left winger played deep in the midfield.

2 Defensive playing style: zone-marking with a libero.

3 Offensive playing style: quick counter-attacks.

4 Results: in 32 games against other teams in the European Cup between 1964 and 1967, Internazionale won 20 games, tied 7, and lost 5.

Conclusion

Whereas England, Brazil, and Hungary were sup-porters of the developed three back line, Germany and Italy refined and improved the two back model. This is the case even today. Italy and Germany are still using man-to-man marking with libero cover. It seems, however, that more initiative is given to individual players, when it comes to the classic problem in defense: either to follow the opponent or stay in position in the team formation.

The British style of play has come closer to the Italian/German one, since the former now tries to play with a numerical superiority in defense. Therefore, most contemporary British-style teams play with a three back line against the two top forwards, with the wing halfbacks covering along the sidelines and the two inside forwards and the withdrawn center forward responsible for the central mid-field area.

The development according to the two models will continue, but they probably will come closer and finally melt together.

(8.4 ± 1.8) or defenders (6.3 ± 2.0), the fullbacks and center backs being undifferentiated in the latter study. These frequencies suggest that whilst jump-endurance training may not be important for football players, strikers and center backs in particular do need to possess a high anaerobic power output and an ability to jump well vertically.

The work-rate profile of outfield players is highly reproducible from game to game as far as individual players are concerned, with occasional exceptions due to tactical reasons already mentioned. Ekblom (1986) commented that the distance covered by a fullback was between 9.1 and 9.6 km in six different games. For a midfield player the range was 10.2–11.1 km and for one forward over five games it was 9.8–10.6 km. It does seem that outfield players do pace themselves relatively consistently and that the average overall pace may be set by aerobic fitness as well as playing position and state of play.

The goalkeeper covers approximately 4 km in the course of a game, 10% of which was in possession of the ball in the 1970s (Reilly & Thomas 1976). This latter figure is likely to have been reduced by subsequent rule changes relating to transport of the ball by the goalkeeper and the rule introduced in 1992 prohibiting pick-up of a back-pass. Of the total distance covered, jogging comprises 27.4%, walking 33.7%, cruising 12.5%, sprinting 0.8%, and moving backward 25.6%. Sprints were found to range in distance from 1 to 12 m. Time spent stationary is much greater than for outfield players, amounting to 776 s comprised of 252 separate pauses. Much of the lower level activity of the goalkeeper may be an involuntary mechanism to maintain arousal and concentration on the game rather than a direct imposition of game demands. It may also help to maintain thermoregulation within the thermal comfort zone in winter conditions. The critical demands on the goalkeeper are anaerobic in nature, in jumping to catch the ball and diving to save. The timing with which these tasks are executed is the hallmark of a good goalkeeper.

Aerobic fitness

Motion characteristics may be influenced by physical fitness. The ability to sustain a high work-rate for 90 min is likely to be determined by aerobic factors. These would include both aerobic power ($\dot{V}_{O_{2}max.}$)

and a high fractional utilization of $\dot{V}_{O_{2}max.}$. It is estimated that football match-play calls for an average oxygen uptake of about 75% of $\dot{V}_{O_{2}max.}$, a level comparable with the energy expenditure in marathon racing (Reilly 1990). It is probable that the so-called "anaerobic threshold" which is thought to represent the upper limit of exercise that can be sustained for 60–120 min, is close to this relative oxygen consumption in top football players.

Midfield players, who tend to have the highest work-rates of English League footballers, also had the highest values for aerobic power (Reilly 1990). The central defenders were found to have significantly lower relative values than the other outfield players, while the fullbacks and strikers had intermediate values. Indeed the significant correlation between $\dot{V}_{O_{2}max.}$ and distance covered in a game ($r = 0.67$; $n = 31$) demonstrates the need for a high work-rate and a high aerobic fitness level in midfield players who act as a link between defense and attack. Smaros (1980) confirmed the strong correlation ($r = 0.89$; $n = 8$) between $\dot{V}_{O_{2}max.}$ and distance covered in a match but added that the $\dot{V}_{O_{2}max.}$ also influenced the number of sprints that players attempted. Research on Danish players has shown that not only $\dot{V}_{O_{2}max.}$ ($r = 0.64$; $n = 20$), but also performance in a continuous field test over 2.16 km ($r = 0.68$; $n = 14$) and the $\dot{V}_{O_{2}max.}$ corresponding to 3 mmol·l^{-1} blood lactate level ($r = 0.59$; $n = 20$) were significantly correlated to match distance (Bangsbo & Lindquist 1992).

Fatigue

Fatigue may be defined as a decrement in performance due to the necessity to continue performing. This is reflected in a decline in work-rate in football toward the end of a game. This fatigue effect has been examined by comparing work-rates between the first and the second halves of matches.

Van Gool et al. (1988) reported that their university players covered 444 m more in the first half than in the second. Reilly and Thomas (1976) noted that in 32 out of 44 English professional football matches more distance was covered in the first half than in the second, the difference being significant. A similar finding was reported for Danish League matches, a 5% greater distance being covered in the first compared to the second half (Bangsbo et al. 1991).

Aerobic fitness may protect against a fall in work-rate towards the end of a game. Reilly and Thomas (1976) noted that the decrement in work-rate was related to fitness in that the players with the higher $\dot{V}_{O_{2max}}$ values, in midfield and fullback, did not have a significant drop in distance covered in the second half. In contrast all seven center backs and 12 out of 14 strikers had higher figures for the first half, the difference between halves being significant.

The fatigue effect can also be related to nutritional state as reflected in muscle glycogen stores. Saltin (1973) found that players with a low glycogen content in their thigh muscles at the start of a game covered 25% less distance than the others. An even more marked difference was noted for running speed; players with low glycogen content covered 50% of the total distance walking and 15% at top speed compared with 27% walking and 24% sprinting for the players with initially high muscle glycogen levels. The preparation for important matches should ensure that glycogen stores are not reduced at the start of the game in order that a high work intensity can be sustained.

The ultimate indicator of performance is the match result and this depends on the balance of goals scored to goals conceded. It is noteworthy that more goals are scored toward the end of a game than at any other time (Fig. 3.2). This is evident from analysis of goals scored in the three divisions of the Scottish League over successive weeks in the 1991–1992 season. There are many possible reasons for this. The phenomenon cannot simply be explained by a fall in work-rate which should balance out between the two contestant teams. It might be related to the generally superior aerobic fitness of attackers compared to central defenders which gains the forwards the advantage toward the end of a game. It may be linked with "mental fatigue," lapses in concentration promoting tactical errors that open up goal-scoring opportunities. The phenomenon may be inherent to the game, with the losing team or the home team "chasing" a result as the end of the match approaches. Whatever the explanation a strategy that maintains team performance to the end to the 90 min of play is bound to be effective long term.

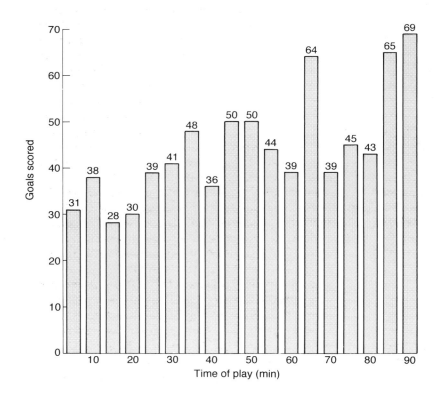

Fig. 3.2 Goals scored in Scottish League football during the major part of the 1991–1992 season.

Styles of play

The style or system of play may determine both the overall work-rate and the detailed work-rate profile. The "total football" exemplified by the Dutch National team of the 1970s called for an ability to interchange positional roles among outfield players. Footballers must have the versatility in both fitness and skills to implement such a system. This levelling effect in fitness may be achieved both through training and the physiological stimulus of competing at a high work intensity. A characteristic of successful teams in major championships, most notably the German national sides in the 1980s and 1990s, is the high work-rate potential of all outfield players.

The "direct method" of play may also serve to even out work-rate profiles among outfield players. This style of play is more characteristic of British teams than of European continental or South American sides. Known as the Reep system (Reep & Benjamin 1968) the main elements are quick movement of the ball from defense to attaining zones for creating scoring opportunities, use of long passes rather than a lengthy sequence of short passes, exploitation of defensive errors and harrying opponents into mistakes when in possession of the ball. These arise from the observations that the number of passes prior to scoring a goal is generally low; 50% of goals come from passing moves originating in the quarter of the pitch nearest to the goal, half of which come from gaining possession from defenders in that area.

The direct style of play was used to good effect by Wimbledon, Watford, and Cambridge United in the 1980s in the English League and in a modified form by Eire in the 1990 World Cup finals. The style has a levelling effect on work-rate of outfield players since all players are expected to work hard off the ball to dispossess opponents. In consequence it makes increased demands on aerobic fitness, irrespective of designated positional role.

Environmental factors

The level of competition clearly affects work-rate profiles of football players. Aerobic fitness tends to improve with the competitive performance levels. Without the fitness requirements to work off the ball, players will be unable to compete at the higher levels of competition.

The behavioral pattern may also be affected by weather conditions. Work-rate is likely to be adversely affected on icy or water-logged surfaces and execution of skills such as turning, accelerating, decelerating, tackling, and so on, impaired. In contrast work-rate will be promoted by firm surfaces. Whilst this applies to grass pitches, and running speed is likely to be enhanced by synthetic surfaces, it is questionable whether these artificial pitches offer any physiological advantage to players.

The major hazard in cold conditions is likely to be associated with the condition of the pitch and its implications for safety. There are consequences also for the risk of injury to muscle unless the active muscles are warmed up prior to match-play. It is established that muscle performance deteriorates as muscle temperature falls (Åstrand & Rodahl 1986) and that injury is more likely to occur if the warm-up is inappropriate (Reilly & Stirling 1993).

Major tournaments, such as the World Cup finals in Spain 1982, Italy 1990, and the USA 1994, have been played in hot conditions with ambient temperatures around 30°C. Performance over 90 min of play is likely to be affected when such conditions are combined with high humidity. Work-rate efforts should be distributed carefully when playing in the heat since the rise in body temperature and the dehydration due to sweat losses are functions of the exercise intensity. Acclimatization prior to tournaments in the heat and adequate hydration pre-exercise and during the intermission are likely to promote work-rate capability. A good adaptation may be secured within $10-14$ days of the initial exposure. Further adaptations will enhance the player's ability to perform well under heat stress. The work-rate is most likely to be impaired toward the end of the game and particularly in extra time when matches are drawn. Muscle cramp, commonly noted when play is extended into extra time, will severely restrict activity, especially off the ball.

The work-rate profile may also be altered in matches played at altitude. Two World Cup finals have been played in Mexico (1970 and 1986), the altitude in Mexico City being 2.3 km. At this altitude maximum oxygen uptake ($\dot{V}_{O_{2}max}$) is impaired by about 15%, and running performance over 5 km by 9%. After a month at altitude the $\dot{V}_{O_{2}max}$ is still depressed by about 9% compared to its sea-level value and the 5 km running time is 6% less. At a given running speed the blood lactate is increased, the rise being a function of the fall in $\dot{V}_{O_{2max}}$. A consequence is that the work-rate preferred in matches at sea-level cannot be realized at conditions of altitude. Players will therefore need to pace their high-intensity efforts with a greater than customary discretion. Whilst some teams may have suffered due to inexperience of altitude exposure at the 1970 finals, most teams were able to cope well with the conditions in 1986. This was largely attributable to the fact that the teams used acclimatization regimens in the build-up to the finals. Whilst patterns of play in the Mexico finals have been thoroughly investigated, there have been no definitive investigations to determine whether work-rate was seriously compromised by the selection of Mexico City as a venue for World Cup finals.

The home venue is generally regarded as offering an advantage to a football team. The home team obtains about 64% of all points gained in the English Football League and home advantage has not changed since the formation of the League in 1888. The advantage is less marked in local derbies but is more pronounced in European Cup matches (Pollard 1986). Players are more anxiety prone when playing at home, as indicated by pre-exercise emotional tachycardia (Thomas & Reilly 1975). This does not translate into work-rate alterations since Reilly and Thomas (1976) failed to show any difference in distance covered per game between home and away matches. Pre-match anxiety may have more subtle effects on competitive behavior in critical incidents. The links between anxiety and injury proneness, culminating in tentative and mis-timed tackles that lead to injury, have been outlined by Sanderson (1981).

Physiology of game-related activities

The distance covered in a game under-represents the energy expended because of the extra demands of game skills which are not accounted for. These include the frequent accelerations and decelerations, angular runs, changes of direction, jumps to contest possession, tackles, avoiding tackles, and all the manifold aspects of direct involvement in play. Some attempts have been made to quantify the additional physiologic demands of game skills over and above the physiologic cost of locomotion.

Dribbling the ball is an example of a game skill amenable to physiologic investigation in a laboratory context. Reilly and Ball (1984) examined physiologic responses to dribbling a football on a treadmill at speeds of 9, 10.5, 12, and 13.5 km·h^{-1}, each for 5 min. A rebound box on the front of the treadmill returned the ball to the player's feet after each touch forward. The procedure allowed precise control over the player's activity while expired air, blood lactate level, and perception of effort were measured. The energy cost of dribbling, which entailed one touch of the ball every 2−3 full stride cycles, was found to increase linearly with the speed of running. The added cost of dribbling was constant at 5.2 kJ·min^{-1}. This value is likely to vary in field conditions according to the closeness of ball control the player exerts.

When dribbling with tight control of the ball, the stride rate increases and the stride length shortens compared with normal running at the same speed; these changes are likely to contribute to the additional energy cost. Increasing or decreasing the stride length beyond that freely chosen by the individual increases the oxygen consumption for a given speed (Cavanagh & Williams 1982). The energy cost may be further accentuated in matches as the player changes stride characteristics irregularly or feigns lateral movements while in possession of the ball in order to outwit an opponent. A reduction in stride length when dribbling is perhaps needed to effect controlled contact with the ball and propel it forward with the right amount of force by the swinging leg. The muscle activity required for kicking the ball and the action of synergistic and stabilizing muscles to facilitate balance while the kicking action is being executed are also likely to contribute to the added energy cost.

Perceived exertion also increases while dribbling in parallel with the elevation in metabolism (Reilly & Ball 1984). All-out efforts are likely to be limited by attaining the ceiling in perceived exertion and so top running speeds may not be attained in dribbling practices unless the frequency of ball contact is reduced. This in effect is what happens when a player kicks the ball ahead to allow enough space to accelerate past a stationary opponent.

Blood lactate levels are also elevated as a consequence of dribbling the ball, the increased concentrations being disproportionate at high speeds. In the study of Reilly and Ball (1984) the lactate inflection threshold was estimated to occur at 10.7 km·h^{-1} for dribbling but not until 11.7 km·h⁻¹ in normal running. This indicates that the metabolic strain of fast dribbling will be underestimated unless the additional anaerobic loading is considered.

About 16% of the distance covered by players in a game is in moving backward or sideways. The percentage is highest in defenders who may, for example, have to back quickly under high kicks forward from the opposition's half or move sideways in jockeying for position prior to tackling. The added physiological costs of unorthodox directions of movements have been examined by measuring nine football players running on a treadmill at speeds of 5, 7, and 9 km·h⁻¹, running normally, running backward, and running sideways (Reilly & Bowen 1984). The extra energy cost of the unorthodox modes of running increased disproportionately with speed. Running backward and running sideways did not differ in terms of energy expenditure or ratings of perceived exertion (Table 3.4). Clearly improving the muscular efficiency in these unorthodox modes of movement would benefit the player.

There is a myriad of other actions and alterations in activity during play that are superimposed on the requirements to cover distance. Although the extra energy cost of isolated actions is small, the additional energy expended may have considerable impact when all the added loads are aggregated. An analysis of 20 Australian football players showed that on average each player was engaged in 13 (± five) tackles, 10 (± six) headers, 26 (± 12) ball contacts with the foot, 51 (± 11) total ball contacts, 50 (± 13) turns, and nine (± six) jumps. Such activities provide an extra perturbation to the physiologic responses to motion.

Conclusion

The movement patterns imposed by football competition on its players have implications for the physiologic capacities of those players. The physiologic demands vary with the level of competition, the playing style, the positional role, and environmental factors. Nevertheless all outfield players must be mobile, capable of covering ground quickly to contest possession, play the ball, or support team-mates in defense and attack. They may need to sustain runs and recover quickly to move into positions supporting the player on the ball or maintain defensive lines.

Many aspects of football performances are aleatory or dependent on chance. Nevertheless patterns of movement behavior and work-rate profiles during competition provide useful information in delineating the physiologic demands of the game. These profiles form a basis for establishing physical training regimens and for modelling experimental protocols whereby the physiologic stresses associated with the exercise intensity of football can be investigated.

References

Agnevik G. (1970) *Fotboll. Rapport Idrottsfysiologi* (Football. A Report in Sports Physiology). Trygg-Hansa, Stockholm.

Åstrand P.O. & Rodahl K. (1986) *Textbook of Work Physiology*. McGraw-Hill, New York.

Bangsbo J. & Lindquist F. (1992) Comparison of various exercise tests with endurance performance during soccer in professional players. *Int. J. Sports Med.* **13**, 125–132.

Bangsbo J., Nørregaard L. & Thorsøe F. (1991) Activity profile of competition soccer. *Can. J. Sports Sci.* **16**, 110–116.

Cavanagh P.R. & Williams K.R. (1982) The effect of stride length variations on oxygen uptake during distance running. *Med. Sci. Sports Exerc.* **14**, 30–35.

Coghlan A. (1990) How to score goals and influence people. *New Scientist* **126** (No. 1715), 54–59.

Ekblom B. (1986) Applied physiology of soccer. *Sports Med.* **3**, 50–60.

Hughes M. (1988) Computerized notation analysis in field games. *Ergonomics* **31**, 1585–1592.

Knowles J.E. & Brooke J.D. (1974) *A movement analysis of player behaviour in soccer match performance.* Paper presented at the 8th Conference, British Society of Sports Psychology, Salford.

Mayhew S.R. & Wenger H.A. (1985) Time–motion analysis of professional soccer. *J. Hum. Movement Studies* **11**,

Table 3.4 Mean (± SD) for energy expended (kJ·min⁻¹) and ratings of exertion at three speeds and three directional modes of motion (n = 9) (from Reilly & Bowen 1984)

Speed (km·h⁻¹)	Forward	Backward	Sideways
Energy expended			
5	37.0 ± 2.6	44.8 ± 6.1	46.6 ± 3.2
7	42.3 ± 1.7	53.4 ± 3.5	56.3 ± 6.1
9	50.6 ± 4.9	71.4 ± 7.0	71.0 ± 7.5
Perceived exertion			
5	6.7 ± 0.1	8.6 ± 2.0	8.7 ± 2.0
7	8.0 ± 1.4	11.2 ± 2.9	11.3 ± 3.2
9	10.2 ± 2.1	14.0 ± 2.0	13.8 ± 2.5

49—52.

Ohashi J., Togari H., Isokawa M. & Suzuki S. (1988) Measuring movement speeds and distances covered during soccer match-play. In Reilly T., Lees A., Davids K. & Murphy W.J. (eds) *Science and Football*, pp. 329—333. E. & F.N. Spon, London.

Ohta T., Togari H. & Komiya Y. (1969) Game analysis of soccer (in Japanese). In *Soccer*, pp. 31—43. Japan Football Association, Tokyo.

Pollard R. (1986) Home advantage in soccer: a retrospective analysis. *J. Sports Sci.* **4**, 237—248.

Reep C. & Benjamin B. (1968) Skill and chance in Association Football. *J. Roy. Stat. Soc. Series A* **131**, 581—585.

Reilly T. (1990) Football. In Reilly T., Secher N., Snell, P. & Williams C. (eds) *Physiology of Sports*, pp. 371—425. E. & F.N. Spon, London.

Reilly T. & Ball D. (1984) The net physiological cost of dribbling a soccer ball. *Res. Q. Exerc. Sport* **55**, 267—271.

Reilly T. & Bowen T. (1984) Exertional costs of changes in directional modes of running. *Percept. Motor Skills* **58**, 149—150.

Reilly T. & Holmes M. (1983) A preliminary analysis of selected soccer skills. *Phys. Educ. Rev.* **6**, 64—71.

Reilly T. & Stirling A. (1993) Flexibility, warm-up and injuries in mature games players. In Duquet W. & Day J.A.P. (eds) *Kinanthropometry IV*, pp. 119—123. E. & F.N. Spon, London.

Reilly T. & Thomas V. (1976) A motion analysis of work-rate in different positional roles in professional football match-play. *J. Hum. Movement Studies* **2**, 87—97.

Saltin B. (1973) Metabolic fundamentals in exercise. *Med. Sci. Sports* **5**, 137—146.

Sanderson F.H. (1981) The psychology of the injury-prone athlete. In Reilly T. (ed.) *Sports Fitness and Sports Injuries*, pp. 31—36. Faber & Faber, London.

Smaros G. (1980) Energy usage during a football match. In Vecchiet L. (ed.) *Proceedings of the 1st International Congress on Sports Medicine Applied to Football*, vol. 11, pp. 795—801. D. Guanello, Rome.

Thomas V. & Reilly T. (1975) The relationship between anxiety variables and injuries in top-class soccer. In Alderson G.J.K. & Tyldesley D. (eds) *Proceedings of the European Sports Psychology Conference*, Edinburgh, pp. 213—222.

Togari H. (1967) Asian elimination round for Mexico Olympics from a scientific veiwpoint (in Japanese). *Soccer Mag.* **12**, 86—89.

Van Gool D. (1987) *De fysieke belasting fijdens een voetbalwedstrijd: Studie van apgelegde afstand, hartfreykintie, energieverbruck en lactaatbepulinyer*. PhD thesis, University of Leuven, Belgium.

Van Gool D., Van Gervan D. & Boutmans J. (1988) The physiological load imposed on soccer players during real match-play. In Reilly T., Lees A., Davids K. & Murphy W.J. (eds) *Science and Football*, pp. 51—59. E. & F.N. Spon, London.

Vinnai G. (1973) *Football Mania*. Ocean Books, London.

Wade A. (1962) The training of young players. *Med. Sport Torino* **3**, 1245—1251.

Withers R.T., Maricic Z., Wasilewski S. & Kelly L. (1982) Match analysis of Australian professional soccer players. *J. Hum. Movement Studies* **8**, 159—176.

Yamanaka K., Haga S., Shindo M. *et al.* (1988) Time and motion analysis in top class soccer games. In Reilly T., Lees A., Davids K. & Murphy W.J. (eds) *Science and Football*, pp. 334—340. E. & F.N. Spon, London.

Zelenka V., Seliger V. & Ondrej O. (1967) Specific function testing of young football players. *J. Sports Med. Phys. Fit.* **7**, 143—147.

Chapter 4

Physiological demands

Energy production in football

During exercise muscles use energy, which is provided from either aerobic (aero: air) or anaerobic (an: non; aero: air) processes. The anaerobic energy is released from breakdown of adenosine triphosphate (ATP), which is stored within the muscle or produced either by splitting creatine phosphate (CP) or by degrading carbohydrate (CHO) to pyruvate (glycolysis) which leads to the formation of lactate. A minor anaerobic energy contribution can also occur by the degradation of adenosine diphosphate (ADP) to adenosine monophosphate (AMP) and further to inosine monophosphate (IMP) and ammonia (NH_3). The aerobic energy is produced in special compartments (mitochondria) in the muscle cell by using oxygen, which is taken up from the blood. The substrates for these reactions are formed through glycolysis (utilization of CHO), catabolism of fat and, to a lesser extent, amino acids (protein). The rate of ATP production during exercise and, thus, utilization of substrates is controlled by the intensity of the activity. In most cases, the anaerobic processes are so rapid, and the aerobic system has such a capacity that the muscles are able to maintain ATP at a high level during exercise.

The CHO for glycolysis is primarily glycogen stored within the exercising muscles, but glucose taken up from the blood can also be used. The glucose is taken up from the gut and released to the blood from the liver, which forms the glucose from breakdown of glycogen (glycogenolysis) or from precursors such as glycerol, pyruvate, lactate, and amino acids (gluconeogenesis). The substrates for fat oxidation are triglycerides (TG) stored within the muscles and fat carried in the blood, primarily free fatty acids (FFA) released from adipose tissue and to a lesser extent TG. The different processes related to energy production are summarized in Fig. 4.1, where some of the key enzymes in the different reactions are also given.

In football, players perform many different types of exercise, and the intensity can alternate at any time and range from standing still to maximal running. Thus, besides having a well-developed ability to exercise with a high power output the players should also be able to work for a long time (endurance). This separates football from sports in which continuous exercise is performed with either a very high or moderate intensity during the entire event, such as a 400 m and a marathon run, respectively. This chapter will focus on how much energy is provided from the aerobic and the anaerobic reactions and which substrates are used during a football match.

Aerobic energy production

There have been several attempts to determine the aerobic contribution by measuring oxygen uptake ($\dot{V}_{O_2}$) during match-play, but none of these seem to have been successful in getting realistic values. The major problems are that the determination of $\dot{V}_{O_2}$ interferes with normal play and that only minor parts of a match can be analyzed.

Another way to obtain information about the aerobic energy expenditure during football is by measuring heart rate (HR) continuously during a match and estimating energy expenditure from the $HR-\dot{V}_{O_2}$ relation determined in the laboratory. As HR determinations can be performed without any restrictions on the player, it might represent a more exact picture of the contribution of the aerobic system in football. Seliger (1968) found that the mean HR during a match was 165 beats·min^{-1} (80% of maximal HR) for Czechoslovakian football players, and later Agnevik (1970) observed a mean value of 175 beats·min^{-1} (93% of maximal HR) for a single Swedish player during a match. Smodlaka (1978) reported that HR for Russian players was above 85% of maximal HR (171 beats·min^{-1}) for 57% of the playing time, and Reilly (1986) found a mean HR of 157 beats·min^{-1} when investigating English League players in friendly games. Slightly higher values were recorded for a Belgian University team also participating in a non-competition match, namely 169 and 165 beats·min^{-1} for the first and second half, respectively (Van Gool *et al.* 1988). Measurements have also been performed during com-

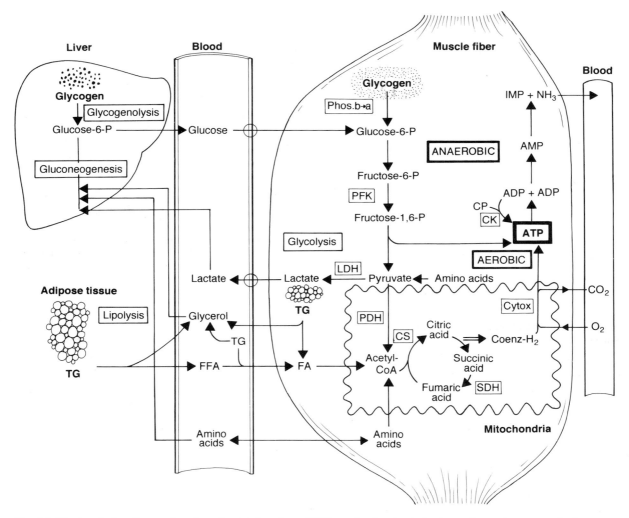

Fig. 4.1 Biochemical pathways for adenosine triphosphate (ATP) production in skeletal muscles and sources of substrates. The flux through a pathway is among other factors regulated by the activity of enzymes involved in the reactions. Some of the key enzymes are given in the figure. ADP, adenosine diphosphate; AMP, adenosine monophosphate; CK, creatine kinase; CP, creatine phosphate; CS, citrate synthase; Cytox, cytochrome oxidase; FA, fatty acids; FFA, free fatty acids; IMP, inosine monophosphate; LDH, lactate dehydrogenase; NH_3, ammonia; PDH, pyruvate dehydrogenase; PFK, phosphofructokinase; Phos. a, b, phosphorylase a and b; SDH, succinate dehydrogenase; TG, triglycerides.

petitive matches. In a league match the mean HR for six Danish players was 164 beats·min^{-1} during first half and about 10 beats·min^{-1} lower during the second half (Bangsbo 1994). Similar findings were obtained by Rhode and Espersen (1988) by observing six other Danish football players in four First Division games. They found further, that the HR during a match was below 73% of maximal HR for 10 min (11% of the playing time), between 73 and 92% for 57 min (63%), and higher than 92% for 23 min (26%).

Based on individual relationships between HR and $\dot{V}_{O_2}$ obtained during standardized exercise tests in the laboratory, the HR determinations during match-play can be transformed to oxygen uptake. An example of this conversion is shown on Fig. 4.2. By such esti-mations mean values about 75% of $\dot{V}_{O_{2max.}}$ have been

Table 4.1 Lactate concentration (mmol·l^{-1}) in blood*
taken from a fingertip or an arm vein during or after a
football match. Data presented as mean ± SD or range
(in brackets)

| Study | Players | First half | | Second half | |
		During	End	During	End
Agnevik (1970)	First Division (Sweden)	—	—	—	10.0 (−15.5)
Smaros (1980)	Second Division (Finland)	—	4.9 ± 1.9	—	4.1 ± 1.3
Ekblom (1986)	First Division (Sweden)	—	9.5 (6.9−14.3)	—	7.2 (4.5−10.8)
	Second Division (Sweden)	—	8.0 (5.1−11.5)	—	6.6 (3.1−11.0)
	Third Division (Sweden)	—	5.5 (3.0−12.6)	—	4.2 (3.2−8.0)
	Fourth Division (Sweden)	—	4.0 (1.9−6.3)	—	3.9 (1.0−8.5)
Rhode & Espersen (1988)	First and Second Division (Denmark)	—	5.1 ± 1.6	—	3.9 ± 1.6
Gerisch et al. (1988)	Top amateur league (Germany)	—	5.6 ± 2.0	—	4.7 ± 2.2
	University match (Germany)	6.8 ± 1.0	5.9 ± 2.0	5.1 ± 1.6	4.9 ± 1.7
Smith et al. (1993)	College matches	—	—	5.2 ± 1.2	—	—
Bangsbo et al. (1991)	First and Second Division (Denmark)	4.9 (2.1−10.3)	—	3.7 (1.8−5.2)	4.4 (2.1−6.9)
Bangsbo (1994)	League match (Denmark)	4.1 (2.9−6.0)	2.6 (2.0−3.6)	2.4 (1.6−3.9)	2.7 (1.6−4.6)
	League match (Denmark)†	6.6 (4.3−9.3)	3.9 (2.8−5.4)	4.0 (2.5−6.2)	3.9 (2.3−6.4)

* Lactate analysis was performed using whole blood except in the case marked with (†), where plasma was used.

Energy turnover during specific match activities

Supplementary to measurements performed during
match-play, the energy cost of different simulated
match activities has been determined in laboratory
conditions. Reilly and Ball (1984) examined players
dribbling a football on a treadmill at four different
speeds, each of a duration of 5 min. They found that
the additional $\dot{V}O_2$ due to dribbling was about 0.3 l·
min^{-1}, which was the same at the four speeds. At the
high speeds blood lactate concentrations were also
higher than dribbling. The increased energy demand
during dribbling can to some extent be explained by a
greater need to maintain balance, by a shorter stride

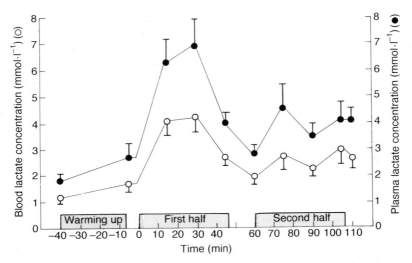

Fig. 4.6 Whole blood (○) and plasma (●) lactate concentration for six players before, during, and after a competitive football match. Blood was taken from an arm vein, and in order to collect the samples the match was stopped for 1 min twice in each half. Heart rate (HR) was recorded continuously during the match, and the mean HR 5 min prior to each blood sampling for the first half was 166 (15 min), 163 (30 min), and 163 (45 min) beats·min⁻¹ and the corresponding values for the second half were 161, 160, and 166 beats·min⁻¹, respectively. Note that the plasma lactate values were about twice as high as the whole blood values. Thus, erythrocytes are only of minor importance as a "lactate titration space," and plasma lactate reflects better the concentration in the exercising muscles (Juel *et al.* 1990). Means ± SE are given.

length and by a higher stride frequency than used in running, which is known to decrease running efficiency (Cavanagh & Williams 1982). During treadmill running, the ball was touched once every two or three full strides. The additional energy cost of dribbling is probably higher during a match, since the ball is often touched more frequently in order to protect it from the opponent. However, as the total time of ball contact for an individual player averages about 1 min during a match, the extra energy cost for dribbling only to a minor extent influences the total energy expenditure.

The energy cost of sideway and backward movements has also been examined (Reilly & Bowen 1984). Nine football players were required to run forwards, sideways, and backwards at three different treadmill speeds. The extra energy consumption for sideway and backward running was of a similar magnitude, and it was increased with enhanced treadmill speed. The difference in $\dot{V}_{O_2}$ was about 0.6 (23% of the total energy expenditure) and 1.0 l·min⁻¹ (29%) at 5 and 9 km·h⁻¹, respectively. These values should be related to the occurrence of sideway and backward move-

ments during a football match. Reilly and Thomas (1976) found for English players that the total distance covered by these activities was about 1400 m performed during 16% of the total playing time, while observations of Danish players have shown corresponding values of 230 m and 1.3% for backward running (Bangsbo *et al.* 1991). The difference between the two observations was partly due to the fact that Reilly and Thomas (1976), in contrast to the study by Bangsbo *et al.* (1991), included backward walking in the category of backward movements. Apparently, the total distance covered by backward and sideway running at high speed is small. Thus, the total extra energy consumption due to sideway and backward movements seems to play a minor role in football.

Metabolism

Substrate utilization

The large aerobic energy production in football and the pronounced anaerobic energy turnover during periods of a match are associated with a large consumption of substrates. The dominant substrates are CHO and fat either stored within the exercising muscle or delivered via the blood to the exercising muscles (see Fig. 4.1). The role of protein in football is unclear, but studies with continuous exercise at a mean work-rate and duration similar to football have shown that oxidation of proteins contribute less than 10% of the total energy production (Wagenmakers *et al.* 1989).

Carbohydrate consumption

CHO is stored as glycogen in the muscles (300−500 g) and in the liver (50−100 g) (see Fig. 4.1). In addition, a small amount (about 5 g) is circulating in the blood as glucose. During exercise, the CHO used is primarily the glycogen stored within the exercising muscles, but glucose from the blood is also taken up and utilized by the muscles. Figure 4.7 shows the blood glucose concentrations during a competitive match. During the entire match blood glucose was higher than at rest and no player had values below 4 mmol·l⁻¹. Glucose concentrations after matches have also been obtained in other studies. The mean values for Danish and Swedish élite players were 4.5 and 3.8 mmol·l⁻¹, respectively, with a few measurements below 3.2 mmol·l⁻¹ (Ekblom 1986). Thus, it appears that the liver, under most circumstances, is able to release enough glucose to maintain, and even at times elevate, the blood glucose concentration during a match.

Information about muscle glycogen utilization during a football match can be obtained from determinations of glycogen in muscle biopsies taken before and after a football match. The difference in glycogen content represents the net use of muscle glycogen, but it does not indicate the absolute amount of glycogen used, since resynthesis of glycogen probably occurs during the rest and low-intensity exercise periods during a match (Nordheim & Vøllestad, 1990). In a Swedish study the average thigh muscle glycogen concentrations of five players were 96, 32, and 9 mmol·kg⁻¹ wet weight (w.w.) before, at half-time, and after a non-competitive match, respectively (Saltin 1973). Four other players started the same match with low muscle glycogen levels (45 mmol·kg⁻¹ w.w.) as a result of extensive physical exercise the day prior to the game, and for these players, the muscle glycogen storage was almost depleted by half-time. Another Swedish study has shown that the muscle glycogen stores are not always totally emptied at the end of a match, since the mean glycogen concentration in the quadriceps muscle for 15 players was 46 mmol·kg⁻¹ w.w. (Jacobs *et al.* 1982). Unfortunately, the change in muscle glycogen could not be determined in the latter study, since no samples were taken before the match. It has to be emphasized that the glycogen level varies between muscle fibers and it is possible that a considerable number of fibers are depleted, even though the average concentration of glycogen is quite high.

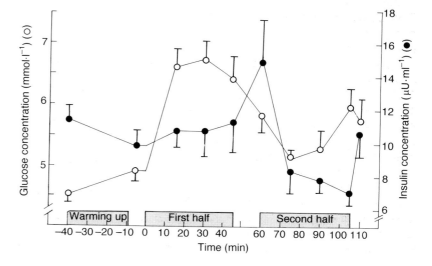

Fig. 4.7 Blood glucose (○) and insulin (●) concentration for six players before, during, and after a competitive football match. The same players and match as referred to in Fig. 4.6. Note that the lowered insulin concentration in the second half is associated with a decrease in blood glucose concentration. Mean ± SE are given.

Fat oxidation

Fat oxidized in the exercising muscles during a football match is either provided from the intramuscular stores of TG or delivered to the muscle via the blood as FFA or TG (see Fig. 4.1). The FFA is, together with glycerol, released from the adipose tissue after the breakdown of TG (lipolysis). As shown in Fig. 4.8 blood FFA concentration increased during a football match and more so during the second half. The concentration in the blood is the net result of the uptake of FFA in various tissues and release of fatty acids, which is influenced by the lipolytic activity in the adipose tissue. The release of fatty acids is also related to the perfusion of the adipose tissue, and as the blood supply probably is elevated in the rest periods during a football match, it favors a high blood FFA concentration. This is also illustrated by the high blood FFA 5 min after the match (Fig. 4.8), which is probably a combination of decreased utilization of FFA and elevated blood flow to the adipose tissue. In contrast to observations for continuous exercise, only a minor increase in glycerol was found during the match (Fig. 4.8). This indicates a high uptake of glycerol in various tissues. The most important is likely to be the liver, which presumably has a larger uptake of glycerol than observed during continuous exercise due to an elevated blood flow in the rest periods. Thus, it appears that glycerol might represent a significant gluconeogenic precursor during a football match. It is very difficult to determine the uptake of FFA and the amount of fat oxidized during a football match from the blood FFA and glycerol concentrations, as they reflect the balance between release to and removal from the blood. Furthermore, studies of repeated intense exercise bouts suggest that intramuscular TG is a major source of the fat oxidized in the recovery periods in between the exercises, and thus probably also during football (Essén 1978).

Another method of evaluating fat oxidation is to determine the respiratory exchange ratio (R) under steady-state conditions, and use this as an expression of the non-protein respiratory quotient (RQ). This is difficult during a football match, but can be done during standardized intermittent exercise simulating the activity pattern of football. Measurements during this type of exercise resulted in R values of 0.85, 0.87, and 0.91 at work-rates corresponding to 55, 71, and 81% of $\dot{V}_{O_2max.}$, respectively. This relationship between the R value and the relative work-rate is comparable to the relationship obtained during long-term intermittent exercise (Essén 1978, Bangsbo *et al.* 1992b). Based on these determinations and HR measurements during a football match, from which the $\dot{V}_{O_2}$ is estimated, the mean R value during a match can be calculated to be 0.88. This corresponds to a contribution from CHO and fat of 60 and 40%, respectively, to the total oxidation. With the use of these numbers, combined with assumed values which seem reasonable in football, the total oxidation of CHO and fat during a match can

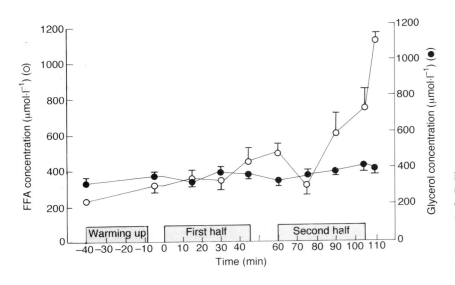

Fig. 4.8 Free fatty acid (FFA) (○) and blood glycerol (●) concentration for six players before, during, and after a competitive football match. The same players and match as referred to in Fig. 4.6. Mean ± SE are given.

then be calculated. If a player with a body mass of 75 kg has a $\dot{V}_{O_{2max.}}$ of 60 ml·kg^{-1}·min^{-1}, and the mean $\dot{V}_{O_2}$ for this player during a football match is 70% of $\dot{V}_{O_{2max.}}$, the total oxidation of CHO and fat would be about 1140 (205 g) and 230 (56 g) mmol, respectively. Part of the CHO oxidized is glucose taken up from the blood, which might account for about 200 mmol glycosyl units, released from the liver via glycogenolysis and gluconeogenesis. This leaves about 940 mmol to be supplied by muscle glycogen, which also should provide substrate for anaerobic glycolysis. The net muscle glycogen utilization for the latter process may be estimated to be 60 mmol glucosyl units, if it is assumed that the lactate removed from the blood is oxidized either as lactate or glucose formed in the liver. Then, the total net muscle glycogen use is about 1000 mmol glucosyl units. This value can be compared with the observed decline in muscle glycogen of about 85 mmol·kg^{-1} w.w. during a match for players with normal muscle glycogen concentrations prior to the match (Saltin 1973). From these calculations the mean muscle mass, which was glycogen depleted to the same extent as the biopsied muscle, can be estimated to approximately 12 kg. This value does not appear unrealistic for a player with a body mass of 75 kg. It has to be emphasized that these calculations are based on several assumptions, mean values are used and there are likely to be large inter-individual differences.

Hormones

Both the hormones epinephrine and norepinephrine are elevated during a football match as illustrated in Fig. 4.9. The considerable increase in norepinephrine shows that the sympathetic nervous system is stimulated, which also enhances the secretion of norepinephrine and in particular epinephrine from the adrenal medulla. As the norepinephrine concentration exceeds that of epinephrine about sevenfold, it appears that most of the circulating norepinephrine originates from sympathetic release (Fig. 4.9). Neither the epinephrine or norepinephrine values were close to the upper limit of about 2 and 10 ng·l^{-1}, respectively, observed during maximal exercise (Kjær 1989), Nevertheless, they are likely to have a pronounced influence on metabolism.

The elevated epinephrine affects blood glucose and CHO metabolism, as it stimulates glycogenolysis in the muscles. In addition, both epinephrine and norepinephrine increase lipolysis in the adipose tissue, and thus, the release of fatty acids into the circulation. Insulin has the opposite effect and high blood lactate also suppresses mobilization of fatty acids from the adipose tissue. Thus, the unaltered insulin (see Fig. 4.7) and elevated lactate concentration during the first half have probably counteracted the effects of elevated epinephrine and norepinephrine on the release of fatty acids. This can partly explain the only moderate

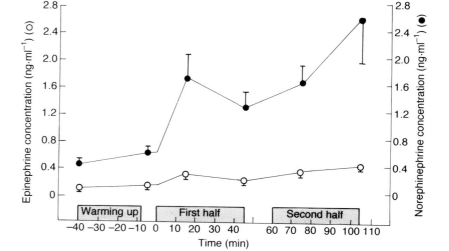

Fig. 4.9 Blood epinephrine (○) and norepinephrine (●) concentration for six players before, during, and after a competitive football match. The same players and match as referred to in Fig. 4.6. Mean ± SE are given.

increases in the FFA concentration in the early stage of the match (see Fig. 4.8). Correspondingly, the lowered insulin and lactate concentrations in the second half and the progressively increased epinephrine and norepinephrine concentrations might have increased the FFA concentrations towards the end of the match (see Fig. 4.8). Also growth hormone (GH) has a stimulating effect on lipolysis and it appears to be elevated during a football match (Carli *et al.* 1986). It has been demonstrated that GH increases as exercise progresses (Kjær *et al.* 1988). Therefore, it is likely that the increased FFA concentration at the end of the match is also caused by a progressively elevated GH concentration. FFA provide an alternative fuel to blood glucose and muscle glycogen, and increasing uptake of FFA in the muscles probably delays the time when muscle glycogen stores become critically low. In addition, the decrease in circulating insulin level during a match slow the uptake of glucose by most tissues, sparing the remaining glucose for active muscle and other tissues (e.g. brain) with an essential requirement for glucose. Other hormones also influence the blood glucose concentration. Glucagon may be important in the control of hepatic glycogenolysis and gluconeogenesis, which is also stimulated by cortisol (with amino acids as precursor). While cortisol appears to be elevated, it is likely that only minor changes occur in the glucagon concentration during a football match (Carli *et al.* 1986, Kjær *et al.* 1988).

Temperature regulation

The high energy turnover in football causes a large heat production, which has to be removed in order to avoid overheating and subsequent deterioration of performance. Most of the heat produced is released from the body by evaporation, which is associated with loss of body fluid. In addition, water lying on the surface of the skin may be absorbed by the clothes or may fall to the ground without any accompanying heat loss.

Under extreme conditions the decrease in body water has been observed to be higher than 3.5 l for individual players (Mustafa & Mahmoud 1979). Weight loss is increased by elevated air temperature and humidity as observed by Mustafa and Mahmoud (1979). They found that fluid loss (3.1% of body weight) during a match at an air temperature of 33°C and a humidity

of 40%, was similar to a loss during a match where the corresponding values were 26.3°C and 78%, respectively. In a third match with an air temperature of 13.2°C and a humidity of 7%, the fluid loss was reduced to 1.2% of body weight. Under normal weather conditions the decrease in body fluid during a match is approximately 2 l, a magnitude that can have a negative influence on performance at the end of a match (Saltin 1964). Thus, it is important for players to take in fluid during a game. Besides reducing the net loss of fluid the intake of fluid can supply the body with CHO. For a further discussion of this topic see Chapter 11.

In spite of the considerable release of heat via evaporation, the body temperature rises during a football match. For environment temperatures between 20 and 25°C, Ekblom (1986) found, that the mean rectal temperature after matches was 39.5°C for Swedish First Division players, while the levels were between 39.0 and 39.2°C for players from lower divisions. Some players were found to have a temperature higher than 40°C. Similar values were reported by Smodlaka (1978).

Rectal temperature is another indirect measure of energy production during exercise, since a linear relationship between rectal temperature and relative work-rate during prolonged continuous exercise has been demonstrated (Saltin & Hermansen 1966). At a room temperature of about 20°C the rectal temperature was 38.7°C at a work-rate corresponding to 70% of $\dot{V}_{O_{2max}}$. The ratio between relative energy expenditure and rectal temperature is probably lower in football, since it has been demonstrated that intermittent exercise increases body temperature more than continuous exercise at a given oxygen uptake (approximately 0.3°C at a relative work-rate of 60%; Ekblom *et al.* 1971). A loss of fluid during a match also elevates body temperature without a concomitant increase in energy consumption (Ekblom *et al.* 1970). Thus, the rectal temperatures of 39.0–39.5°C for the Swedish élite players indicate a relative work-rate of 70–80% of $\dot{V}_{O_{2max.}}$, which is in accordance with the determinations from HR measurements during football matches as discussed at the beginning of this chapter ('Aerobic energy production').

Fatigue

Fatigue during intense periods of a match

During a football match, a player might be fatigued after a period of high-intensity exercise, i.e. not being able to perform maximally in a subsequent exercise bout. The question is what causes deterioration in performance during and after severe exercise.

During intense exercise there is a large production of lactate with a subsequent acidity of the active muscles, as lactate dissociates hydrogen ions (H^+). Skeletal muscles have a high buffering capacity (neutralize H^+), which limits the increase in free hydrogen ions. Nevertheless, decreases in muscle pH from 7.1 to 6.4–6.8 can be observed during very intense, exhaustive exercise; and pH in individual fibers, particularly fast twitch (FT) fibers, might be even lower (Juel *et al.* 1990, Vandenborne *et al.* 1991). The low pH at the end of intense exercise may affect the function of the muscle cells, and it is generally believed that lactic acid accumulation and the concomitant elevation in H^+ concentration cause fatigue. However, in recent studies an exclusive role of lactate and acidity as "fatigue factors" has been questioned. In one of these studies exhaustion occurred at a significant lower muscle lactate concentration when intense exercise was repeated after 1 h of recovery (Bangsbo *et al.* 1992a). In another study, Sahlin and Ren (1989) showed that despite a persistently high muscle lactate level (probably lowered muscle pH), contraction force was completely restored 2 min after intensive isometric muscle contractions (Fig. 4.10).

If muscle lactate and pH are not causally linked with a deterioration in muscle tension, what then is the cause of fatigue? It is difficult to identify a single factor responsible for the reduction in performance during intense exercise. It appears not to be related to lack of energy, since muscle ATP is relatively high at exhaustion. Fatigue may be caused by a failure in the propagation of electrical impulses (action potential) due to ion disturbances over the muscle fiber membranes or an inability of the nervous system to activate the muscle fibers. It is well known that muscle fibers release potassium (K^+) during contractions, and that K^+ accumulates around the muscle fibers despite an elevated activity of the Na^+/K^+ pumps, which brings K^+ back to the muscle cell. It has been speculated that

K^+ stimulates a reflex inhibition from the muscles (Bangsbo *et al.* 1992a). This is supported by the finding of the same interstitial K^+ concentrations at exhaustion when intense exercise is repeated, and by the observation that the time course of changes in muscle force and K^+ in recovery from exhaustive exercise are similar, and much faster than the changes in muscle pH (Fig. 4.10).

The scheme which may prevail is that elevated K^+ around the muscle fibers stimulates the sensory input, which causes inhibition of spinal motor nerves. This is likely to be a gradual phenomenon, and can at first be overcome by the drive from the motor cortex as new motor units are activated (recruiting other muscle fibers), if the player is able to tolerate the pain of concomitant intense exercise. However, a point is reached when the number of new muscle fibers which could be activated is considerably reduced and the reflex inhibition causes such a reduction in spinal motor activity output that the muscles are unable to reach the target force and maintain running speed. It might not only be the physical capacity that is influenced under these conditions, but the technical performance, even at lower exercise intensities, may also be reduced.

Fatigue during match-play is temporary and might last for several minutes, but in most cases it is much shorter. Nevertheless, fatigue of a player might be crucial for the final result of the match. Thus, it is very important that the players recover as fast as possible. The time needed to return to normal levels after intense exercise is dependent on a variety of factors such as the fitness level of the subject, the activity in the recovery period, and the intensity and duration of the preceding exercise. The latter is illustrated by the findings of Balsom *et al.* (1991). They observed that running time (approximately 5.5 s) was progressively increased when a 40-m all-out sprint was repeated 15 times, whereas performance was unaltered in 40 sprints of 15 m (approximately 2.5 s). In both cases the sprints were separated by a 30-s rest period. Thus, it appears that 30 s was long enough to recover from approximately 3 s of maximal exercise, but not when the duration of the maximal exercise was about 6 s. Fatigue can be postponed by training which among other things develops the player's ability to tolerate the discomfort of fatigue and to recover from intense exercise (see Chapter 10).

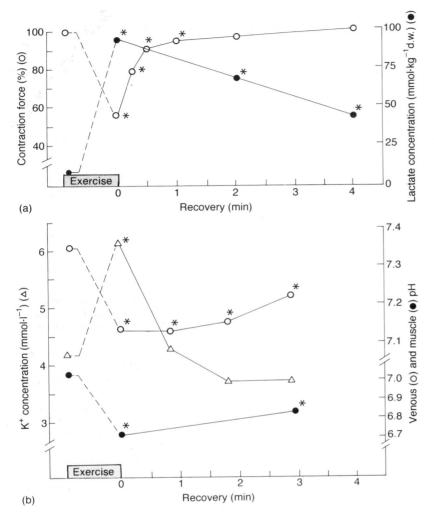

Fig. 4.10 (a) Force development (○) and muscle lactate concentration (●) after exhaustive isometric contraction (data from Sahlin & Ren 1990). (b) Femoral venous blood pH (○) and K⁺ (△) and further muscle pH (●) after exhaustive knee-extensor exercise (data from Bangsbo & Saltin 1993). * Significantly different from the resting value.

Fatigue at the end of a match

Toward the end of a football match fatigue might not only be related to very intense exercise, but it can also be an effect of a general muscle exhaustion as a result of the exercise previously in the match. The players may be able to exercise at low intensities and perform maximally for a short while, but their ability to exercise at a high intensity for a longer time can be reduced. It is often related to reduction in muscle glycogen. The muscles utilize their glycogen stores in selected patterns. The muscle fibers that are most frequently recruited and have the lowest capacity to rebuild glycogen in the rest period during the match may become depleted of glycogen. This reduces the number of fibers that are capable of generating enough tension for the exercise and fewer fibers can be recruited to compensate for the loss in muscle force. In agreement with this is the observation of an improved long-term intermittent exercise performance when muscle glycogen was elevated prior to testing by a CHO rich diet (Bangsbo et al. 1992b). Apparently, optimal preparation for a football match should also include intake of a proper diet (for details see Chapter 11).

Conclusion

The aerobic energy cost during a football match can be

estimated from measurements performed during or immediately after the match, e.g. HR and rectal temperature. Based on such determinations the aerobic energy production for élite players was estimated to be about 70% of maximum oxygen uptake. It is difficult to quantify the anaerobic energy turnover during match-play as the exercise intensity alternates frequently, but the energy production from this system appears only to account for a minor part of the total energy yield during a match. Nevertheless, the anaerobic system is very important during match-play, since it is associated with the intense exercise periods during a match, which, in turn, appear to be closely related to the competitive level of football (Ekblom 1986, Bangsbo 1992). Thus, it seems important that a player is able to repeatedly perform high-intensity exercise during match-play. It has to be emphasized that there are large individual differences in both the relative and absolute energy turnover.

Fatigue during intense exercise is probably due to a complex series of events, and it is difficult to identify any one factor responsible for the reduction in force development. On the other hand, it appears that the sensation of fatigue in the late stages of a match may coincide with the depletion of muscle glycogen.

References

Agnevik G. (1970) *Fotboll. Rapport Idrottsfysiologi* (Football. A Report in Sports Physiology). Trygg-Hansa, Stockholm.

Balsom P.D., Seger J.Y. & Ekblom B. (1991) A physiological evaluation of high intensity intermittent exercise. *Abstract from the 2nd World Congress on Science and Football*, 22–25 May 1991. Veldhoven, the Netherlands.

Bangsbo J. (1992) Time motion characteristics of competition football. *Sci. Football* **6**, 34–42.

Bangsbo J. (1994) Physiology of soccer — with special reference to intense intermittent exercise. *Acta Physiol. Scand.* **151**, Suppl., 619.

Bangsbo J., Graham T.E., Kiens B. & Saltin B. (1992a) Elevated muscle glycogen and anaerobic energy production during exhaustive exercise in man. *J. Physiol.* **451**, 205–222.

Bangsbo J., Nørregaard L. & Thorsøe F. (1991) Activity profile of competition soccer. *Can. J. Sport Sci.* **16**, 110–116.

Bangsbo J., Nørregaard L. & Thorsøe F. (1992b) The effect of carbohydrate diet on intermittent exercise performance. *Int. J. Sports Med.* **13**, 152–157.

Bangsbo J. & Saltin B. (1993) Recovery of muscle from exercise, its importance for subsequent performance. In Macleod D.A.D., Maughan R.J., Williams C., Madeley C.R., Sharp J.C.M. & Nutton R.W. (eds) *Intermittent High Intensity Exercise. Preparation, Stresses and Damage Limitation*, pp. 49–69. E. & F.N. Spon, London.

Boobis L.H. (1987) Metabolic aspects of fatigue during sprinting. In Macleod D., Maughan R., Nimmo M., Reilly T. & Williams C. (eds) *Exercise, Benefits, Limits and Adaptations*, pp. 116–143. E. & F.N. Spon, London.

Carli G., Bonifazi M., Lodi L., Lupo C., Martelli G. & Viti A. (1986) Hormonal and metabolic effects following a football match. *Int. J. Sports Med.* **7**, 36–38.

Cavanagh P.R. & Williams K.R. (1982) The effect of stride length variation on oxygen uptake during distance running. *Med. Sci. Sports Exerc.* **14**, 30–35.

Davis J.A. & Brewer J. (1991) Physiological characteristics of an international female soccer squad. *Abstract from the 2nd World Congress on Science and Football*, 22–25 May 1991. Veldhoven, the Netherlands.

Ekblom B. (1986) Applied physiology of soccer. *Sports Med.* **3**, 50–60.

Ekblom B., Greenleaf C.J., Greenleaf J.E. & Hermansen L. (1970) Temperature regulation during exercise dehydration in man. *Acta Physiol. Scand.* **79**, 475–483.

Ekblom B., Greenleaf C.J., Greenleaf J.E. & Hermansen L. (1971) Temperature regulation during continuous and intermittent exercise in man. *Acta Physiol. Scand.* **81**, 1–10.

Essén B. (1978) Studies on the regulation of metabolism in human skeletal muscle using intermittent exercise as an experimental model. *Acta Physiol. Scand.* **454**, Suppl., 1–32.

Gerisch G., Rutemoller E. & Weber K. (1988) Sports medical measurements of performance in soccer. In Reilly T., Lees A., Davids K. & Murphy W.J. (eds) *Science and Football*, pp. 60–67. E. & F.N. Spon, London.

Hultman E. & Sjöholm H. (1983) Substrate availability. In Knuttgen, H.C., Vogel J.A. & Poortmans J. (eds) *Biochemistry of Exercise*, pp. 63–75. Human Kinetics, Champaign, Illinois.

Jacobs I., Westlin N., Karlsson J., Rasmusson M. & Houghton B. (1982) Muscle glycogen and diet in élite soccer players. *Eur. J. Appl. Physiol.* **48**, 297–302.

Jensen K. & Larsson B. (1993) Variations of physical capacity in a period including supplemental training of the Danish soccer team for women. In Reilly T., Clarys J. & Stibbe A. (eds) *Science and Football II*, pp. 114–117. E. & F.N. Spon, London.

Juel C., Bangsbo J., Graham T. & Saltin B. (1990) Lactate and potassium fluxes from skeletal muscle during intense dynamic knee-extensor exercise in man. *Acta Physiol. Scand.* **140**, 147–159.

Kjær M. (1989) Epinephrine and some other hormonal responses to exercise in man: with special reference to physical training. *Int. J. Sports Med.* **10**, 2–15.

Kjær M., Bangsbo J., Lortie G. & Galbo H. (1988) Hormonal response to exercise in humans: influence of hypoxia and physical training. *Am. J. Physiol.* **23**, R197–R203.

Lindquist F. & Bangsbo J. (1993) Do young soccer players need specific physical training? In Reilly T., Clarys, J. & Stibbe A. (eds) *Science and Football II*, pp. 275–280. E. & F.N. Spon, London.

Mustafa K.Y. & El-Din Ahmed Mahmoud N. (1979) Evaporative water loss in African soccer players. *J. Sports Med. Phys. Fit.* **19**, 181–183.

Nordheim K. & Vøllestad N. (1990) Glycogen and lactate metabolism during low intensity exercise in man. *Acta Physiol. Scand.* **139**, 475–484.

Reilly T. (1986) Fundamental studies on soccer. In Andresen R. Hamburg (eds) *Sportswissenshraft und Sportspraxis*, pp. 114–121. Verlag, Ingrid Czwalina.

Reilly T. & Ball D. (1984) The net physiological cost of dribbling a soccer ball. *Res. Q. Exerc. Sport* **55**, 267–271.

Reilly T. & Bowen T. (1984) Exertional costs of changes in directional modes of running. *Percep. Motor Skills* **58**, 149–150.

Reilly T. & Thomas V. (1976) A motion analysis of work-rate in different positional roles in professional football match-play. *J. Hum. Movement Studies* **2**, 87–97.

Reilly T. & Thomas V. (1979) Estimated daily energy expenditures of professional association. *Ergonomics* **22**, 541–548.

Rohde H.C. & Espersen T. (1988) Work intensity during soccer training and match-play. In Reilly T., Lees A., Davids K. & Murphy W.J. (eds) *Science and Football*, pp. 68–75. E. & F.N. Spon, London.

Sahlin K., Harris R.C. & Hultman E. (1979) Resynthesis of creatine phosphate in human muscle after exercise in relation to intramuscular pH and availability of oxygen. *Scand. J. Clin. Lab. Invest.* **39**, 551–558.

Sahlin K. & Ren J.M. (1989) Relationship of contraction capacity changes during recovery from a fatiguing contraction. *J. Appl. Physiol.* **67**(2), 648–654.

Saltin B. (1964) Aerobic work capacity and circulation at exercise in man. With special reference to the effect of prolonged exercise and/or heat exposure. *Acta Physiol. Scand.* **230**, Suppl., 62.

Saltin B. (1973) Metabolic fundamentals in exercise. *Med. Sci. Sports Exerc.* **5**, 137–146.

Saltin B. & Hermansen L. (1966) Esophageal, rectal and muscle temperature during exercise. *J. Appl. Physiol.* **21**, 1757–1762.

Seliger V. (1968) Heart rate as an index of physical load in exercise. *Scripta Medica*, Vol. 41, pp. 231–240. Medical Faculty, Brno University.

Smaros G. (1980) Energy usage during football matches. In Vecchiet L. (ed.) *Proceedings of the First International Congress on Sports Medicine Applied to Football*, pp. 795–801. D. Guanello, Rome.

Smith M., Clarke G., Hale T. & McMorris T. (1993) Blood lactate levels in college soccer players during match-play. In Reilly T., Clarys J. & Stibbe A. (eds) *Science and Football II*, pp. 129–134. E. & F.N. Spon, London.

Smodlaka V.J. (1978) Cardiovascular aspects of soccer. *Physiol. Sports Med.* **18**, 66–70.

Van Gool D. (1987) *De fysieke belasting tijdens een voetbalwedsfrifd: Studie van afgelegde afstand, hartfrequintie, energieverbruck en lactaatbepalingen.* PhD thesis, University of Leuven, Belgium.

Van Gool D., Van Gerven D. & Boutmans J. (1988) The physiological load imposed on soccer players during real match-play. In Reilly T., Lees A., Davids K. & Murphy W.J. (eds) *Science and Football*, pp. 51–59. E. & F.N. Spon, London.

Vandenborne K., McCully K., Kakihira H. *et al.* (1991) Metabolic heterogeneity in human calf muscle during maximal exercise. *Biochemistry* **88**, 5714–5718.

Wagenmakers A.J.M., Brookes J.H., Coakley J.H., Reilly T. & Edwards R.H.T. (1989) Exercise-induced activation of the branched-chain 2-oxo acid dehydrogenase in human muscle. *Eur. J. Appl. Physiol.* **59**, 159–167.

Chapter 5

Biomechanical aspects

Biomechanical analysis of football aims to provide recommendations concerning:

1 The training, teaching and coaching methods needed to improve performance.

2 Factors relating to performance and safety (the interrelationships between player, motion, and environment).

3 The evaluation of performance and traumas associated with football activities.

4 Therapeutic methods used in the treatment of foot-

io-
own
tions.
ent of
ance

idons
stem
cle
iade,
ystem
sary
or-
e

de-
per-

have
n also
arded.
ercep-
icinity.
de
not, or
iation.

The relevant information is then processed in the central nervous system.

Individual skills in football

This chapter aims to review the concept of individual skills in football: the relationships between individual skills, basic movements, physical fitness, and psychological features in football; an analysis of individual skills and basic movements in high-level games; to discuss the development of individual skills and basic movements in players; and to draw conclusions about the methodology of teaching individual skills and basic movements to players.

Individual skills range from the fundamental basis for possession of the ball, for keeping it under control in difficult match situations, and for using it to good advantage. Good technical skill adapted to any particular situation enables the player to avoid losing the ball too frequently and then having to expend more energy in trying to regain it. Individual skill is not a singular element which can be explained in conclusive terms; in fact, it is constantly developing.

There is no form of individual skill acquisition which is universally valid, however there are a few basic rules for the trainer to follow. The important point is for the trainer to perceive each player's own individual technical qualities and the ways in which these skills may be developed further. Technically gifted young players are able to learn more skills, and at a faster rate, than the ordinary player.

The trainer must ensure that a training session works on all the interdependent motor faculties of the players, such as speed and strength together, or speed and agility. The physiologic effects of the training are thus bound to complement each other rather than cancel each other out. Additionally, individual skills depend upon perceptual, and maybe intellectual, abilities of the players. Motivation in the individual skill training depends on how complex or simple, and how real or artificial, the training is.

Basic movements in football

Little attention has been focused on the total skill and basic movement analysis of football players. Permanent records by means of videotape and film-recording give a more detailed total skill analysis in football concerning individual skill analysis, locomotion, and tactical behavior of players. It has therefore been possible to obtain information about technique or skill frequencies (ball contacts, passes, dribbling, tackles, jumps, turns, etc.), the distances and times for high-intensity work (striding and sprinting; with or without the ball), and the times for the intervening periods of low-intensity work (walking, jogging, forward, backward, sideways, etc.). As discussed in Chapter 3, the average distance covered in a match has been calculated to be about 10–12 km.

In top-level football, 900–1000 actions with the ball will be executed per match, 350 passes with one touch, 150 with two touches, and the rest with several touches and after dribbling the ball. The successful top teams need an average of 16–30 attacks and 7–10 shots to score one goal. The attacks which produce a goal take less than 25 s. Two to six players take part in these attacks and one to six passes will be needed to score one goal. The distance covered and the type of movement by players depends on the players' position and role in the game. During a game of 90 min, players move without the ball approximately 98% of the total distance covered. On average, small differences exist in these ratios between the matches of seniors and juniors (Luhtanen 1990b).

The relationships between individual skills have been studied in match and test conditions, as well as understanding of the game, team skills, and physical and psychomotor tests in junior football players

(Luhtanen 1988b, 1990a). The framework of these studies is presented in Fig. 5.1.

Twelve junior teams participated in this study. The players who completed all the tests and games totalled 117. All actions with the ball during matches were recorded with a videocamera. The technical skills examined were receiving, passing, dribbling, shooting, scoring, tackling, and dead ball situations for all players. These were analyzed with respect to the team, player, position, location on the field, time spent in a single maneuver, technique used, speed, and direction of the maneuver. The skill tests included ball control, dribbling, passing, combined dribbling–passing–shooting, and heading tests. The total skill index was calculated. The physical tests included maximal starting speed, maximal running velocity, and vertical jumping height. The psychomotor tests included simple reaction and choice reaction time measurements to light signal responding with fingers. In the game-understanding test, the purposefulness of action of one player and player group were measured. Additionally, knowledge of the rules and ball movements were noted. The total index of understanding was calculated.

The total number of actions with the ball in the match analysis was 4800. On average in one game the players executed 29 passes, tried 34 receiving actions, executed five dribbles, two shots on goal, tried 20 interceptions, and executed four dead balls. A goalkeeper executed on average 13 saves. Relatively, the

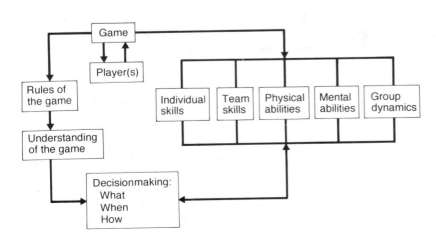

Fig. 5.1 A structured model to study the relationships between game actions and player abilities in football.

players succeeded in their attempts as follows: passing 50%, receiving 69%, dribbling 38%, shooting technically 66% and scoring 8%, interceptions 59%, dead balls 58%, and goalkeeper's saves 82%. The average duration of actions with the ball was 0.9 s. The mean distance covered in one action (pass or dribbling) was 15 m. An analysis between the winners and losers was completed using all the tested variables and actions in game situations. The total goals for the winners vs. losers 2.0 vs. 0.4. The winners accomplished the successful actions as follows: successful receiving 23.0 vs. 16.8, passes 13.9 vs. 9.0, dribbles 3.2 vs. 1.2, and shots 1.6 vs. 0.4. In skill tests the losers scored less than the winners as follows: bouncing the ball 15%, dribbling 6%, passing 4%, combined dribbling–passing–shooting 8%, and total skills 8%. The losers were better than the winners in the heading test. The losers scored less than the winners in the physical tests by 3–8%. By contrast, in the game-understanding test the losers scored better than the winners by 8%. Selected correlation coefficients between the total technical skills, understanding, running, jumping, and successful actions in match situation are shown in Table 5.1. The correlation coefficient between the total skills and different technical skills with feet ranged from 0.877 to 0.938 ($P < 0.001$).

The meaning of the individual football skills, psychomotor skills, physical abilities, and tactical understanding of the game have been speculated about often in the practical coaching of football. It has been shown clearly that at junior level the age, physical abilities,

psychomotor skills, and game-like skills influence success in matches.

In the present study the relationships between the tested skills, game understanding, and physical abilities (e.g. running speed and jumping height) were higher than the corresponding correlations between the successful actions in passing, receiving, dribbling, and shooting (Table 5.2). This could mean that overall training programs have not been well balanced for the total development of the players. It could be suggested that when coaches are planning future programs a better balance between skill, tactical, and physical training should be kept in mind.

Table 5.2 shows how in the study under discussion the successful maneuvers in match conditions were dependent on the player's abilities in test conditions.

It could be argued that the players with better running skills, decision-making skills, ball control, and understanding have more experience in the game situation and so can execute better decisions than the players with less ability in these areas.

Control of skilful movement

Biomechanics as applied to football includes all the domains which are dependent on the control system of humans. The player makes decisions relative to all the perceptual stimuli coming from various sources. Tactically, the players make selections between relevant and irrelevant information, and between all the relevant elements of information. All the perceptual elements which might provide signs for decision-making (i.e. whether to kick the ball or not) are accepted information.

For learning skills, the actions of external and internal feedback loops are important (Fig. 5.2). The mechanisms in the internal loop include:
1 The nerve endings in the skin which tell the player about the touch of the ball.
2 Kinesthetic receptors in the joints which control the joint angle.
3 Muscle spindles which control possible length changes in the muscle.
4 The Golgi apparatus which controls tension in the tendon.

The quality of this mechanism is hereditary. In the external feedback system the visual and auditive systems play the most important roles.

Table 5.1 Selected correlation coefficients between the tested skill, understanding, physical and successful actions in match conditions ($n = 117$)

Variable	1	2	3	4
Total skills	1.000			
Total understanding	0.686	1.000		
Maximal velocity	0.851	0.600	1.000	
Jumping height	0.818	0.630	0.892	1.000
Successful passes	0.500	0.281	0.357	0.324
Successful receiving	0.422	0.202	0.239	0.275
Successful dribbling	0.478	0.339	0.464	0.394
Successful shooting	0.270	< 0.200	< 0.200	< 0.200

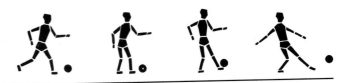

Table 5.2 Relationship between successful maneuvers in match and test conditions (Luhtanen 1989)

Percentage of successful maneuvers in match conditions	Tested player abilities				
	Skills	Speed	Understanding of the game	Leg strength	Choice reaction speed
Receiving skills	++	++	−	−	−−
Passing skills	++	0	−	+	−
Dribbling skills	0	+	0	0	0
Shooting skills	+	+	+	0	0
Dead balls	+	+	−	−	0
Interception skills	+	+	0	−−	−−
Total skills	++	++	−	−−	−−

++, strong positive effect on playing skills.
+, weak positive effect on playing skills.
0, no effect on playing skills.
−, weak negative effect on playing skills.
−−, strong negative effect on playing skills.

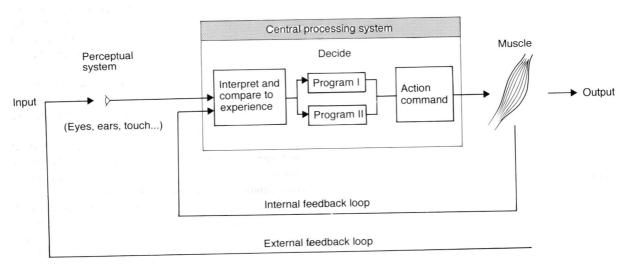

Fig. 5.2 A model of the human control system.

Higher levels of skills

The content of skills can be defined as a product of four different biomechanical elements as follows:

skill = force × velocity ×
 accuracy × purposefulness.

In skillful performance as well as in kicking and jumping this means that all four biomechanical variables must exist at the same time in exactly the right combination. In general, the total force is a sum of several forces produced by internal (muscular force) and external (reaction force, impact force, air resistance, etc.) forces.

In the human body, the velocity of the distal body parts (foot, hand, head) is produced through the lever system and joints. The linear velocity of the distal body part is dependent on the length and angular velocity of the respective lever (shank, thigh, etc.). The relative angular velocities for each body part will be produced through the respective muscle group (knee extensors, dorsiflexors, etc.). Accuracy means a certain space which can be time dependent because of the moving players on the field. Purposefulness means the final output of an execution relevant to the match situation.

Most of the actions and maneuvers in match situations are executed with submaximal force and velocity, but with great accuracy and purposefulness. Fewer maneuvers will be executed with maximal force and speed. The most successful actions in games are seen when the purposefulness of an action is unique and the accuracy, speed, and utilization of force are at a maximum.

Kicking

Ball velocity

The release velocity of the ball in the instep kick for skilled football players has been reported by several investigators as $17-28 \text{ m·s}^{-1}$ (Roberts & Metcalfe 1968, Roberts *et al.* 1974, Asami *et al.* 1976, Asami & Nolte 1983, Luhtanen 1984, Robertson & Mosher 1985, Isokawa & Lees 1988, Luhtanen 1988a, Narici *et al.* 1988). It has been suggested (Roberts & Metcalfe 1968) that foot speed just before contact is approximately $18-24 \text{ m·s}^{-1}$, and when contact is good ball speed

may be up to 7 m·s^{-1} faster than the foot. Calculations from the 1990 World Cup in Italy on television indicated that the velocities produced by the top professional players could reach the speed of $32-35 \text{ m·s}^{-1}$.

Biomechanics of kicking

The kicking movement in football is a relatively easy series of rotational movements. In this movement, the aim is to produce, through the kinematic chain of the body segments, high angular velocity to the foot. The length of the body segments or the radius of rotational movements influences the linear velocity of the rotating foot. Thus the body height and lengths of different body segments can be an advantageous feature for players, because the linear velocity of rotating levers can be expressed as a product of the radius of rotational movement and angular velocity.

The support foot remains firmly planted as the kicking foot makes contact with the ball. As the support foot is planted, the kicking leg is left well behind the body, with the hip hyperextended and the knee maximally flexed. The trunk is also rotated backward and sideways toward the kicking leg, to increase the length of the backswing and to add the force of trunk rotation forward into the kick. The arms are extended out to the sides of the body to aid in maintaining balance.

From the point of view of biomechanical principles in kicking the ball, the velocity production of the ball can be evaluated according to the conservation of the linear momentum in collision.

Horizontal ball displacement is primarily a result of the transfer of momentum to the ball, which is a function of the interaction of both leg strength and motor co-ordination (Hoshizaki 1984). The momentum of the kicking foot and leg is the product of the mass of the leg and the velocity of the foot at impact, plus the velocity of the body as the player approaches the ball. The greater the mass of the leg, and the greater the velocity of the foot at impact, the greater the resultant velocity of the ball at impact. The acceleration of the kicking leg, and the resultant velocity at impact, is determined by the muscle forces being applied by the kicker. It has been reported that the speed of the ball at impact was directly related to the measured strength of the subjects (Hoshizaki 1984).

The release velocity of the ball with respect to timing had the strongest relationship to the maximal torque produced during the (a) hip flexion; (b) knee extension; and (c) short ankle stabilizing in the kicking leg. Also the relationship between the maximal resultant forces of the thigh and shank and the release velocity of the ball was strong (Luhtanen 1988a). The relationships between the release velocity of the ball and age was high but less than with weight or height. Thus an increase in body mass means an increase in the mass of the foot and this automatically increases the release velocity of the ball in the kick. The player can also influence the effective mass of the foot by instantaneously changing the muscle tension in the muscles around the ankle. The regulation of the effective mass in the kicking foot might play an important role for getting a high release velocity to the ball.

Skilled senior football players performed slow, medium, and fast kicks. When their foot velocity was on average $20.1 \, m \cdot s^{-1}$ the release velocity of the ball was $27.4 \, m \cdot s^{-1}$ (Zernicke & Roberts 1978). In these fast kicks the evaluated peak muscle force produced in knee extensors could be about 2000 N (200 kg).

The skillful football player produces high ball velocity by maximizing angular velocities of the thigh and shank. The accuracy of kicks depends mainly on the contact area of foot with the ball. The bigger the ball, the better the accuracy. Accuracy in kicking was the highest when the velocity of the ball was 80% of the maximal velocity (Asami *et al.* 1976). Mechanically, the kicker can produce a small extra velocity to the foot and ball by a rotational movement of the support leg. The acquisition of the biomechanical principles of movement, countermovement, and balance increase still further the release velocity of the ball in kicking. Additionally, the utilization of muscular elasticity of hip flexors and knee extensors with correct timing means higher ball velocity.

The instep kick

In submaximal kicking and passes players prefer a linear movement of the foot to the ball, while in maximal kicks the foot pathways are curvilinear. Figure 5.3 shows the typical moments of the proximal ends of the thigh (hip), shank (knee), and foot (ankle) in the kicking leg. The maximal torques varied in the hip of the kicking leg from 55 to $232 \, N \cdot m^{-1}$, in the knee from

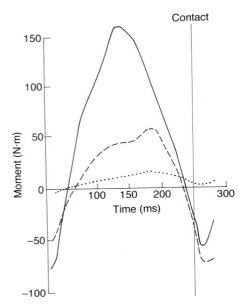

Fig. 5.3 Typical moments of a selected instep kick in the hip (——), knee (– – –), and ankle (. . . .) (Luhtanen 1988a).

24 to $108 \, N \cdot m^{-1}$, and in the ankle from 7 to $24 \, N \cdot m^{-1}$, respectively.

The direction angles between the arrows of the resultant forces decreased when foot to ball contact was approached (Fig. 5.4). Before this contact, the direction of the moments turned, except for the moment of the foot. The average timing for the three selected phases of the moments applied to the joints was similar in all the groups. The difference between age groups was mainly in the magnitude of force production. The results may mean that in all age groups the pattern in skilled kicking movements was similar in type and timing when the contact of the foot and ball occured. The pattern had more variation in the first phases of the leg swing. In the MKA phase (the phase when the knee angle was at its minimum), the forces applied to the hip might be directed slightly forward or backward (Fig. 5.4). In the CKL phase (the kicking phase when the contact of foot and ball occurred), the directions of the forces, both in the hip and knee, were slightly backward, which means proper timing is needed to get high linear velocity for the foot and ball.

The kick with run-up produces longer and more powerful kicks than the standing kick (Opavsky 1988).

Fig. 5.4 The range of directions of the resultant forces and moments of kicking in selected phases (CSL, the phase when the first contact of the support leg occurred; MKA, the phase when the knee angle was in its minimum; CKL, the phase when the contact of kicking with foot and ball occurred) (Luhtanen 1988a).

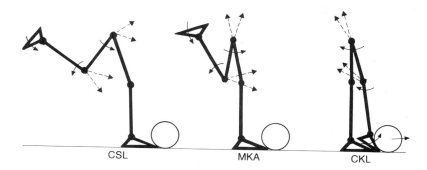

CSL　　　　MKA　　　　CKL

This is due to the increased momentum of the kicker at impact. If the kicker is moving forward horizontally at $4 \, \text{m·s}^{-1}$ at impact with the ball, this velocity is added to that imported by the kicking leg as it moves about the hip joint. However, some of the horizontal velocity is lost at the time of placement of the support foot, as the center of gravity must be slowed down to allow time for the full leg swing of the long kick.

Knee linear velocity reaches its peak between 40 and 70 ms after peak hip velocity is reached (Isokawa & Lees 1988). The angular motion on the thigh segment stops when the knee is approximately in position over the ball. The thigh is almost stationary at impact, while the leg and foot have reached peak velocity and zero acceleration (Huang *et al.* 1982). The phenomenon of the thigh slowing down or stopping before impact with the ball prior to speeding up in the follow-through may not be well known, since the time during which this occurs is so short it is difficult to observe visually. The exchange of angular velocities between the proximal and distal segments would suggest that there may be some transfer of angular momentum between the larger thigh and the smaller leg (Huang *et al.* 1982). Recent findings suggest that the thigh slows down due to the action of the shank as it accelerates toward the ball (Dunn & Putnam 1988). It was concluded that in a kicking movement the thigh deceleration is primarily influenced by the motion of the lower leg, and not by the resultant joint moment about the hip.

Following the deceleration of the thigh, the shank then continues to accelerate until impact, so that the peak velocity of the shank and foot segment occurs just before the ball is contacted. It has been reported that the maximal angular velocity of the shank is reached on average 9 ms before the contact of the foot and ball (Luhtanen 1988a). Ankle and toe velocities

reached their peak just before impact, and from 40 to 50 ms after the peak velocity of the knee (Isokawa & Lees 1988).

Swing time is the time from the landing of the support leg until the contact with the ball. The range of times for this portion of the kick has been reported to be between 0.13 and 0.15 s. It has been suggested that there may be two types of kicking pattern within the instep kick: (a) one using a long backswing which has a longer kicking time, and (b) the other using a small backswing, moving the lower leg sharply by knee extension resulting in a shorter kicking time (Isokawa & Lees 1988).

Maximizing the release velocity of the ball

In performing kicking movements the dominant extremity functions as an open kinetic chain system. In this segmental link system the internal muscle torques act between the individual links, which in football kicking are thigh, shank, and foot. These body segments move by rotating around an imaginary axis of rotation that passes through the articulation of the segments. The motion of rotating body segments in kicking can be described in terms of angular position, displacement, velocity, or acceleration. The linear velocity of the rotating foot hitting the ball is directly proportional to the sum of both the angular velocity and the radius of rotation of the consecutive segments. The timing of these consecutive rotational movements is important in relation to the impact of the foot with the ball when maximizing the release velocity of the ball in kicking. The linear momentum of the kicking leg transfers to the ball according to the relationship between the force impulse and the change of linear momentum. The angular acceleration of the segmental link system in the kicking leg depends on the external torque of the muscles producing the rotation of the thigh, shank, and foot, and on the resistance provided by the rotational inertia of these leg segments being moved by the motive moment. Mobility of the joints is a precondition for optimal shooting skill. The inertial resistance of the thigh, shank, and foot is determined by the distribution of the mass relative to the axis of rotation.

There are many practical benefits in increasing the release velocity of the ball. This can be done by increasing the velocity of the foot mechanically, by leaning the body away from the ball, and balancing the body with extended arms during the kicking movement.

The moment arm is defined as the perpendicular distance from the axis of rotation (usually through a body joint), to the center of gravity of the resistance, in this case the ball. The greater the distance from the center of the ball to the center of the active joints in the kick, the longer the lever system acting and the faster the speed of the kick. By fully extending the leg at impact, and leaning away from the ball, the kicker will increase the speed at the end of the foot.

Muscle activity in football kicking

An important aspect of the football kick is the interplay between the various muscle groups. The agonists contract to initiate the movement at each of the joints, but these muscles become the antagonists to slow the rapid angular movements at the joints just prior to or following release of the ball (De Proft *et al.* 1988). The hip flexor muscles are dominant during the majority of the swing to the ball. They are initially contracting eccentrically, to stop the leg's backswing; then their activity becomes concentric to accelerate the thigh toward the ball (Robertson & Mosher 1985).

Just prior to ball contact the hip extensors (e.g. the hamstrings) become dominant, causing the thigh and knee joint to slow down or even stop in some players. The follow-through is characterized by a flexor concentric contraction, followed by an eccentric contraction. The knee extensors (the quadriceps group) are the dominant muscles during the backswing and downswing. These muscles act eccentrically initially to reduce the rate of knee flexion caused by the leg's backswing and the hip flexor shortening moment. The knee extensors then act briefly to shorten and cause

some degree of knee extension. The knee flexors quickly become dominant just prior to ball contact, acting eccentrically to actually reduce the rate of knee extension. This is an interesting finding, as one would expect knee extensor activity throughout contact. However, no knee extensor activity was found just prior to ball contact (Robertson & Mosher 1985), and in fact the flexors were dominant, eccentrically, causing a reduction in the rate of knee extension. The knee flexors, especially the hamstring group, may be acting to prevent hyperextension and possible damage to the knee.

Skilled players showed greater muscle relaxation of the antagonistic muscles in the swinging phase than less skilled players (Bollens *et al.* 1987). There was also greater peak muscle activity in the knee extensors during the swinging phase in the skilled players.

Receiving the ball

Receiving the ball consists of gaining control of the ball from a pass or header, so that the ball can be controlled, shot, or passed. The key to controlling the ball is relaxation of the body parts used to control the ball. The player must give with the impact of the ball by moving the body parts backward in the direction of the oncoming ball, to absorb the momentum of the ball (inelastic collision).

Heading the ball

Heading is an important skill in football for advancing the ball downfield, intercepting a pass, or as a shot at goal. In élite football matches, a large percentage of the goals are scored from headers.

Heading the football has some risk for the less skilled or younger football player. The ball has a relatively high mass (0.425 kg), which increases considerably when wet. It has been suggested that the injury risk is minimal for skilled adults, who have the head and body mass and skill to withstand high impact forces. However, in children's football the mass of the impacting body has to be adjusted to the reduced head mass of the child. Children should therefore only use smaller footballs to avoid risk of head injury.

The head is more susceptible to injury from angular acceleration than from linear acceleration. If the neck muscles are weak, the angular acceleration from a hard ball impact will be greater. With strong neck muscles firmly contracted at impact, the angular acceleration of the head will be less, and the risk of injury to the brain or neck will be less.

The best part of the head to use is the middle zone of the forehead as this is the thickest portion of the skull. The forehead is also the flattest portion of the skull, so the margin for error is greater.

The distance of the header will be determined by the force provided by the player at impact, the velocity of the ball at impact, direction angle of the ball in the release phase, and the height of ball contact. There are three main types of header: (a) from a position standing on the ground; (b) when jumping from a stationary position; and (c) when jumping with an approach run. Several modifications of the header can be applied depending on the direction and movement of the ball and players. The force applied by the player at impact will be determined by the speed of the run-up, as well as by the number of joints used to produce velocity of the head, and may include the legs, trunk, arms, and shoulders. The neck should remain relatively fixed with both the flexors and extensors of the neck strongly contracted isometrically to fix the head as a firm impact surface. If the neck muscles are not strongly contracted, the ball may produce some backward movement of the head at impact, decreasing the control of the player over the ball. If the ball is contacted at the top of the jump, the vertical velocity of the body is close to zero, so velocity will have to be generated by the trunk muscles.

The action of the body in heading has been compared to that of a catapult with the principle of movement and countermovement, in which both the upper and lower halves of the body are extended backward after leaving the ground. Trunk extension is an important factor in achieving greater trunk velocity in the standing jump technique, and works like a bow. The further back the trunk extends, the greater the maximum forward velocity of the upper trunk and head. Force is produced by strong contraction of the trunk flexors, hip flexors, and knee extensors prior to impact. The role of the trunk flexors is very important and they need to be strengthened. The force of the header can be increased by using more body parts through a greater range of motion during the airborne phase of the jump and during take-off. A longer run-up prior to the take-off will generate more momentum at take-off.

Moving header

Very few headers are taken in a game in which the feet are in contact with the ground — usually the player has jumped into the air and is contacting the ball at the top of the jump. The ability to jump and to make contact with the ball above other defending players is a key aspect of heading. There is often forceful body contact with surrounding players while trying to head the ball, so strength and mass are important for success. Although the take-off for the header is often taken from a stationary jump, it is usually taken from a running approach. The running approach enables the player to attain greater upward velocity which will give greater momentum to the ball at impact.

As the player approaches the peak of the jump, the knees are flexed, and the hips and trunk hyperextended (Fig. 5.5). The arms remain in a position extended horizontally in front of the body. Just prior to impact, the knees are extended and the hips are flexed, producing a reaction consisting of forward trunk flexion. The action of the hip flexors was found to be the dominant muscle action during forward motion in heading. This forceful flexion forward of the trunk is assisted by strong contraction of the abdominal and trunk muscles. The arms are horizontally extended around long axes through the shoulder joints to increase resistance to twisting movements and decrease the tendency for the trunk to rotate around a long axis through the spine.

Throwing the ball

The range of throwing depends on the initial velocity and release angle of the ball. The initial velocity of the ball will be produced by the consecutive rotational movements of the body segments. Maximizing the release velocity of the ball, v_b, can be reached by lengthening the radius of motion and/or increasing the angular velocity in the rotation of the throwing

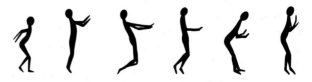

Fig. 5.5 The sequence of a moving header.

movement. The length or radius (r) of body parts and relative angular joint velocities (w) will influence the velocity of the ball in respect to the hip (h) through trunk (t), upper arm (u), shoulder (s), forearm (f), elbow (e), hand (h), and wrist (w) as follows:

$$v_b = r_t w_h + r_u w_s + r_f w_e + r_h w_w.$$

In the successful throw, the pattern could work like a whip from the center of action (hip) to the distal segments (hands). Mechanically, the traditional throw-in relies on rapid trunk flexion, shoulder extension, elbow extension, and wrist flexion to provide force for ball release. The backswing movements consist of trunk hyperextension, hip extension, and knee flexion, as well as elbow flexion and wrist hyperextension. The player leans well back and brings the ball back as far as possible behind the body. The elbows (24 rad·s^{-1}) and wrists (7.7 rad·s^{-1}) reach their peak angular velocity at the instant of release of the ball (Levendusky *et al*. 1985).

The handspring throw-in was developed in an attempt to produce greater release velocities of the ball, by generating greater angular momentum during the run-up movements. The player holds the ball in two hands, and performs a short run-up before diving forward onto the ball, and performs a front handspring flip over the ball. The thrower rotates at very high speeds and lands on both feet, and using both hands performs a legal throw-in rotating over the feet (Levendusky *et al*. 1985, Messier & Brody 1986). The handspring throw-in technique has the potential to generate greater release velocities and longer throws, possibly enhancing scoring opportunities during throw-in situations. The disadvantage of this technique, aside from the obvious difficulty of requiring some skill in the handspring, is that the ball is released from a much lower point, requiring a higher trajectory and angle of release to achieve comparable distances. Since a higher trajectory gives the defense some advantage in reaching the landing point, this may offset any advantages in speed of release.

Speed

Velocity in football depends on the foreshadowing of the game, reaction, choice reaction and movement time, starting position and velocities, and maximal speed in final phases (Fig. 5.6). The experienced high

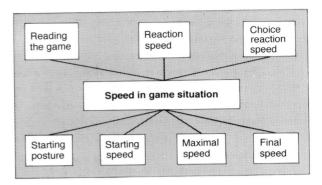

Fig. 5.6 Factors influencing the velocity in the game situation.

caliber players are able to read the game well and react quickly. Running and maximal velocities depend on muscular and reaction force production and mass of the player. In different phases of running it is important to analyze the changes of velocity — decrease and/or increase — and to think about the reasons for these changes from the point of view of running economy (Luhtanen & Komi 1978a).

Running velocity (v) can be evaluated by the following method (Luhtanen & Komi 1978b, Luhtanen *et al*. 1989):

$$v = f \times l$$

where f = stride frequency and l = stride length.

The primary factors influencing high velocity in running are the high stride frequency and stride length. In most players, stride frequency provides the dominant role, especially in the start. In practice, the stride frequency means short support phase and fast movement of the recovery leg under the trunk but not too much forward movement in respect to the center of gravity of the total body. All decelerating and resisting forces should be minimized.

Basic movements in football

Basic movements on the field without the ball include starts, runs, jumps, twists, turns, feints, and stops. Video and film-recordings facilitate a more detailed skill and running analysis in football. How can this information be used in football training and coaching?

There is no form of individual running skill which is universally valid for everyone. There are, however, a few basic rules for the trainer to follow. The importance for the trainer is to perceive each player's own individual technical qualities and the ways in which these skills may be developed further.

It is useful for coaches to understand the biomechanical structure of players, including their mass, height, center of gravity, and moment of inertia; and additional biomechanical forces between players and the environment: weight or gravitational force, ground reaction force, friction, muscle force produced, elasticity forces, and so on.

Reaction time and starting speed

The start in football sprints includes both the reaction and movement time. The simple reaction and choice reaction times to light signals in top players can be 0.15−0.20 s and 0.17−0.22 s, respectively. The starting velocity in a sprint of 30 m is related to a player's age.

Jumping

In jumping, the player is producing vertical velocity for the center of gravity through plantar flexion in the ankle, knee extension, hip extension, and trunk, head and arm movements. During take-off, a key factor is to utilize all positive net impulse effects for a high vertical release velocity of the center of gravity of the player. Timing of the segmental movements is a real skill factor in jumping.

Jumping skills are most important for the field player in the moving header and for goalkeepers in all take-off actions. The goalkeeper must be a skilled jumper, as many saves require a maximum jump to reach the ball. The majority of the jumps made by the goalkeeper will be performed using a one-legged take-off because it is faster, as the goalkeeper is often moving toward the ball at take-off. However, since a higher jump can usually be attained using a two-legged take-off, this take-off is recommended for high shots near the crossbar. As soon as the ball has been released and a high shot is anticipated, the goalkeeper should assume a deepened crouch position, and prepare for the jump by lowering the arms. From this position, the arms accelerated upward in the direction of the jump, and the trunk is also extended upward. The legs then forcefully extend in the direction of the jump, to project the goalkeeper as high as possible in the direction of the ball. Maximizing the impulse at take-off will increase both the force applied at take-off and the time over which that force is applied. The range of the arm swing, trunk extension, and depth of crouch will all determine the height attained on the jump. As the goalkeeper's center of gravity and arms are lowered prior to take-off, by flexing the legs and flexing the trunk forward, then the forces applied to the ground increase acceleration upward.

Segmental contributions to the rise of the center of gravity in vertical jumps is highest in knee extension (55%) followed by plantar flexion of the ankles (25%). The role of trunk extension and arm movement has been measured at about 10% from both (Luhtanen & Komi 1978c). For the coach it is important to recognize the priority of different joint and segment movements. If any of these joint actions are not used, the output of jumping performance will not be maximal.

Starting, changing direction, and turning

For fast starting in a good position, the vertical line of the center of gravity must be as close as possible to the edge of the support area in the direction of intended motion. In stopping, the body lean causes deceleration. Then the gravity line is taken as far as support friction permits from the edge in the direction of the motion. A balance principle appropriate for running-type linear acceleration and deceleration situations is as follows. For maximum stability in motion the base of support must be enlarged in the direction of momentum and in the direction of intended acceleration or deceleration. The greater the momentum and the greater the acceleration or deceleration, the larger the base of support should be in that direction. Any change in the direction of running and in linear momentum is caused by an external impulse in the direction of that change. The greater the direction change desired, the greater must be the push and ground reaction force. In abrupt direction changes the ground−foot friction needs to be high enough to prevent slipping when the foot push is made. In wet conditions because of lowered friction massive players are not so quick in chancing direction, accelerating or decelerating, running and maintaining balance. In turning around 180° it is important to keep the mass distribution as close to the turning axis as possible so that the moment of inertia is small and the turning fast. Any extra steps during turning need to be avoided.

Progression in skill training

It is difficult to produce a progressive classification of individual skills in football. This classification has to be multidimensional and include factors which are always influencing the total performance. For example, highly skilled players can predict ball-contact points with such precision that successful plays and strikes at the ball can be made without looking at it just before ball contact. The question is how to develop a talented junior player to become a highly skilled senior player? A progressive training plan should include primary and secondary factors, as listed in Table 5.3. Striking skill can be defined as a combination of four variable factors in the game:

$$\text{striking skill} = \text{player} \times \text{ball} \times \text{environment} \times \text{target}.$$

Table 5.3 Classification of the factors influencing the striking skill performance in football

Primary factors	Secondary factors

Player	Age
	Preferred foot
	Run-up
	  stationary to moving
	  constant speed (low–high)
	  accelerating or decelerating

Ball	Stationary to moving On the ground or in the air Pathway Bouncing or non-bouncing Low speed or high speed Backward or forward To the right or to the left
Environment	Surface Wind Rain Opponent, etc.
Target	Stationary (goal) Moving (player) To the foot or to the free space Speed Direction, etc.

There is little objective data available on the best methods of teaching, training, or learning individual skills in football. Theories of motor learning have been applied and methodologies built up. The objective comparison of achieved results has been impossible to date. However, success in different international championship competitions can be achieved when a total educational system is adopted. Elements in this total educational system include selection of talented players, good organization in football schools and clubs, league system, education of coaches, quantity and quality of both general and specific individual training, and so on.

Each player, for each skill, will exhibit a different pattern of movement dependent upon that player's morphology together with external environmental and functional factors. Only in single and simple movements does the pattern stay consistent. Additionally, the level of skill for each player and type of skill will influence the total pattern of movement. Systematic analysis of skills (individual skills and basic movements in football) should lead to the development of skills.

Selected biomechanical principles in football

In terms of individual skills, the aim of the players is to generate precise and accurate performances consistently, with maximum speed and force. There are a number of mechanical principles which should produce maximal accuracy, speed, and force (Table 5.4). In performances with maximal force, speed, and accuracy, all of these principles are working simultaneously. Biomechanics as applied to football should include:

1 Application of biomechanics to teaching and coaching of motor skills.
2 Teaching of the basic biomechanical principles when practising football skills.
3 How to identify errors in motor performances.
4 Identification of the motor patterns of technically skilled performances.
5 Simple qualitative analysis of individual skills.
6 How the mechanism of error correction works in practice.
7 Qualitative studies to enhance the future progress of the game.

8 Interpretation of research results of sports studies and their application to football.

A basic structure of football training for different age ranges is given in Table 5.5.

Testing

There are more suitable times for testing a team than others. This depends on the age and skill level of the teams. Possible times include the following:
1 When the training season starts.
2 When the playing season starts.
3 When the playing season is in the middle.

Table 5.4 Goals of movements and principles associated with the performance

Goal	Principle
Production of accuracy	Stable basis of support
	Stable body support
	Active use of distal segments (foot, head) associated the proximal segments (shank, trunk)
	Consistency of pattern and movement (pass, heading)
	Large contact surface with ball, if possible
Production of speed	Successive generation of each link from the proximal one to the lateral one
	Small initial radius in link chain; all participating muscle groups begin contraction from maximum length including eccentric and concentric muscle contraction
Production of force	Successive use of body segments from initiation of movement through the action phase
	Summation of muscle forces transferred from the large to small muscle groups through action phase
	Stable base of support: wide, lowered
	Application of generated forces in desired direction

4 When playing season is over.
Excess testing should be avoided. For testing, the coaches need assistance from professionals or laboratory services. For interpreting test results and synthesizing individual training programs coaches need sport-science experts to help them, give feedback, and construct new training programs for the teams and players.

Skills

Matches are the best skill tests for the coaches. Each action with the ball can be considered as a random test. In match conditions the coaches are evaluating the number and percentage of successful actions in different specific skills. For individual skills and team skills the following type of qualitative recordings can be chosen:
1 Scores (number of passes, etc.).
2 Effectiveness (percentage of successful passes, etc.).
3 Efficiency of goal accomplishment.
4 Consistency of outcome.
Scoring can be selected from the following items:
1 Accuracy scores.
2 Error scores.
3 Time on target scores.
4 Variability.
5 Game understanding scores.
The specific skill tests in field conditions play an important role for junior players and coaches. The skill tests can include individual skills as follows:
1 Kicking.
2 Passing.
3 Dribbling.
4 Heading.
5 Bouncing.
6 Throwing.
Receiving, feigning, and tackling skills can also be measured. Advanced skill tests may include any combinations of individual basic skills. Skill tests have not been standardized universally.

Perceptual abilities

In a match situation, factors are constantly changing and players have to see and read the game in an efficient way, and they have to react quickly according to the decision they have made. Tests which could be

Table 5.5 A basic structure of football training at different age ranges

Age (years)	Technique	Tactics	Condition
< 6	Individual skills	Mini game	—
6–8	Basic skills	Ball possession	Speed, flexibility
8–10	Advanced skills	Attack, defense	Speed, flexibility
10–12	Competitive skills	Principles of the game	Speed, flexibility
12–14	Match-like with opponent	Stationary Individual tactics	Speed, flexibility Endurance
14–16	Match-like with opponent	Team Individual Stationary	Speed, flexibility Endurance Strength
16–18	Match-like with opponent	Team Individual Stationary	Speed, flexibility Endurance Strength
> 18	Match-like with opponent	Team Individual Stationary	Speed, flexibility Endurance Strength

useful in an early selection phase of talent searching are as follows:

1 Vision (field of vision).
2 Reaction time.
3 Choice reaction time.
4 Decision-making speed (relevant to football).

Figure 5.7 shows an example.

Running speed

According to match analysis the maximal sprinting distance is on average 20–30 m (Withers *et al.* 1984). A player performs about 100 sprinting spurts per match, though this number is probably increasing. A player will reach maximal speed on average after a distance of 30 m, maintaining maximal speed on average for about another 30 m. Then the speed starts to decrease. It is useful to test both the starting and maximal speed of the players.

Starting speed

A run of 20 or 30 m is used to measure starting speed. The time for the starting speed can be measured with a photocell timer system with an automatic timing device (Digitime, Ergorun, Bosco system) after each 10 m. The speed can be calculated by dividing the respective distance by the respective time (Fig. 5.8). For the best training in improving starting speeds, it is necessary to film the individual sprints of all players by video, to analyze them with experts, and to plan a technical program to correct running technique in starts.

Maximal speed

It is useful to evaluate the maximal running speed over 30 m with a flying start. The time for the maximal speed can be measured with a photocell timer system with an automatic timing device for a distance of

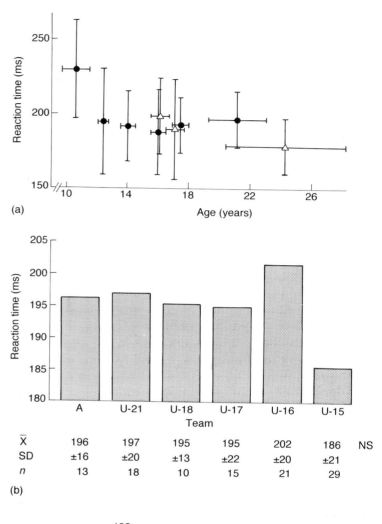

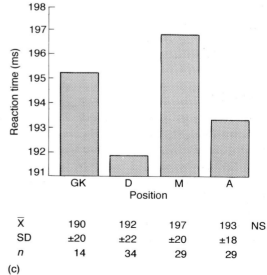

Fig. 5.7 (a) Average development of simple reaction time with age in two player categories (●, junior club players; △, national team players); (b) average reaction time in different national teams (A, adults; U-21, under 21s; etc.); and (c) average reaction time in respect to player position. A, attack; D, defense; GK, goalkeeper; M, midfield.

(b)

	A	U-21	U-18	U-17	U-16	U-15	
$\overline{X}$	196	197	195	195	202	186	NS
SD	±16	±20	±13	±22	±20	±21	
n	13	18	10	15	21	29	

(c)

	GK	D	M	A	
$\overline{X}$	190	192	197	193	NS
SD	±20	±22	±20	±18	
n	14	34	29	29	

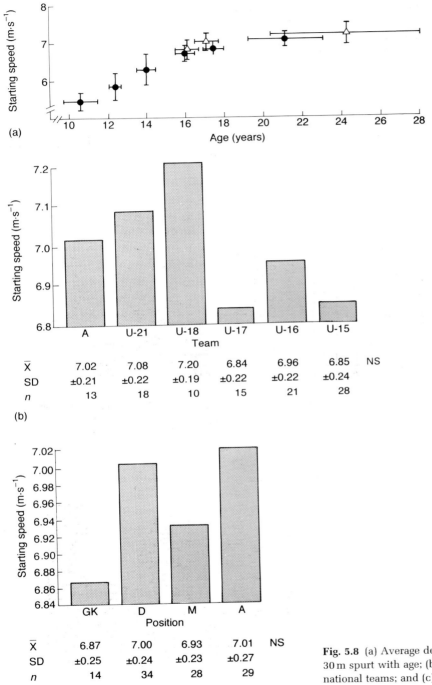

$\overline{X}$	7.02	7.08	7.20	6.84	6.96	6.85	NS
SD	±0.21	±0.22	±0.19	±0.22	±0.22	±0.24	
n	13	18	10	15	21	28	

(b)

$\overline{X}$	6.87	7.00	6.93	7.01	NS
SD	±0.25	±0.24	±0.23	±0.27	
n	14	34	28	29	

(c)

Fig. 5.8 (a) Average development of the starting speed in 30 m spurt with age; (b) average starting speed in different national teams; and (c) average starting speed in respect to player position. Abbreviations as in Fig. 5.7.

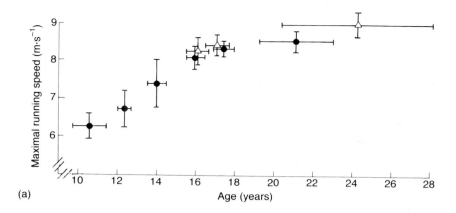

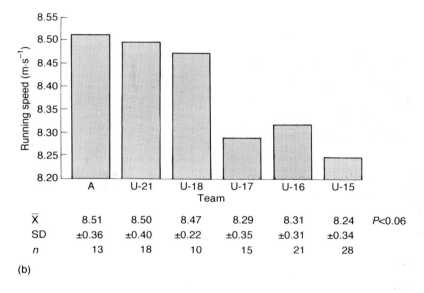

$\overline{X}$	8.51	8.50	8.47	8.29	8.31	8.24	$P<0.06$
SD	±0.36	±0.40	±0.22	±0.35	±0.31	±0.34	
n	13	18	10	15	21	28	

(b)

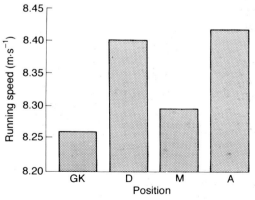

Fig. 5.9 (a) Average development of the maximal running speed in 30 m with flying start with age; (b) average final speed of 30 m in different national teams; and (c) average final speed in respect to player position. Abbreviations as in Fig. 5.7.

$\overline{X}$	8.26	8.40	8.30	8.42	NS
SD	±0.41	±0.34	±0.36	±0.33	
n	14	34	28	29	

(c)

30 m. The speed can be calculated by dividing 30 m by the respective time (Fig. 5.9). Again, for the best possible development in maximal running speed it is necessary to film the individual runs of all players by video, to analyze them with experts, and to plan a technical program to correct running technique in maximal running.

Conclusion

In the 1990s, a coach can have too much information on the players and team, and he or she may have difficulty managing it. All the available data should be used in an optimum way for success of the team and individual players. Sport scientists and coaches have co-operated in developing practical and modern microcomputer-based tools to control the relevant information in developing coaching (Luhtanen *et al.* 1990). This team-manager coaching system covers almost the whole field of data-processing relating to football coaching. The management system includes aspects of coaching such as:

1 Basic information: players, their statistics, and selected characteristics.
2 Year plan: coaching objectives and goals, and competition objectives and goals.
3 Training: seasonal, weekly, and daily planning, follow-up and analysis of training including technique, tactics, etc.
4 Testing: testing plans, goals to be achieved in different aspects of the player's characteristics, test results and their graphic presentation.
5 Games: planning of the games, follow-up and analysis of the team selection, team-play characteristics, individual evaluation of players, and team performances.
6 Specialist expertise: testing and problem-solving alternatives of team play, developing physical fitness, individual skills, and mental aspects.

Each coach has their own coaching philosophy, in which priorities are made. The computer-based management systems have an unlimited capacity for coaches to apply their own ideas to the program.

References

Asami T. & Nolte V. (1983) Analysis of powerful ball kicking. In Matsui M. & Kobayashi K. (ed.) *Biomechanics VIII—B*, pp. 695–699. Human Kinetics, Champaign, Illinois.

Asami T., Togari H., Kikuchi T. *et al.* (1976) Energy efficiency of ball kicking. In Komi P.V. (ed.) *Biomechanics V—B*, pp. 135–140. University Park Press, Baltimore.

Bollens E.C., De Proft E. & Clarys J.P. (1987) The accuracy and muscle monitoring in soccer kicking. In Jonsson B. (ed.) *Biomechanics X—A*, pp. 283–288. Human Kinetics, Champaign, Illinois.

De Proft E., Clarys J.P., Bollens E. & Dufour W. (1988) Muscle activity in the soccer kick. In Reilly T., Lees A., Davids K. & Murphy W.J. (eds) *Science and Football*, pp. 434–440. E. & F.N. Spon, London.

Dunn E. & Putnam C.A. (1988) The influence of the lower leg motion on thigh deceleration in kicking. In de Groot G., Hollander A.P. & Huijing P.A. (eds) *Biomechanics XI—B*, pp. 787–790. Free University Press, Amsterdam.

Hoshizaki T.B. (1984) Strength and coordination in the soccer kick. In Terauds J. (ed.) *Sport Biomechanics: Proceedings of International Conference of Sport Biomechanics*, pp. 271–275. Academic Publishers, Del Mar.

Huang T.C., Roberts E.M. & Youm Y. (1982) The biomechanics of kicking. In Ghista D.N. (ed.) *Human Body Dynamics*, pp. 409–443. Oxford University Press, New York.

Isokawa M. & Lees A. (1988) A biomechanical analysis of the instep kick motion in soccer. In Reilly T., Lees A., Davids K. & Murphy W.J. (eds) *Science and Football*, pp. 449–455, E. & F.N. Spon, London.

Levendusky T.A., Clinger C.D., Miller R.E. & Armstrong C.W. (1985) Soccer throw-in kinematics. In Terauds J. & Barham J. (eds) *Biomechanics in Sports II*, pp. 258–269. Academic Publishers, Del Mar.

Luhtanen P. (1984) Development of biomechanical model of in-step kicking in football players (in Finnish). *Report of the Finnish FA* 1/1984. Helsinki, Finland.

Luhtanen P. (1988a) Kinematics and kinetics of maximal in-step kicking in soccer. In Reilly T., Lees A., Davids K. & Murphy W.J. (eds) *Science and Football*, pp. 441–448. E. & F.N. Spon, London.

Luhtanen P. (1988b) Relationships of individual skills, tactical understanding and team skills in Finnish junior soccer players. *Scientific Olympic Congress Proceedings*, vol. II, pp. 1217–1221. Seoul, South Korea.

Luhtanen P. (1989) Developmental levels of young players. In *Proceedings of the 3rd Course of UEFA for National Youth Coaches*, pp. 30–35. Union des Associations Europeennes de Football, UEFA, Bern.

Luhtanen P. (1990a) Relationships between successful skill manoeuvres in match conditions and selected test variables in soccer players. In Santilli G. (ed.) *Congress Proceedings of the International Conference Sports Medicine Applied to Football*, p. 437. CONI, Rome.

Luhtanen P. (1990b) Video analysis of technique and tactics. In Santilli G. (ed.) *Congress Proceedings of the International Conference Sports Medicine Applied to Football*, pp. 77–84. CONI, Rome.

Luhtanen P., Eskelinen J., Kauppinen T. & Madsen D. (1990)

Team management system for quality coaching. In Nozek M. Sojka D., Morrison W.E. & Susanka P. (eds) *Proceedings of the VIIIth International Symposium of the Society of Biomechanics in Sports*, pp. 363–366. Conex Company, Prague.

Luhtanen P. & Komi P.V. (1978a) Mechanical energy states in running. *Eur. J. Appl. Physiol.* **38**, 41–48.

Luhtanen P. & Komi P.V. (1978b) Mechanical factors influencing running speed. In Asmussen E. & Jörgensen K. (eds) *Biomechanics VI–B*, pp. 23–29. University Park Press, Baltimore.

Luhtanen P. & Komi P.V. (1978c) Segmental contribution to forces in vertical jump. *Eur. J. Appl. Physiol.* **38**, 181–188.

Luhtanen P., Mero A. & Bosco C. (1989) Step length, frequency, velocity and power relationships in running and jumping. In Gregor R.J., Zernicke R.F. & Whiting W.C. (eds) *Congress Proceedings of XII International Congress of Biomechanics*, p. 82ab. UCLA, Los Angeles.

Messier S. & Brody M. (1986) Mechanics of translation and rotation during conventional and handspring soccer throw-ins. *Int. J. Sports Biomech.* **2**, 301–315.

Narici M.V., Sirtori M.D. & Mognoni P. (1988) Maximal ball velocity and peak torques of hip flexor and knee extensor muscles. In Reilly T., Lees A., Davids K. & Murphy W.J.

(eds) *Science and Football*, pp. 429–433. E. & F.N. Spon, London.

Opavsky P. (1988) An investigation of linear and angular kinematics of the leg during two types of soccer kick. In Reilly T., Lees A., Davids K. & Murphy W.J. (eds) *Science and Football*, pp. 456–459. E & F.N. Spon, London.

Roberts E.M. & Metcalfe A. (1968) Mechanical analysis of kicking. In Wartenweiler J., Jokl E. & Hebblinck M. (eds) *Biomechanics I*, pp. 315–319. University Park Press, Baltimore.

Roberts E.M., Zernicke R.F., Youm Y. & Huang T.C. (1974) Kinetic parameters in kicking. In Nelson R.C. & Morehaus C.A. (eds) *Biomechanics IV*, pp. 157–172. University Park Press, Baltimore.

Robertson D.G.E. & Mosher R.E. (1985) Work and power of the leg muscles in soccer kicking. In Winter D.A. (ed.) *Biomechanics IX–B*, pp. 533–538. Human Kinetics, Champaign, Illinois.

Withers R.T., Maricic Z., Wasilewski S. & Kelly L. (1984) Match analysis of Australian professional soccer players. *J. Hum. Movement Studies* **8**, 159–176.

Zernicke R.F. & Roberts E. (1978) Lower extremity forces and torques during systematic variation of non-weight bearing motion. *Med. Sci. Sports* **10**, 21–26.

Chapter 6

Physiological profile

of the player

Football places physical and physiological demands on its participants, which become more pronounced the higher the level of competition. The physical demands are related both to technical aspects of the game and its physical contact elements. The physiological demands are linked in the main with the intensity at which the game is played. Without the necessary attributes, the individual will not be able to cope with the stresses of play at the top level. Certain anthropometric features may be desirable for all players although positional roles may dictate their dispersion throughout the team as a whole.

Success in a team sport such as football depends on how individual characteristics are blended within the team to form a coherent playing system. This makes the interpretation of physiological profiles of individual players more difficult than in individual sports such as athletics, cycling, and swimming where the relationship between physiological capacities and sport performance can be outlined more precisely. Nevertheless the determination of physiological profiles of football players can provide useful information both for the team as a whole and for the individuals that comprise it.

A physiological profile of the team provides detail on the overall state of fitness of the squad. This may vary according to the physical training regimens employed, the frequency of competition, the stage of the competitive season, and so on. It can help also in identifying strengths and weaknesses of individual players within the team. Physiological attributes may be depressed in players without adequate fitness training, on return to play after injury, and at times of overtraining. They may also be inadequate after transfer to a new team organized on a different tactical basis. Identification of individual weak points will allow trainers and coaches to take remedial action.

In presenting fitness profiles of the team, average values are used for reference purposes. In football, where game requirements are multifactorial, these are best seen as guidelines, rather than rigid standards. For parameters such as maximal oxygen uptake, for example, the acceptable range of variation is lower than for a linear measure such as height since specific ensembles of skills rather than physical size determine the performance capability of the player. Nevertheless linear anthropometric measures may determine the ways in which these skills can be exploited by the team.

Group measures, mean and variance or SD, are useful in locating the individual within the team's profile. The individual's values may also provide a reference: the effectiveness of an individually tailored training program may be gauged by measuring changes in aerobic power and capacity or muscular strength and power of the player in question. It may also be relevant to use muscle performance in one limb as reference: for example, measurement of muscle strength and its rehabilitation is best gauged by referencing the improvements to the status of the uninjured leg.

This chapter reviews the literature on anthropometric characteristics of football players and the implications for performance at different levels of play. Muscle function, strength, and anaerobic power are also considered and their relations to fitness and to football skills performance described. The relevance of flexibility and agility to football are also noted. Special attention is given to the characteristics of the oxygen transport system of football players. Psychophysiological attributes are also described. The effects of positional role, performance level, training effects, and seasonal changes are taken into account where appropriate.

Anthropometry

Age

Most professional football players have an active playing career of about a decade, with peak performance spanning approximately half of those years. Top football teams tend to be comprised of players with an average age of about 25 years and a typical SD of 2 years or so (Reilly 1979). Players 20 years of age or less do feature in the top club teams, and occasionally at international level, but they tend to reach the pinnacle of their own playing careers some years later. Most professional players are in their twenties and the few who continue to play at a high level until well into their thirties are exceptions. Some years ago Hirata (1966) concluded from his study of entrants at the Tokyo Olympic Games in 1964, that success in ball games such as football, hockey, basketball, and volleyball is mainly achieved in the period 24–27 years, football being the earliest of these. This probably still holds true, the average age of the highly successful German national side in the 1970s and 1980s falling within this range. Goalkeepers seem to have longer playing careers than outfield players and it is not unusual to find players at international level in their late thirties in this position. Indeed Dino Zoff (Italy), Pat Jennings (Northern Ireland), and Peter Shilton (England) competed in World Cup finals when they were 40 years of age. This prolongation of career may be related to a lower incidence of chronic injuries and degenerative trauma in goalkeeping compared to outfield positions but also to the fact that players mature in this position with experience in the game. A loss of motivation to continue playing and training hard or a reluctance of management to renew contracts of the older players may contribute to an earlier than necess-

ary retirement from playing professional football. Active athletes can maintain fitness levels well into their thirties before physiological functions begin to show signs of deterioration. That football can be played at ages later than that at which professionals normally retire is evidenced by the growth of veteran's football in recent years.

Height and weight

Data on height and weight of football teams (Table 6.1) suggest that players vary widely in body size and that size is not necessarily a determinant of success. Multivariate analysis of fitness data of English League First Division players showed that 23% of the total variance among individuals was accounted for by a component related to body size, while a further 10% was explained by a component related to body density (Reilly & Thomas 1980). Lack of height is not in itself a bar to success in football, though it might determine the choice of playing position.

Of course mean values have only limited use for comparative purposes when the variability is large. A coach may modify the team formation and style of play to accommodate individuals without the expected physical attributes of conventional positional roles

Table 6.1 Mean (± SE) height and weight of football teams in a sample of reports in the literature

	Height (cm)	Body mass (kg)	Reference
English League, First Division	180.4 ± 1.7	76.7 ± 1.5	White *et al.* (1988)
English League, First Division	176.0 ± 1.1	73.2 ± 1.5	Reilly (1979)
Tottenham Hotspur	178.5 ± 1.3	77.5 ± 1.3	Reilly (1979)
Aberdeen FC	174.6 ± 0.9	69.4 ± 2.1	Williams *et al.* (1973)
Dallas Tornados	176.3 ± 1.2	75.7 ± 1.9	Raven *et al.* (1976)
South Australian representatives	178.1 ± 3.6	75.2 ± 2.2	Withers *et al.* (1977)
Italian professionals	177.2 ± 0.9	74.4 ± 1.1	Faina *et al.* (1988)
Ujpesti Dozja, Budapest	176.5 ± 1.7	70.5 ± 1.3	Apor (1988)
Honved, Budapest	177.6 ± 1.1	73.5 ± 1.6	Apor (1988)
Danish national squad	183.0 ± ?	77.0 ± ?	Bangsbo *et al.* (1988)

but who compensate by superior skills and motivation. Ethnic or racial influences also affect the average body size of a team, for example the North African and the Korean teams playing the World Cup final matches have tended to be smaller than their European and South American rivals. Japan's team in the 1964 Olympic Games was described as especially small and light for playing at that level (Hirata 1966) and illustrated characteristic ethnic differences from others, Asians on the whole being smaller than non-Asians. The Danish World Cup side of 1986 was the largest of the teams reviewed in Table 6.1 (Bangsbo *et al.* 1988). Many top European teams contain players of different ethnic backgrounds and this can confound the interpretation of anthropometric profiles.

Height is an advantage to the goalkeeper, the center backs and to the forward used as "target player" for winning possession of the ball with the head. Thus a particular stature may orientate players toward specific positional or tactical roles. The defenders tended to be the tallest and heaviest players among the Australian national squad studied by Cochrane and Pyke (1976) whereas the midfield players were well below the overall squad means for height and weight. A study of British college players confirmed that the goalkeepers (mean 180 cm) were the tallest while the midfield players (mean 173 cm) were the smallest (Bell & Rhodes 1975). A similar trend was noted among professional English League players, the center backs being taller than the fullbacks with midfield players being the smallest of those playing outfield (Reilly 1979).

A general trend in the population is that the lower the level of play the greater is the body size of football players. When Yugoslav players were classified according to the level of performance, those of top-class ability tended to be slightly smaller and lighter than those of moderate ability (Medved 1966). Nevertheless this trend in body size brings no guarantee of success in the game. A particular body size may encourage the acquisition of certain skills and force a gravitation toward a specific playing position: this is likely to occur before maturity so that the individual will tend to favor one positional role before playing at senior level.

Body composition

Body composition is an important aspect of fitness for football as superfluous body fat acts as dead weight in activities where body mass is lifted repeatedly against gravity in running or jumping during play. The amount of adipose tissue in an adult male in his mid-twenties averages about 16% of body weight; for a female this value is 25%. Lowest values among athletic groups are found in distance runners with mean levels 4–7% for males. Values as low as 8.3% have been reported for attacking and defending backs in American football (Wilmore & Haskell 1972). Football players, even at the highest level, tend to have depots of body fat that seem higher than optimal. Hirata (1966) concluded that Olympic Games players were "a little stout" as well as rather small. Professional players studied by others have shown values between 9 and 19%, including 14.9% for Aberdeen FC players (Reid & Williams 1974) and 9.6% for members of the Dallas Tornado FC team (Raven *et al.* 1976). Brazilian players were reported to have mean values of 10.7%, the national level players being just below 10% (De Rose 1975). The 12 players of the Dallas Sidekicks, an indoor professional team in the USA, had a mean ($\pm$ SE) value of 7.1 $\pm$ 0.4). The average for college players in outfield roles was found to be 14.7% (Bell & Rhodes 1975). Higher values are found in goalkeepers than in outfield players, probably because of the lighter metabolic loading imposed by match-play and training on goalkeepers.

Football players accumulate body fat in the off-season: a mean percentage of body fat as high as 19.3% was noted for a top English League team starting pre-season training (White *et al.* 1988). The energy expended during weekly training in English League professionals was found to be moderate compared with other endurance sports (Reilly & Thomas 1979). Thus the habitual activity of players at the time of measurement, their diet, and the stage of competitive season should be considered when body composition is evaluated. The observations may depend on the methods of measuring or estimating percentage of body fat and the scale of measurement error should be recognized when results are being compared.

Somatotype

Football players tend to be well developed muscularly especially in the thigh muscles and this produces a characteristic body shape or physique. Somatotyping offers a convenient method of describing the physique of players according to three dimensions — endomorphy, mesomorphy, and ectomorphy. English college players seem to vary a little around the basic 3 : 5 : 2.5 somatotype profile (Bell & Rhodes 1975); professional players also tend to occupy a similar area of the somatochart when average values for the team are plotted (White *et al.* 1988). Mean rating of the Australian football squad was 3 : 5 : 3, again emphasizing a tendency towards mesomorphy (Cochrane & Pyke 1976). Top Czech players averaged ratings of 2.5 : 4.6 : 2.5 (Chovanova & Zrubak 1972) and 3 : 5.1 : 2.5 (Stepnicka 1977), these players meriting the description of middle to strong mesomorphs. The mean profile of the 1982 Kuwait World Cup squad was 2.1 : 4.5 : 2.1, the goalkeepers having significantly higher mesomorphy and endomorphy values than players in outfield roles (Ramadan & Byrd 1987). The somatotype of top Hungarian players was found to be 2.1 : 5.1 : 2.3, the players with only a few exceptions belonging to the balanced mesomorphy category (Apor 1988). The muscular make-up could be expected to be an advantage in game contexts such as tackling, turning, accelerating, kicking, and so on.

A comparison of top English League players with the 1960 Olympic athletes studied by Tanner (1964) using similar procedures showed that the football players closely resembled the 400-m hurdlers in weight and thigh circumference, but were shorter and had higher skinfold thicknesses and endomorphy ratings (Reilly 1979). Thigh and calf circumferences, endomorphy, and skinfold thicknesses approximated the values of triple jumpers who were lighter and taller. Controlled output of anaerobic power is required in parts of these athletic events and periodically in football play. The English League players were on average heavier and smaller than the Olympic athletes (the 400-m hurdlers and triple jumpers) they most closely resembled in physique but were unlike any of the other track and field athletes.

Muscle function

Muscle strength

Various tests of muscle strength and power have been employed for assessment of football players. These have ranged from performance tests and measurement of isometric strength to contemporary dynamic measures using computer-linked isokinetic equipment. Tests of anaerobic power have also evolved as well as short-term performance on the force platform that have relevance to football play.

Stronger than normal muscular strength would be expected in football players from the trend toward mesomorphy that is apparent in experienced players. Nevertheless the average back strength of the Japanese internationals was 148.8 kg which was equivalent to results obtained for the general population at age 20 years. One repetition maximum bench press was used by Raven *et al.* (1976) as a field test of muscular fitness of the Dallas Tornado professionals, a mean value of 73 ($\pm$ SE = 4) kg being observed. This is not impressive when compared to values produced by weight-trainers or American football specialists. This may reflect a lack of strength training for the upper limbs in football players rather than a specific physiological requirement for the game, except for throw-ins.

Strength in the lower limbs is of obvious concern in football: the quadriceps, hamstrings, and triceps surae groups must generate high forces for jumping, kicking, tackling, turning, and changing pace. The ability to sustain forceful contractions is also important in maintaining balance and control. Isometric strength is possibly important in maintaining a player's balance on a slippery pitch and also in contributing to ball control. For a goalkeeper almost all the body's muscle groups are important. For outfield players the lower part of the trunk, the hip flexors, and the plantar- and dorsiflexors of the ankle are used most exactly. Upper body strength is employed in throw-ins and the strength of the neck flexors could be important in forcefully heading the ball. At least a moderate level of upper body strength should prove helpful in preventing being knocked off the ball.

Football players are generally found to be only a little above average in isometric muscle strength. This may reflect inadequate attention to resistance training in their habitual program. Besides, isometric strength may not truly reflect the ability to exert force in dynamic conditions. It may also be a poor predictor of muscle performance in the game.

Brooke *et al.* (1970) found non-significant correlations between football kick length and static and explosive leg strength. A leg dynamometer was used to measure static strength while a short shuttle run and a vertical jump test were used as indices of "explosive" leg strength. The authors concluded, albeit tentatively, that a degree of learned skill in the applied task of kicking predominated over the degree of basic strength required. The interaction of strength and velocity of the moving limb may also be a relevant factor. Asami and Togari (1968) did find a relation between knee extension power and ball speed in instep kicking, both increasing with experience in the game. Cabri *et al.* (1988) also reported a significant relation between leg strength, measured as peak torque during an isokinetic movement and kick performance indicated by the distance the ball travelled. The relationship was significant for both eccentric and concentric contractions of hip and knee joints in flexion and extension.

The correlation between leg strength and kick performance implies that strength training could be effective in improving the kicking performance of football players. Given a certain level of technique, it seems that strength training added to the normal football training improves both muscular strength and kick performance (De Proft *et al.* 1988). Football players have greater fast speed capabilities than normal (Öberg *et al.* 1986) and this may be an important determinant of technique in kicking the ball.

The relationship between dynamic muscle strength of the knee extensors and kick performance may be dependent on the level of skill already acquired. Trolle *et al.* (1991) measured isokinetic strength of the leg extensors in skilled football players at angular velocities between 0 and 4.18 rad·s^{-1}. No relationship was found between these measures and ball velocity measured during a standardized indoor football kick. Ball velocity was unchanged after 12 weeks of strength training. Motor control may override muscular strength in well-trained football players' performance, whilst the choice of criterion of kick performance may also be a factor.

Strength of shoulder and trunk muscles are engaged in throwing in the ball from the sidelines and a long throw into the opponent's penalty area can be a rich source of scoring opportunities. The throw-in distance of football players has been found to be related to pull-over strength and trunk flexion strength (Togari & Asami 1972). Training methods, using a medicine ball, increased strength measures but without a corresponding increase in throw distance. This demonstrates a degree of specificity in the throwing skill and suggests that individual players should be pre-selected to take tactical long throws.

As the maximal aerobic power tends to be greatest in midfield players and least in goalkeepers and center backs, it is conceivable that the latter might compensate by superior muscle strength. Goalkeepers and defenders were found by Öberg *et al.* (1984) to have higher knee extension torque at 0.52 rad·s^{-1} than midfield players and forwards. The result was attributable to differences in body size since correction for body surface area removed the positional effect. A similar observation was recorded by Togari *et al.* (1988) in their observations on Japanese Football League players. The goalkeepers were significantly stronger than forwards at slow (1.05 rad·s^{-1}) speeds of movement, midfield players being intermediate. The differences tended to disappear when the angular velocity was raised to 3.14 rad·s^{-1}.

It is now common to monitor the muscle strength of football players using isokinetic apparatus such as Cybex, Kin-Com, Bio-Dex, or Lido Inc. systems (Fig. 6.1). These systems offer facilities for determining torque–velocity curves in isokinetic movements and joint–angle curves in a series of isometric contractions. The data provided by Kirkendall (1985) showed the typical torque–velocity curve with performance of USA national players being superior to all other groups at all the angular velocities tested. These included Swedish professionals, USA Olympic trialists, and USA collegiate players.

Isokinetic tests of football players have concentrated almost exclusively on lower limb muscle groups and in concentric contractions. Whilst knee extension strength in concentric contractions is correlated with kick performance, an even higher correlation has been reported for knee flexion strength in an eccentric contraction (Cabri *et al.* 1988). The strength of the hamstrings, particularly in eccentric modes, is an important characteristic for playing football.

The balance between hamstring and quadriceps strength may predispose toward injury in football players (Fowler & Reilly 1993). At slow speeds and under isometric conditions a knee flexor–extensor ratio of 60–65% is recommended (Öberg *et al.* 1986). This ratio is increased at the higher angular velocities of commercially available apparatus, although the reliability of measurement is reduced at fast speeds.

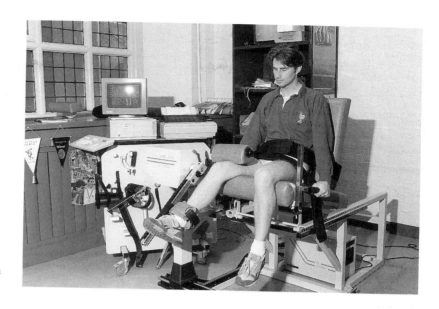

Fig. 6.1 Muscle strength testing on an isokinetic dynamometer.

Isokinetic strength testing allows comparison of left and right legs to identify any muscle imbalance, the weaker side being the one most liable to injury. Test profiles are also important in monitoring regains in muscle strength using the uninjured side as reference. Isokinetic dynamometers can be used for retraining as well as for monitoring purposes during the rehabilitation period (Fowler & Reilly 1993). It should be mentioned that comparisons to identify asymmetry or weakness within an individual player may be more important than comparison between teams. This reservation applies especially to comparisons with data from other laboratories using alternative test protocols.

Anaerobic power

Explosive leg strength has traditionally been measured by means of vertical and standing long jumps (Fig. 6.2). Mean values for the vertical jump have included 49.9 cm for the Australian World Cup team (Cochrane & Pyke 1976), 52.8 cm for North American Football League professionals, and 58 cm for English League professionals (Thomas & Reilly 1979). Observations on USA players have been 55.6 cm at collegiate level, 55.9 cm for the national junior team, 56.4 cm for the national senior team, and 57.6 cm for Olympic trialists (Kirkendall 1985). English League players cleared 219

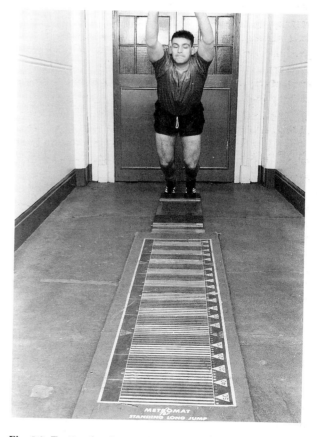

Fig. 6.2 Testing for the standing long jump.

($\pm$ SE = 3) cm in the standing long jump. The superior performances in this and in the vertical jump were found among goalkeepers and center backs and in forwards operating as target players. Midfielders had relatively low scores in both tests. The performances of two center backs and one striker in the vertical jump were similar to results reported for international high jumpers (Reilly 1979).

The splitting of high-energy intramuscular phosphagens contributes along with anaerobic glycolysis to the maximal power a player can develop. These substrates (adenosine triphosphate, creatine phosphate, and glycogen) may be used for combustion by muscle at the onset of exercise and result in a high anaerobic work production. The maximum power output can be calculated from performance on the stair-run test (Margaria *et al.* 1966). Measurement is made of the time taken for the player to run between two steps on the stairs, the vertical distance between which is known. The anaerobic power of Olympic football players measured in this way was found to be less than pentathletes, sprinters, and middle-distance runners (Di Prampero *et al.* 1970). Another research group found higher values in representative football players (mean 16.2 $W \cdot kg^{-1}$) than in basketball players, walkers, and runners at the same competitive level (Withers *et al.* 1977). Caru *et al.* (1970) studied 95 young football players aged 14–18 years and reported mean values ranging from 15 $W \cdot kg^{-1}$ at 14 to 16.1 $W \cdot kg^{-1}$ at 18. These values were significantly higher than in non-athletes of similar ages but no significant differences were apparent among any of the playing positions examined. This may have been due to the number of versatile players at this stage who may not settle into a successful positional role until later in their career.

Bosco *et al.* (1983) described a method for measuring mechanical power output in jumping. It required repeated jumping for a given period, usually 60 s, the flight time and jumping frequency being recorded. Kirkendall (1985) reported values of 23 $W \cdot kg^{-1}$ for professional indoor football players and 21 $W \cdot kg^{-1}$ for collegiate players, results which are in agreement with observations on volleyball and basketball players.

Bosco (1990) employed a 15-s test and found that the mean power output of two football players (27 $W \cdot kg^{-1}$) was superior to that of skiers (22 $W \cdot kg^{-1}$) and endurance runners (24 $W \cdot kg^{-1}$) but was lower than for skaters (28 $W \cdot kg^{-1}$) and sprinters (30 $W \cdot kg^{-1}$). A longer duration of test is needed if the anaerobic capacity is to be taxed. Performance at various parts of the 1-min test (for example) can be compared, the tolerance to fatigue as the test progresses being indicative of the anaerobic glycolytic capacity.

As football players must be prepared to repeat fast bursts supported by anaerobic glycolysis, a high anaerobic capacity is needed in order to play at a high tempo. Anaerobic capacity is measured utilizing the Wingate test which entails 30-s all-out effort on a cycle ergometer. Bergh and Ekblom (1979) reported values of 13.5 $W \cdot kg$ for Swedish national players. These were higher than mean power outputs of top English Rugby Union players in any positional role (Rigg & Reilly 1988). A major limitation of such anaerobic capacity profiles is the mode of exercise. Measurement of power production and anaerobic capacity on a treadmill are likely to constitute such tests for football players in the future.

Muscle fiber types

Football play demands an ability to sustain physical effort, albeit discontinuously, over 90 min, some of which is at high intensity. As the activity profile is compatible with both slow twitch (ST) and fast twitch (FT) muscle fiber characteristics, a balanced combination of muscle fiber types would be expected in top players (Table 6.2). The muscle fibers in the vastus lateralis of the Swedish professional club players was found to be 59.8 ($\pm$ SD = 10.6)% FT. The percentage of FT area was 65.6 ($\pm$ 10.6)%, depicting a FT/ST mean fiber area of 1.28 ($\pm$ 0.22). These figures suggest that the fiber types of football players are closer to sprinters than to endurance athletes in make-up. However, a large range was observed within the squad, the values for FT fibers ranging from 40.8 to 79.1%. It would be expected that the fiber types of the goalkeeper and central defenders, in which an anaerobic profile of physical performance dominates, would be biased towards FT fibers.

This picture changes a little when the oxidative enzymes of the gastrocnemius muscles are considered (Bangsbo & Mizuno 1988). The relative occurrence of ST, STa, and FTb fibers in four Danish professionals was 55.9 (range 48–63.6), 39.8 (33–46.5) and 4.4 (3.0–5.5)% respectively. A reduction in fiber area

Table 6.2 Muscle fiber composition of football players from various sources. Values of $\dot{V}_{O_{2max.}}$ (± SD) are also included

Players	n	Muscle	Fiber type		$\dot{V}_{O_{2max.}}$ (ml·kg^{-1}·min^{-1})	Reference
			FT	ST		
Malmo FC	19	Vastus lateralis	59.8 ± 10.6	40.2	—	Jacobs *et al.* 1982
Danish professionals	4	Gastrocnemius	44 (IIa, IIb)	55.9	66.2	Bangsbo & Mizuno 1988
Finnish Second Division	8	Vastus lateralis	53 (IIa, IIb)	47 ± 13.3	63.6 ± 6.6	Smaros 1980
Spanish and Italian semi-professionals	12	Quadriceps (undefined)	61.2 (type IIa, IIb)	38.8 (type I, IIc)	—	Montanari *et al.* 1990
Japanese university players	12	Vastus lateralis	55.4	44.6	—	Ryushi *et al.* 1979

FT, fast twitch; ST, slow twitch.

with 3 weeks of detraining was observed only in the FTa fibers and the decrease was small (7%). The number of capillaries around the fibers was found to decrease with detraining only in the ST fibers. Mitochondrial activities at the time of full training for oxidative enzymes were similar to those for cross-country skiers in the case of 3-hydroacyl coenzyme A dehydrogenase (HAD). Values for citrase synthase were intermediate between middle-distance runners and non-athletes.

Eight Finnish Second Division players were examined by Smaros (1980). Biopsies taken from the vastus lateralis muscle showed an average fiber type distribution of 47% FT and 53% ST. Moreover, muscle biopsies taken at the end of a game showed that the reduction in glycogen stores occurred mainly in the ST fibers. This reflects the aerobic regimens of match-play.

Ryushi *et al.* (1979) reported fiber type percentages for Japanese university players that were very close to the values found in the Finnish study. They found no relation between percentage of fiber area and isometric strength but the maximal power of the knee extensors per kilogram of body mass was highly correlated ($r = 0.734$) with the percentage of fiber area.

It seems that any inferences about muscle fiber

types and élite football play must be tentative. Fiber type distributions could reflect positional role and so a team may be relatively heterogenous in muscle composition. Fiber type distributions also vary between skeletal muscles. The gastrocnemius has an important function in locomotion whereas the quadriceps comprise the important muscle group in powerful kicking. The observations on football players may therefore reflect a relatively higher FT proportion in vastus lateralis than in the gastrocnemius compared to the ratio noted in other athletic populations.

Agility and flexibility

Muscle performance profiles described so far eminate from tests that involve either static contractions or dynamic contractions in the sagittal plane. The ability to turn quickly, dodge, and side-step calls for motor co-ordination and is reflected in a standardized agility run test. Dallas Tornado players were found to have average times on the Illinois agility run above the 99.95 percentile for the test norms (Raven *et al.* 1976). The test distinguished the football players as a group from the normal population better than any field test used for strength, power, and flexibility.

Muscle strength and joint flexibility are important safety factors in football. Strength imbalance between the limbs increases the likelihood of injury: comparison of strength data between left and right legs can be of benefit in screening for injury predisposition. Factor analysis of a number of strength and muscular power tests on English professional players showed the stronger individuals were the more successful in avoiding injuries throughout the season (Reilly & Thomas 1980). Similar statistical procedures showed that flexibility in a range of movements in the hip joint afforded protection against injury in games players (Reilly & Stirling 1993).

Muscle tightness, particularly in the hamstring and adductor groups, has been linked with increased risk of muscle injury in Swedish professionals (Ekstrand 1982). Two-thirds of the players had flexibility values poorer than non-players. This may be an adaptation, but it could also reflect a lack of attention to flexibility practices in training. Poorer range of motion has also been noted at the ankle joint in Japanese (Haltori & Ohta 1986) and English League (Reilly 1979) players, although the goalkeepers were exceptions among the English professionals. The Japanese players were less flexible than a reference group in inversion, eversion, plantar-, and dorsiflexion. This may reflect an adaptive response of soft tissue around the ankle which improves stability at the joint.

The oxygen transport system

Pulmonary function

Pulmonary function tests are frequently used as measures of the adequacy of the respiratory system (Fig. 6.3). The volume of gas that can be forcibly expired after a maximum inspiration represents the approximate useable capacity of the lungs and is indicated by the vital capacity (VC). The air remaining in the lungs after a complete exhalation is represented by the residual volume (RV). Mean values ($\pm$ SE) for VC (BTPS, body temperature and pressure saturated) were 5.29 ($\pm$ 0.174) l for Dallas Tornado professionals, for RV values were 1.385 ($\pm$ 0.117) l, and for total lung capacity 6.735 ($\pm$ 0.224) l (Raven *et al.* 1976). Mean VC values for English League players were 5.80 ($\pm$ 0.18) l at the start of pre-season training and 5.9 ($\pm$ 0.16) l at the beginning of the competitive season (Reilly 1979). These values were significantly higher than the 5.15 ($\pm$ 0.06) l predicted from height and age using a standard nomogram. It seems that VC represents a structural component of the body, similar to other assessments of body size and this is the basis of predicting pulmonary capacity from body surface area or body size. Several authors have reported that VC is higher in athletes than in non-athletes of similar body size and this superiority seems to be due more to genetic factors than to training.

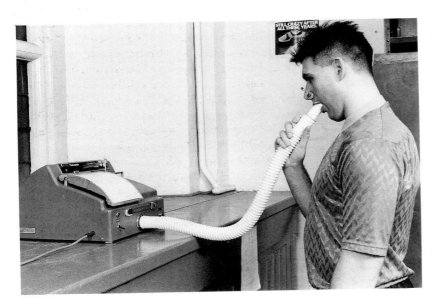

Fig. 6.3 Testing for pulmonary function.

The lung power of English League subjects as indicated by forced expiratory volume in 1 s (FEV_1) was 4.95 (± 0.16) l. This was significantly higher than the predicted value of 4.3 (± 0.04) l. The forced expiratory flow (FEF) rate was 10.6 (± 0.32) $l \cdot s^{-1}$ (Reilly 1979). The FEV_1/VC was 84%, being close to the normal rate of exhalation in a forced single breath. A higher proportion (89.8%) was reported for Hungarian footballers, although mean values ($\pm$ SD) of VC were 5.9 (± 0.37) l for Honved (Budapest) and 5.79 (± 0.42) l for Ujpesti Dozsa (Budapest) players (Apor 1988).

Pulmonary function is not normally a factor limiting the maximal aerobic performance and the main use of single-breath spirometry is in screening for any impairment or lung obstruction. The oxygen transport system in strenuous exercise may be affected by pulmonary ventilation, pulmonary diffusion, the oxygen carrying capacity of the blood, the cardiac output, and the arteriovenous difference in oxygen saturation. Oxygen transport at high exercise intensities may be limited in some well-trained individuals by oxygen desaturation in the lungs but this has not been studied in football players. It is reasonable to expect that the maximum breathing capacity, the maximum rate at which air can be breathed in and out per min, should be high in football players to furnish the oxygen transport system with the necessary supplies of air throughout 90 min of play. More information about dynamic pulmonary function in football players has been obtained from measurements of maximum minute ventilation ($\dot{V}_{E max.}$) during exercise tests designed to assess $\dot{V}_{O2 max.}$

Reported values of $\dot{V}_{E max.}$ of football players exhibit a large variation. These include 108.3 (± 16.9) $l \cdot min^{-1}$ for Aberdeen FC (Williams *et al.* 1973); 125.2 (± 17.8) $l \cdot min^{-1}$ for Honved and 141.2 (± 7.0) $l \cdot min^{-1}$ for Ujpesti Dozsa (Apor 1988); and 153.6 (± 4.1) $l \cdot min^{-1}$ for Dallas Tornado professionals (Raven *et al.* 1976). The $\dot{V}_{E max.}$ of 30 Dutch players in a First Division Club was $149 \pm 9 \, l \cdot min^{-1}$ for 15 players with the higher $\dot{V}_{E max.}$ values and 151 ± 11 for the others (Verstappen & Bovens 1989). The second group was heavier (77.7 $\pm$ 4.8) than the first (72.0 $\pm$ 7) kg, suggesting that $\dot{V}_{E max.}$ is influenced by body size more than aerobic power. To what extent the differences between these studies reflect differences in the protocol used for exercise testing is uncertain. In general the figures are well below those anticipated for top-class middle-distance runners whose $\dot{V}_{E max.}$ values would typically exceed $170 \, l \cdot min^{-1}$.

Cardiac function

The heart responds to strenuous training by becoming larger and more effective as a pump. The chambers (particularly the left ventricle) increase in volume from a repetitive overload stimulus such as endurance running whilst the walls of the heart thicken and may grow stronger as a result of a pressure stimulus. Hypertrophy of cardiac muscle is reflected in a greater stroke volume and a larger ventricular size enables more blood to fill the chamber before the heart contracts. Both are manifested in a lower heart rate at rest and this is apparent in observations on well-trained athletes.

The maximal heart volume of football players is intermediate between well-trained cyclists and long-distance runners at one extreme and sports specialists in golf, gymnastics, and sprinting at the lower extreme. Top players tested at the Cologne Institute (Rost 1987) had higher heart volumes than field hockey players but lower than middle-distance runners. Another study of German footballers demonstrated that national class players ($n = 11$) had higher heart volumes (1010 $\pm$ 107 ml) than regional ($n = 13$) players (955 $\pm$ 114 ml) or performers in the Third Division ($n = 14$; 945 $\pm$ 114 ml) or the Fourth Division ($n = 11$; 969 $\pm$ 117 ml) of the Bundesliga. The lowest heart rates were recorded in the national class players (50 $\pm$ 9 $beats \cdot min^{-1}$) but in the other groups the mean resting heart rate was only marginally higher, ranging from 51 to 53 $beats \cdot min^{-1}$ (Dickhuth *et al.* 1981).

Seventy top players in the Italian League, including 11 who had played for their national teams in the 1986 World Cup, were studied by Pelliccia *et al.* (1990) using echocardiography. Results showed an absence of ventricular hypertrophy, although a moderate enlargement of the left ventricular cavity resembling that found in endurance athletes was acknowledged. The large left ventricular dimension could have been accounted for by body size and state of training of the players at the time of measurement.

Heart rates of top football players at rest tend to be much lower than the general population average of 72 $beats \cdot min^{-1}$. Mean values ($\pm$ SE) reported include 48 (± 1) $beats \cdot min^{-1}$ for English League players (Reilly 1979), 50 (± 1) $beats \cdot min^{-1}$ for Dallas Tornado players (Raven *et al.* 1976), and 52 (± 2) $beats \cdot min^{-1}$ for the Romanian League champions (Balanescu *et al.* 1968). These values suggest a large degree of cardiac adaptation to exercise. Resting circulatory efficiency identified in English League players by means of factor analysis, was also reflected in low diastolic blood pressures, mean blood pressure being 120/70 mmHg (Reilly 1979). The slower heart rate allows extended relaxation time during diastole for the pressure to drop below the normal level of about 80 mmHg. The pulse pressure, the difference between systolic and diastolic pressures, with a value of 50 mmHg for the English League players was superior to the normal 40 mmHg and the 42 mmHg reported for 201 Olympic Games athletes of a previous generation (Berry *et al.* 1949).

On analyzing data from a battery of fitness tests using multivariate methods, Reilly and Thomas (1977) identified resting circulatory efficiency as a principal component of fitness for football. This factor significantly discriminated between levels of playing proficiency. This advantage is likely to be transferred to exercise and post-exercise recovery. The heart rate response to submaximal exercise is used for estimating $\dot{V}_{O_2max.}$ and for measuring the physical working capacity (PWC_{170}). The kinetics of heart rate recovery post-exercise are also related to the state of endurance training.

The ability to recover quickly from strenuous exercise may be important in football which involves intermittent efforts interspersed with short rests. The Harvard step test designed initially for college undergraduates and later used in testing of military conscripts provides a fitness index which is based on the recovery of pulse rates over 3.5 min after a standard work rate. Although easy to administer, the Harvard step test has now lost favor due to the availability of alternatives that can be employed during exercise. Similarly the PWC_{170} test has limited relevance to football as it is usually conducted on a cycle ergometer, an exercise mode unsuitable for football players. A convenient practical test for football players is the multistage shuttle run (Leger *et al.* 1988). The speed is dictated by a rhythm on a tape-recorder, the pulse rate response to each running intensity being monitored. This test is now accepted as a valid method of indirectly estimating the maximal oxygen uptake and is suitable for testing football squads because of its close fidelity to movements in the game. The results may be compared to reference values for $\dot{V}_{O_2max.}$ but are of most value in monitoring changes in fitness at different stages of the season.

Football players have maximal heart rates that are close to the norms for non-athletic populations of similar age and race. Nevertheless there is a large variation in the maximal heart rates reported and this may be due in part to the exercise protocol used for testing as well as true individual variability. The mean values ($\pm$ SE) include 179 ($\pm$ 2) beats·min^{-1} for South Australian representatives (Withers *et al.* 1977); 176 ($\pm$ 8) beats·min^{-1} for the 1984 West German national team (Nowacki *et al.* 1988); 179 ($\pm$ 2) beats·min^{-1} for English League First Division players (White *et al.* 1988); 188 ($\pm$ 2) beats·min^{-1} for USA club professionals (Raven *et al.* 1976); 187 ($\pm$ 7) beats·min^{-1} in USA indoor professionals (Winter *et al.* 1989); 189 ($\pm$ 7) and 185 ($\pm$ 5) in two groups of players in a First Division Dutch team (Verstappen & Bovens 1989); 193 beats·min^{-1} for Danish semi-professionals (Bangsbo & Mizuno 1988); and 198 ($\pm$ 1) beats·min^{-1} for English League football players (Reilly 1979). Indications are that the maximal heart rate does not increase with training but may show a slight reduction as a result of lowered sympathetic drive at maximal effort. Moreover, the values are within the general population norms.

Maximal oxygen uptake

The upper limit of the body's ability to consume oxygen is indicated by the maximal oxygen uptake or $\dot{V}_{O_2max.}$ (Fig. 6.4). The average values of $\dot{V}_{O_2max.}$ for top-level football players tend to be high, supporting the belief that there is a large contribution from aerobic power to playing the game. Nevertheless values do not reach the same levels as in specialist endurance sports such as cross-country running, skiing, distance running, or orienteering where values frequently exceed 80 ml·kg^{-1}·min^{-1}. Values for élite players lie in the region of 55–70 ml·kg^{-1}·min^{-1}, the higher values tending to be found at the top level of play and when players are at peak fitness.

Mean $\dot{V}_{O_2max.}$ reported for 11 members of the Swedish national team was 56.5 ml·kg^{-1}·min^{-1}: the corresponding figure for 50 top Swedish players was 58.6 ml·kg^{-1}·min^{-1} (Åstrand & Rodahl 1986). It was argued that by permitting brief pauses between bursts of physical effort, football does not require the same level of aerobic power in its players as do events calling for long-lasting continuous effort at near maximal

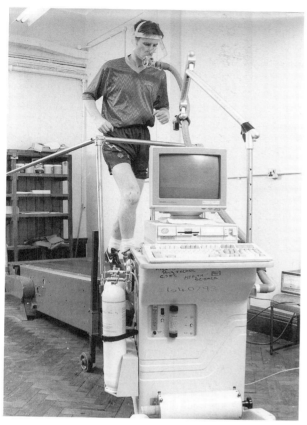

Fig. 6.4 Maximal oxygen uptake testing on the motor-driven treadmill.

intensity. Another report on top Swedish players stated that maximal aerobic power of the national team increased over two decades (Ekblom 1986). The average current value of 61 ml·kg^{-1}·min^{-1} corresponds to that reported for a group of top-level Australian players (62 ml·kg^{-1}·min^{-1}) by Withers *et al.* (1977). The top players in the Swedish squad had values of 65–67 ml·kg^{-1}·min^{-1} with individual values close to 70 ml·kg^{-1}·min^{-1}.

Nowacki *et al.* (1988) reviewed 26 studies of $\dot{V}_{O_{2max.}}$ of German football players at various levels of play. Over half of the studies were conducted using a cycle ergometer which would have underestimated the true $\dot{V}_{O_{2max.}}$ of the players. The highest values reported using a treadmill test were for a German club team, mean 69.2 ($\pm$ 7.8) ml·kg^{-1}·min^{-1}. On the treadmill, the 1978 national German squad ($n = 17$) had a mean

value of 62.0 ($\pm$ 4.5) ml·kg^{-1}·min^{-1} while the Austrian national team ($n = 9$) had poorer values at 58.3 ($\pm$ 4.3) ml·kg^{-1}·min^{-1}.

Values for professional players tend to be higher than for amateurs, though this can depend on the quality of training and the standard of competition. Ekblom (1986) cited values of 45–50 ml·kg^{-1}·min^{-1} for Swedish recreational players. Values of the Ethiopian players competing in the Mexico Olympic Games tournament were 43 ml·kg^{-1}·min^{-1} on average (Di Prampero *et al.* 1970). These unremarkable values could have been due to the altitude conditions under which the tests were performed or to the poor standard of aerobic fitness of the players at that time. Higher standards of fitness were attained by German amateur players, mean values being 50–56 ml·kg^{-1}·min^{-1} in the studies reviewed by Nowacki *et al.* (1988). Top Italian amateurs seem to have higher standards still but this may be connected with their frequency of competition and intensity of training. Faina *et al.* (1988) reported values of 64.1 ($\pm$ 7.2) ml·kg^{-1}·min^{-1} for six amateur players, which were as good as those of 17 professionals and better than the 63.2 ml·kg^{-1}·min^{-1} for a national World Cup star. The Dallas Sidekicks, an indoor professional team in the USA had mean values ($\pm$ SE) of 65.3 ($\pm$ 1.9) ml·kg^{-1}·min, range 51.7–74.0 ml·kg^{-1}·min^{-1} (Kirkendall 1985). Two groups of players (each $n = 15$) in a Dutch First Division club had mean values of 68 ($\pm$ 5) and 63 ($\pm$ 7) ml·kg^{-1}·min^{-1} (Verstappen & Bovens 1989). The $\dot{V}_{O_{2max.}}$ of 19 professional players in the First Division of the Portuguese League was 59.6 ($\pm$ 7.7) ml·kg^{-1}·min^{-1}: the average values for goalkeepers and central defenders, midfield players and forwards were above 60 ml·kg^{-1}·min^{-1} (Puga *et al.* 1993). The mean $\dot{V}_{O_{2max.}}$ of four Danish semi-professionals studied by Bangsbo and Mizuno (1988) was 66 ml·kg^{-1}·min^{-1}: the profile of mitochondrial enzyme activities in the gastrocnemius of the players was closer to that of endurance athletes than to strength-trained individuals.

The $\dot{V}_{O_{2max.}}$ of professional football players does improve significantly in the pre-season period when there is an emphasis on aerobic training (Reilly 1979). Further emphasis on improving the $\dot{V}_{O_{2max.}}$ adds little to the quality of play. When two teams of equal skill meet, the one with superior aerobic fitness would have the edge, being able to play the game at a faster pace throughout. Apor (1988) provided data on Hungarian players which showed perfect rank-order correlation between mean $\dot{V}_{O_{2max.}}$ of the team and finishing position in the Hungarian First Division championship. Mean $\dot{V}_{O_{2max.}}$ for the first, second, third, and fifth teams were 66.6, 64.3, 63.3, and 58.1 ml·kg^{-1}·min^{-1}, respectively. Common factors such as stability in the team, avoidance of injury, and so on, help to maintain both $\dot{V}_{O_{2max.}}$ and team performance independently.

There is evidence that $\dot{V}_{O_{2max.}}$ does vary with positional role, when such roles can be clearly differentiated. When English League players were subdivided into positions according to 4−3−3 and 4−4−2 configurations, the midfielders had significantly higher aerobic power values than those in the other positions. The central defenders had significantly lower relative values than the other outfield players while the fullbacks and strikers had values that were intermediate (Reilly 1979). The significant correlation between $\dot{V}_{O_{2max.}}$ and distance covered in a game ($r = 0.67$) underlines the need for a high work-rate in midfield players who link between defense and attack. The goalkeepers had lower values than the center backs, an observation confirmed by other researchers and reinforced by the highest values for adiposity among goalkeepers. Four goalkeepers in the German national team had values of 56.2 ($\pm$ 1.2) ml·kg^{-1}·min^{-1} compared to 62.0 ($\pm$ 4.5) ml·kg^{-1}·min^{-1} for the squad as a whole (Hollman *et al.* 1981). A study of 95 young non-professional players aged 14−18 years found that goalkeepers had significantly lower $\dot{V}_{O_{2max.}}$ values than outfield players (Caru *et al.* 1970). No differences were observed among outfield positions but players were still at developmental ages and so were unlikely to have been totally specialized in positional roles.

Whilst the $\dot{V}_{O_{2max.}}$ indicates the maximal ability to consume oxygen in strenuous exercise, it is not possible to sustain exercise for very long at an intensity that elicits $\dot{V}_{O_{2max.}}$. The upper level at which exercise can be sustained for a prolonged period is thought to be indicated by the so-called "anaerobic threshold": this is usually expressed as the work-rate corresponding to a blood lactate concentration of 4 mmol·l^{-1}, the onset of accumulation of lactate in the blood (OBLA) or as a deflection in the relation between ventilation and oxygen consumption with incremental exercise (the ventilatory threshold). This has been measured at 77% $\dot{V}_{O_{2max.}}$ in English League First Division players (White *et al.* 1988), a value close to the usual work

intensity in running a marathon. The intermittent nature of football means that frequently players operate at above this intensity although the average fractional utilization of $\dot{V}_{O_{2max.}}$ is deemed to be about 75%.

The oxygen supplied to the tissues largely determines the maximal oxygen consumption and so the maximal cardiac output is an important physiological parameter. High cardiac outputs at maximal exercise are linked with high $\dot{V}_{O_{2max.}}$ values (Åstrand & Rodahl 1986), although there is little specific information about the maximal cardiac output of football players. The oxygen pulse of top football players has been determined by calculating the oxygen consumed per heart beat at maximal exercise. Highest average values reported have been 29.1 ml·beats^{-1} for a German League team, 27.9 ml·beats^{-1} for the 1974 and 1981 national German teams (Nowacki *et al.* 1988), and 25.2 ($\pm$ 4.7) ml·beats^{-1} for Honved (Apor 1988). Since the maximal heart rate differs little between sporting and sedentary populations, these high results are largely attributable to favorable $\dot{V}_{O_{2max.}}$ values.

The oxygen transport capacity of the blood can affect the quantity of oxygen delivered to the active muscle cells, thereby affecting $\dot{V}_{O_{2max.}}$. Studies of professional football players for hemoglobin and hematocrit tend to fall within the normal range. Dallas Tornado players had hemoglobin concentrations of 14.6 ($\pm$ SE = 0.2) g·dl^{-1} and hematocrit levels of 41.9 ($\pm$ SE = 0.5)% (Raven *et al.* 1976). Blood volume and total body hemoglobin tend to be about 20% higher in endurance-trained athletes than in non-athletes. Well-trained athletes tend also to have significantly higher concentrations of 2,3-bisphosphoglycerate in the red blood cells, which would affect oxygen release to the tissues. It is likely that these hematological factors contribute toward the moderately high aerobic power values of top football players, although hematological standards for high levels of play have not been set down.

Psychophysiological characteristics

Simple reaction time gives a measure of how quickly a subject can respond to a stimulus in the immediate environment. This ability is predominantly due to heredity but deteriorates with age. It might be important in football where players have to respond quickly to environmental stimuli. Reaction times of English

League football players to a visual stimulus were found to be faster than the normal values and similar to reaction times of track and field athletes. This result agrees with values for a range of sportspeople and the observation of many investigators that athletes are superior to non-athletes in this measure (Reilly 1979). No significant differences were found between the first team and the reserve team squads nor between goalkeepers and outfield players. The apparently rapid responses of goalkeepers in competitive conditions can be attributed to their trained ability to anticipate the attackers' play from antecedent cues. This ability to predict opponents' maneuvers correctly and to select the appropriate response rapidly from a large array of possible ones is a recognized hallmark of the skilled performer. The highly skilled player has the ability to read and interpret complex situations quickly and to initiate decisive action. The faster the simple reaction time of the individual, the quicker will be the responses to complex situations. It will also give the player an advantage in initiating short, sharp movements. Thus a fast reaction time denotes a general athletic ability whilst fast responses, in a complex or choice reaction time test specific to football characterizes game-related decision-making.

Whole body reaction time (WRT) of football players was studied by Togari and Takahashi (1977). No differences were found in simple WRT between regular and substitute players but the regular players had the faster choice WRTs. No differences were observed between any of the various playing positions, although goalkeepers were generally faster to react in choice WRT. This superiority is likely to be largely a product of training specific to that position.

Fast diving movements are particularly relevant to goalkeeping skills. Suzuki *et al.* (1988) showed that skilled goalkeepers could dive faster than lesser skilled counterparts. The skilled players could generate a faster take-off velocity and turn better to meet the ball compared to less skilled players. Fast reactions in physical activity may be split between reaction time and movement time. Limb movement time should be an important attribute of the successful football player. This measure is independent of reaction time and is quicker in athletic subjects than in non-athletes. It does not, however, appear to have been studied in football players (except when linked with force production at high angular velocities), so that there is

as yet no indication as to whether it discriminates between different levels of playing proficiency or different positional roles in the game. Movement time in a throwing action (football throw-in) has been shown to influence the distance of the throw. The build up of speed in the final phase of the movement was found to be influential (Kullath & Schwirtz 1988).

During a game the player must recognize an array of complex stimuli in a wide range of vision. Peripheral vision would therefore seem to be an important prerequisite for success in football. Singer (1972) cited norms of 84.5° for athletes compared with 71.25° for non-athletes. Visual acuity and depth perception are additional aspects of vision important for football. The need for excellent dynamic visual acuity would apply especially to the goalkeeper because of the correlation of this function with ball catching (Sanderson 1974). Despite the obvious relevance of visual characteristics for success in football play, they do not seem to have been studied in great detail. More attention has in recent years been paid to tracking eye movement in simulated games contexts.

The field dependence/independence construct (Witkin *et al.* 1962) regards perceptual ability as a continuum whose ends represent two contrasting modes of perceiving. This refers to the perception one has of oneself in relation to the surrounding field. Field dependency might be an advantage in performance of team sports in which the performer must relate the skill to the environment. This involves the ability to discriminate among complex visual stimuli. The hypothesis was not supported by the experiments of Barrell and Trippe (1975) who found that 30 English League First Division players were not significantly different from a control group in field dependency. Pargman *et al.* (1976) reported a relationship between visual disembedding and injury in American football players, a finding that has relevance also for football. Individuals who have developed the capability to extract meaningful cues from their surrounding visual fields are less likely to become injured. No relationship was apparent between injury and field dependence as measured with a standardized rod and frame test.

Conclusion

It seems that there are many characteristics that are required for play at top level in contemporary football.

As success is dependent on how individuals are knitted together into a competent unit, the combination of physiological characteristics may vary from player to player. Nevertheless it is possible to generalize on physiological characteristics of specialists in this sport. Anthropometric factors can determine the positional role most appropriate for the player. Body adiposity is highest among players pre-season but players at major international tournaments (with the exception of the goalkeeper) tend to have very little surplus fat. The physique of players generally shows muscular development, reflected in a high mesomorphy and low ectomorphy somatotype profile. Muscular strength, particularly in fast isokinetic movements, does seem to favor game-related performance. Anaerobic power of football players tends toward the profile of sprinters for the goalkeeper and central defenders whereas anaerobic capacity would seem to be more important in the other positions. Imbalanced muscular development (inappropriate flexor−extensor ratios, unilateral weakness, muscle tightness) may predispose toward injury. Leg muscle composition is not extreme, the fiber type distribution favoring fast movements but demonstrating histochemical properties of aerobically trained athletes. This is complemented by the moderately large heart volumes and aerobic power of players. For outfield players values above $60\,\text{ml·kg}^{-1}\text{·min}^{-1}$ would seem desirable for $\dot{V}_{O_{2\text{max}}}$. Sensory physiological mechanisms are also relevant considerations in the make-up of football players. It is likely that central factors in deciding the timing of game-related movements, supported by sufficiently well-developed muscular strength, motor co-ordination, and oxygen transport mechanisms to implement the decisions, are the keys to successful football play.

References

Apor P. (1988) Successful formulae for fitness training. In Reilly T., Less A., Davids K. & Murphy W.J. *Science and Football*, pp. 95−107. E. & F.N. Spon, London.

Asami T. & Togari H. (1968) Studies on the kicking ability in soccer. *Res. J. Phys. Educ.* **2**, 267−272.

Åstrand P.O. & Rodahl K. (1986) *Textbook of Work Physiology*. McGraw-Hill, New York.

Balanescu F., Vokulescu A. & Bobocea A. (1968) The cardiovascular response during exercise in athletes. *Int. Zeit. Angewand. Physiol.* **25**, 361−372.

Bangsbo J., Klausen K., Bro-Rasmussen T. & Larsen J. (1988) Physiological responses to acute, moderate hypoxia in élite soccer players. In Reilly T., Lees A., Davids K. & Murphy W.J. (eds) *Science and Football*, pp. 257−264. E. & F.N. Spon, London.

Bangsbo J. & Mizuno M. (1988) Morphological and metabolic alterations in soccer players with detraining and retraining and their relation to performance. In Reilly T., Lees A., Davids K. & Murphy W.J. (eds) *Science and Football*, pp. 114−124. E. & F.N. Spon, London.

Barrell G.V. & Trippe H. (1975) Field dependence and physical ability. *Percep. Motor Skills* **41**, 216−218.

Bell W. & Rhodes G. (1975) The morphological characteristics of the association football player. *Br. J. Sports Med.* **9**, 196−200.

Bergh U. & Ekblom B. (1979) Influence of muscle temperature on maximal strength and power output in human skeletal muscles. *Acta Physiol. Scand.* **107**, 33−37.

Berry W.T.C., Beveridge T.B., Bainsby E.R. *et al.* (1949) The diet, haemoglobin values and blood pressure of Olympic athletes. *Br. Med. J.* **1**, 300−304.

Bosco C. (1990) Strength elasticity in football. In Santilli G. (ed.) *Sports Medicine Applied to Football*, pp. 63−70. CONI, Rome.

Bosco C.P., Luhtanen P. & Komi P. (1983) A simple method for measurement of mechanical power in jumping. *Eur. J. Appl. Physiol.* **50**, 273−282.

Brooke J.D., Clinton N.M., Cosgrove I.N., Dimple D. & Knowles J.E. (1970) The relationship between soccer kick length and static and explosive leg strength. *Br. J. Phys. Educ.* **1**, XVII−XVIII.

Cabri J., De Proft E., Dufour W. & Clarys J.P. (1988) The relation between muscular strength and kick performance. In Reilly T., Lees A., Davids K. & Murphy W.J. (eds) *Science and Football*, pp. 106−153. E. & F.N. Spon, London.

Caru B., Le Coultre L., Aghemo P. & Pinera Limas F. (1970) Maximal aerobic and anaerobic muscular power in football players. *J. Sports Med. Phys. Fit.* **10**, 100−103.

Chovanova E. & Zrubak A. (1972) Somatotypes of prominent Czechoslovak ice-hockey and football players. *Acta Facult. Rerum Nat. Universit. Comen. Anthropol.* **21**, 59−62.

Cochrane C. & Pyke F. (1976) Physiological assessment of the Australian soccer squad. *Aust. J. Health Phys. Educ. Rec.* **75**, 21−25.

De Proft E., Cabri J., Dufour W. & Clarys J.P. (1988) Strength training and kick performance in soccer players. In Reilly T., Lees A., Davids K. & Murphy W.J. (eds) *Science and Football*, pp. 108−113. E. & F.N. Spon, London.

De Rose E.H. (1975) Determination of the ideal body weight and corporal composition of 16 professional soccer players. In *Questions of Athletes Nutrition: Abstracts of the Reports of the International Symposium*. Leningrad, Leningrad Institute of Physical Culture.

Dickhuth H.H., Simon G., Bachl N., Lehman M. & Keul J. (1981) Zur Hochst- und Dauerleistungsahigkeit von Bundesligafussballspiern (Peak and endurance capacity of Bundesliga players). *Leistrungssport* **11**, 148–152.

Di Prampero P.E., Pinera Limas F. & Sassi G. (1970) Maximal muscular power, aerobic and anaerobic, in the athletes performing at the XIXth Olympic Games in Mexico. *Ergonomics* **13**, 665–674.

Ekblom B. (1986) Applied physiology of soccer. *Sports Med.* **3**, 50–60.

Ekstrand J. (1982) *Soccer injuries and their prevention.* Medical dissertation No. 130, Linköping University, Sweden.

Faina M., Gallozzi C., Lupo S., Colli R., Sassi R. & Marini C. (1988) Definition of the physiological profile of the soccer player. In Reilly T., Lees A., Davids K. & Murphy W.J. (eds) *Science and Football*, pp. 158–163. E. & F.N. Spon, London.

Fowler N.E. & Reilly T. (1993) Assessment of muscle strength asymmetry in soccer players. In Lovesey E.J. (ed.) *Contemporary Ergonomics*, pp. 327–333. Taylor & Francis, London.

Haltori K. & Ohta S. (1986) Ankle joint flexibility in college soccer players. *J. Hum. Ergol.* **15**, 85–89.

Hirata K. (1966) Physique and age of Tokyo Olympic champions. *J. Sports Med. Phys. Fit.* **6**, 207–222.

Hollmann W., Liesen H., Mader A. *et al.* (1981) Zur Hochstund Dauerleistungsfahigkeit der deutschen Fussball-Spitzenspieler (High endurance performance of German élite football players). *Deut. Zeit. Sportsmed.* **32**, 113–120.

Jacobs I., Westlin N., Karlsson J., Rasmusson M. & Houghton B. (1982) Muscle glycogen and diet in élite soccer players. *Eur. J. Appl. Physiol.* **48**, 297–302.

Kirkendall D.T. (1985) The applied sport science of soccer. *Phys. Sportsmed.* **13**, 53–59.

Kullath E. & Schwirtz A. (1988) Biomechanical analysis of the throw-in. In Reilly T., Lees A., Davids K. & Murphy W.J. (eds) *Science and Football*, pp. 460–467. E. & F.N. Spon, London.

Leger L.A., Mercier D., Gadoury C. & Lambert J. (1988) The multistage 20 metre shuttle run test for aerobic fitness. *J. Sports Sci.* **6**, 93–101.

Margaria R., Aghemo P. & Rovelli E. (1966) Measurement of muscular power (anaerobic) in man. *J. Appl. Physiol.* **21**, 1661–1664.

Medved R. (1966) Body height and predisposition for certain sports. *J. Sports Med. Phys. Fit.* **6**, 89–91.

Montanari G., Vecchiet L. & Recoy Campo J.R. (1990) Structural adaptments of the muscle of soccer players. In Santilli G. (ed.) *Sports Medicine Applied to Football*, pp. 169–179. CONI, Rome.

Nowacki P.E., Cai D.Y., Buhl C. & Krummelbein U. (1988) Biological performance of German soccer players (professionals and juniors) tested by special ergometry and treadmill methods. In Reilly T., Lees A., Davids K. & Murphy W.J. (eds) *Science and Football*, pp. 145–157. E. & F.N. Spon, London.

Öberg B., Ekstrand J., Moller M. & Gillquist J. (1984) Muscle strength and flexibility in different positions of soccer players. *Int. J. Sports Med.* **5**, 213–216.

Öberg B., Moller M., Gillquist J. & Ekstrand J. (1986) Isokinetic torque levels in soccer players. *Int. J. Sports Med.* **7**, 50–53.

Pargman D., Sachs M. & Deshaies P. (1976) Field dependence-independence and injury in college football players. *Am. Corr. Ther. J.* **30**, 174–176.

Pellicia A., Sportaro A., Granato M., Alebiso A., Marcello G. & D'Arcangelo E.D. (1990) Doppler and color doppler echocardiography in the cardiological evaluation of soccer players. In Santilli G. (ed.) *Sports Medicine Applied to Football*, pp. 312–317. CONI, Rome.

Puga N., Ramos J., Agostinho J., Lomba I., Costra O. & de Freitas F. (1993) Physical profile of a First Division Portuguese professional soccer team. In Reilly T., Clarys J. & Stibbe A. (eds) *Science and Football II*, pp. 40–42. E. & F.N. Spon, London.

Ramadan J. & Byrd R. (1987) Physical characteristics of élite soccer players. *J. Sports Med. Phys. Fit.* **27**, 424–428.

Raven P., Gettman L., Pollock M. & Cooper K. (1976) A physiological evaluation of professional soccer players. *Br. J. Sports Med.* **109**, 209–216.

Reid R.M. & Williams C. (1974) A concept of fitness and its measurement in relation to Rugby football. *Br. J. Sports Med.* **8**, 96–99.

Reilly T. (1979) *What Research Tells the Coach about Soccer.* AAHPERD, Washington.

Reilly T. & Stirling A. (1993) Flexibility, warm-up and injuries in mature games players. In Duquet W. & Day J.A.P. (eds) *Kinanthropometry IV*, pp. 119–123. E. & F.N. Spon, London.

Reilly T. & Thomas V. (1977) Applications of multivariate analysis to the fitness assessment of soccer players. *Br. J. Sports Med.* **11**, 183–184.

Reilly T. & Thomas V. (1979) Estimated energy expenditure of professional association footballers. *Ergonomics* **22**, 541–548.

Reilly T. & Thomas V. (1980) The stability of fitness factors over a season of professional soccer as indicated by serial factor analyses. In Ostyn M., Beunen G. & Simons J. (eds) *Kinanthropometry 11*, pp. 245–257. University Park Press, Baltimore.

Rigg P. & Reilly T. (1988) A fitness profile and anthropometric analysis of first and second class Rugby Union players. In Reilly T., Lees A., Davids K. & Murphy W.J. (eds) *Science and Football*, pp. 194–200. E. & F.N. Spon, London.

Rost R. (1987) *Athletics and the Heart.* Year Book Medical Publishers, Chicago.

Ryushi T., Asami T. & Togari H. (1979) The effect of muscle fibre composition on the maximal power and the maximal isometric strength of the leg extensor muscle. *Proceedings* of the Department of Physical Education, College of General Education, No. 13. University of Tokyo, 11−15 March.

Sanderson F.H. (1974) *Dynamic visual acuity and ball games ability.* PhD thesis, University of Leeds, UK.

Singer R.N. (1972) *Coaching, Athletics and Psychology.* McGraw-Hill, New York.

Smaros G. (1980) Energy usage during football match. In Vecchiet L. (ed.) *Proceedings 1st International Congress on Sports Medicine Applied to Football*, Vol. 11, pp. 795−801. D. Guanillo, Rome.

Suzuki S., Togari H., Isokawa M., Ohashi J. & Ohgushi T. (1988) Analysis of the goalkeeper's during motion. In Reilly T., Lees A., Davids K. & Murphy W.J. (eds) *Science and Football*, pp. 468−475. E. & F.N. Spon, London.

Stepnicka J. (1977) Somatotypes of Czechoslovak athletes. In Eiben O. (ed.) *Growth and Development*, Vol. 20, pp. 357−364. Physique Symposia Biology, Hungary.

Tanner J.M. (1964) *The Physique of the Olympic Athlete.* Allen & Unwin, London.

Thomas V. & Reilly T. (1979) Fitness assessment of English League soccer players throughout the competitive season. *Br. J. Sports Med.* **13**, 103−109.

Togari H. & Asami T. (1972) A study of throw-in in soccer. In *Proceedings of the Department of Physical Education*, Vol. 6, pp. 33−38. College of General Education, University of Tokyo.

Togari H., Ohashi J. & Ohgushi T. (1988) Isokinetic muscle strength of soccer players. In Reilly T., Lees A., Davids K. & Murphy W.J. (eds) *Science and Football*, pp. 181−185. E. & F.N. Spon, London.

Togari H. & Takahashi K. (1977) Study of "whole-body reac-

tion" in football players. In *Proceedings of the Department of Physical Education*, Vol. 11, pp. 35−41. College of General Education, University of Tokyo.

Trolle M., Aagard P., Simonsen E.B., Bangsbo J & Klausen K. (1991) Effects of strength training on kicking performance in soccer. *Communication to 2nd World Congress on Science and Football.* Eindhoven, the Netherlands.

Verstappen F. & Bovens F. (1989) Interval testing with football players at a laboratory. *Sci. Football* **2**, 15−16.

White J.E., Emery T.M., Kane J.L., Groves R. & Risman A.B. (1988) Pre-season fitness profiles of professional soccer players. In Reilly T., Lees A., Davids K. & Murphy W.J. (eds) *Science and Football*, pp. 164−171. E. & F.N. Spon, London.

Williams C., Reid R.M. & Couttes R. (1973) Observations on the aerobic power of university Rugby players and professional soccer players. *Br. J. Sports. Med.* **7**, 390−391.

Wilmore J.H. & Haskell W.L. (1972) Body composition and endurance capacity of professional football players. *J. App. Physiol.* **33**, 564−567.

Winter F.D., Snell P.G. & Stray-Gunderson J. (1989) Effects of 100% oxygen on performance of professional soccer players. *J. Am. Med. Assoc.* **262**, 227−229.

Withers R.T., Roberts R.G.D. & Davies G.J. (1977) The maximum aerobic power, anaerobic power and body composition of South Australian male representatives in athletics, basketball, field hockey and soccer. *J. Sports Med. Phys. Fit.* **17**, 391−400.

Witkin H.B., Dyk R.B., Faterson H.F., Goodenough D.R. & Kamp S.E. (1962) *Psychological Differentiation.* John Wiley, New York.

Chapter 7

The female player

Football has traditionally been viewed as a game dominated by male participation. Females have had little encouragement to participate in the sport, and have often encountered resistance and open hostility. Indeed the English Football Association banned women from playing football in 1921, and only rescinded this decision as recently as 1971. This is despite the fact that in 1920, over 50 000 spectators watched a game played between two female sides in Liverpool, and large audiences were a regular occurrence at female matches (Fig. 7.1). Scenarios similar to this are common for many other countries, and it is true to say that women's football still has considerable potential for further development. However, the first female European Championships were held in 1982, and in 1991 China staged the inaugural female World Cup, which was won by the USA. Many countries now have regional and national leagues for women's teams (Fig. 7.2), some of which contain a number of professional players. The women's game is being taken more and more seriously, and as such, has established its own niche in an otherwise male-dominated game.

This chapter attempts to examine some of the physiological demands of the female game, the physiological characteristics of the players, and to establish guidelines on diet, the nature of training, and suggested match strategies for female players.

Match analysis

There is a general lack of data analyzing the pattern and demands of women's football, almost certainly due to the relatively recent growth of the sport. From the data that is available, it would appear that there are remarkably little differences between the men's and women's games. B. Ekblom and P. Aginger (unpublished data) studied players of an élite Swedish team,

during several games and found that these players on average covered just under 8500 m during a game. The females studied by Ekblom and Aginger performed over 100 discrete sprints per game, at an average distance of 14.9 ($\pm$ 5.6) m. Their blood lactate levels were found to be 5.1 ($\pm$ 2.1) mmol/l and 4.6 ($\pm$ 2.1) mmol/l at half- and full-time respectively, whilst mean heart rates of 177 ($\pm$ 11) beats·min^{-1}, 174 ($\pm$ 11) beats·min^{-1}, and 173 ($\pm$ 10) beats·min^{-1} were reported for three separate matches. These values are between 89 and 91% of the squad's mean peak heart rate, which was 195 ($\pm$ 9) beats·min^{-1}. Ekblom (1986) reported that male players achieve heart rates in excess of 85% of their maximum heart rate for approximately two-thirds of a match.

B. Ekblom and P. Aginger (unpublished data) recorded a decrease in the body mass of female players during a 90-min game of 0.9 kg, from 62.7 ($\pm$ 6.7) kg pre-match, to 61.8 ($\pm$ 6.6) kg post-match, whilst the amount of fluid consumed was 1.4 l. This would suggest that the actual body weight change was in the region of 2.3 kg, most of which is likely to be due to a loss of fluid. Despite the large intake in fluid, the players in this study still finished the match in a state of near hypohydration. These figures emphasize the importance of fluid intake before, during, and after matches.

Physiological characteristics

As with the male game, considerable variation in the height and body mass of female players has been reported, a factor which is likely to be a reflection of the varying demands of different playing positions. Indeed, the nature of the game of football is such that it does not prevent individuals of different statures competing effectively. This must be one factor behind the worldwide popularity of the men's game, and should therefore enhance the future development of the women's game.

Studies reporting values of body fat percentages in female football players are remarkably consistent. At the end of a competitive season, Australian female players were reported to have an average of 20.8 ($\pm$ 4.7) percentage of body fat and a lean body mass of 43.8 kg (Colquhoun & Chad 1986). A further study on Australian players by Withers *et al.* (1987) reported a mean body fat percentage of 22.0 (+ 6.8) %

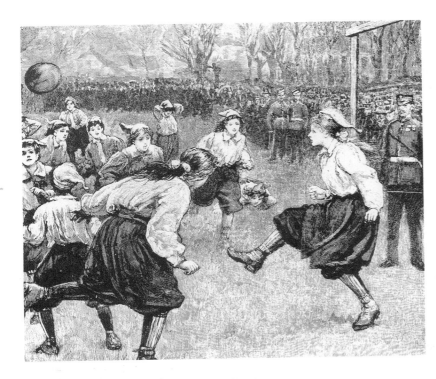

Fig. 7.1 A large crowd assembled to watch the first match played by the British Ladies Football Club in 1895. © Popperfoto, UK.

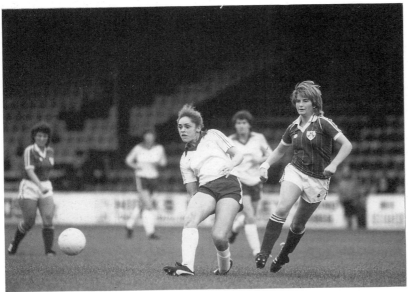

Fig. 7.2 International female football is gaining more recognition. UEFA Competition for Women, England vs Republic of Ireland, September 1983. © Bob Thomas Sports Photography, UK.

and a lean body mass of 47.4 kg. In an estimation of body fat percentage using skinfold measurements on the England Womens International squad, Davis and Brewer (1992) reported values of 21.5 and 21.1% before and after a 12-month period of training. Obviously these values are considerably higher than those observed in male players.

Ekblom (1986) reported a strong positive relationship between work-rate and maximum oxygen uptake ($\dot{V}_{O_{2max.}}$) during a game of male football, and it is likely that a similar relationship exists in the women's game. Hence measurements of maximum oxygen uptake in female football players are of interest and importance to the coach, scientist, and player. Rhodes and Mosher (1992) directly measured the $\dot{V}_{O_{2max.}}$ of 12 élite Canadian collegiate players, recording a mean value of 47.1 ml·kg^{-1}·min^{-1}. This is similar to the mean value of 47.9 ml·kg^{-1}·min^{-1} found in Australian players, but below the $\dot{V}_{O_{2max.}}$ of 52.2 ml·kg^{-1}·min^{-1} measured in English players after a period of concentrated training (Davis & Brewer 1992). These values are less than those reported in élite male players of approximately 60–65 ml·kg^{-1}·min^{-1}, which would tend to suggest that females should be unable to cover the same distances as male football players during matches.

Hematological status

The incidence of sports anemia in both males and females is well recognized, and has been reported by Watts (1989). However, in an investigation of a group of 30 female football and field hockey players during the course of a competitive collegiate season, Douglas (1989) found that hematological parameters (including hemoglobin, hematocrit and red blood cell count) were all normal at the start of the season, and had increased by the end of the season. Furthermore, Davis and Brewer (1992) found an increase in hemoglobin concentration in a female international football squad after a 12-month period of intensive training. These results would suggest that female football players are generally able to maintain their hematological status whilst training and playing, although it is suggested that regular monitoring will assist in the identification of players who develop abnormal values.

The menstrual cycle

Female football players will be as prone to disruptions in performance due to phases of the menstrual cycle as any other female sports competitor. In an investigation of players from the Danish First, Second, and Third Divisions, Møller-Neilsen and Hammar (1989) reported a significantly greater risk of traumatic injury during the premenstrual and menstrual phases of the cycle, particularly in those women experiencing premenstrual and menstrual feelings of discomfort. However, those players using the contraceptive pill were found to sustain significantly fewer traumatic injuries than those using other methods of contraception. This tends to imply an hormonal link with the incidence of injury, and is an area requiring further investigation. Disruption of the menstrual cycle and amenorrhea tends to be more common in endurance sports, and in particular those sports where a low body weight is perceived to be advantageous. Coaches of female football teams should be advised to undertake a sensitive investigation into the occurrence of this condition within their team, since amenorrheic female athletes are more prone to stress fractures and bone fragility. It is also recommended that coaches should keep records of the menstrual phases of their players, and bear these in mind when prescribing individual training loads.

Nutrition

Correct nutrition is as important for female football players as it is for any other sports competitor. Whilst the total calorific intake may be less than that of male players, dietary regimens should still be based on a high carbohydrate intake (50–65% of total calorific intake) and a low-fat intake (not more than 35% of total calorific intake). Protein intake need not be excessive, and should be based on a guideline quota of approximately up to 1.5 g·kg^{-1} of body weight per day.

Glycogen is fundamental to playing, to recovery, and as a fuel for training. Whilst female players who start matches with full stores of muscle glycogen may not totally deplete these by the end of the game, players who start matches with less than full muscle glycogen stores are likely to exhaust these (and thus experience extreme fatigue) before the end of a game. A high-carbohydrate diet is therefore essential to replace glycogen stores, and this should be consumed on a daily basis, not just on the day before a match. Carbohydrates are also vital immediately after a match in order to replace muscle glycogen stores, and to assist in the process of recovery. Among male football players, slow rates of post-exercise muscle glycogen replacement have been linked to poor diet (Jacobs et al. 1982), and good player and coach education is vital if similar circumstances are to be avoided in the female game.

Implications for training

Female football places demands on both the aerobic and anaerobic systems, and as such, successful players need to develop in both these areas. In addition, players need to have a high degree of flexibility, agility, and strength. Thus female players need to adopt a training regimen that focuses on a number of areas, providing a solid foundation upon which match fitness can ultimately be developed. Unlike the élite male game, where the majority of players are full-time professionals, almost no female players are professionals and, thus, train and play on a part-time basis, often combining their sport with a full-time occupation. This obviously means that less time can be devoted to training, so the emphasis of the work done should be on quality training specific to the needs of the individual.

Jensen and Larsson (1992) suggested that Danish female players generally train on two or three occasions each week, with each session lasting approximately 90 min. Danish international standard players supplement this with between two and four running sessions per week, each lasting for 20–30 min, plus one or two weight training sessions. In the training study reported by Davis and Brewer (1992), players were prescribed three physical training sessions (either running or circuit training) each week, supplementary to their technical football training. Nevertheless, the intensity and volume of training undertaken by female football players is likely to be varied, and generally higher with players competing at the élite level.

It is suggested that the close or off-season period is best spent recovering from the demands of the season, whilst maintaining aerobic fitness and flexibility. Activities such as tennis, swimming, and cycling should form part of the "active recovery" which is crucial during this phase of the year. The latter stages of the close season and the early part of the pre-season should be spent consolidating aerobic fitness, with the introduction of specific muscular conditioning work in the form of circuit training. More advanced methods of muscular conditioning, such as weight-training and plyometric work, should only be introduced to females who have completed their physical growth, and who already have a good standard of general conditioning. One area that should not be omitted is the development of knee flexion strength (related to the strength of the hamstring muscle group). This is an often neglected area, and imbalances in lower limb strength have been linked to an increased risk of injury in female football players (Knapik *et al.* 1991).

If aerobic fitness has been maintained during the close season period, more intensive anaerobic training and speed work should be introduced toward the middle of the pre-season period. However, if this form of more intensive training is started before a solid aerobic foundation to fitness has been developed, it is likely that players will be more susceptible to injury and fatigue. Ultimately, match fitness will be developed from competitive games. However, the standard of match fitness which a female player attains is likely to be closely linked to the level of fitness achieved during the close and pre-season conditioning periods.

During the season, matches alone will be unlikely to retain a high standard of basic fitness, and regular supplementary training sessions should be included in the weekly program. The frequency of these sessions will depend on the number of matches being played; if one competitive match is played each week, players should look to supplement this with two or three additional fitness sessions. The nature of the players' training should be specific to individual needs, and to assess these, regular monitoring of players' fitness is essential (see Chapter 9).

Implications for strategy

On the evidence of the available physiological data, it is suggested that female players are more predisposed towards a style of play that entails the patient sequencing of passing, rather than one based on high rates of physical work. Although female players are likely to be able to cope with high rates of work for periods of a game, attempts to sustain this for the entire duration of a 90-min match, played on a full-sized pitch, will almost certainly result in high rates of fatigue before the end of the game. Coaches of female teams should, perhaps, base their strategies on periods of intermittent high-intensity play, separated by "recovery periods" of containment and passing to retain possession.

Conclusion

Female football is a rapidly developing game, and as such the amount of scientific investigation into the sport is limited. There is considerable potential for further research into many aspects of female football, and this is needed to provide the coach, player, and scientist with a greater in-depth knowledge of the game. The evidence that does exist suggests that female players have a high standard of physical fitness, which is similar to that found in many other female team sports. Female football players sustain high relative exercise intensities during matches, but may be best advised to adopt strategies based on intermittent periods of high-intensity play, interspersed with periods of recovery and containment. The limited time available for training female football players, the majority of whom play on a part-time basis, means that female players' training programs need to focus on individual requirements. Regular monitoring of fitness is vital, as is the structured planning of the annual training cycle. Essential to the further successful expansion and development of female football is good coach and player education in the areas of sports science and sports medicine.

References

Colquhoun D. & Chad K.E. (1986) Physiological characteristics of Australian female soccer players after a competitive season. *Aust. J. Sci. Med. Sport* **18**(3), 9–12.

Davis J.A. & Brewer J. (1992) Physiological characteristics of an international female soccer squad (abstract). *J. Sports Sci.* **10**, 142–143.

Douglas P.D. (1989) Effect of a season of competition and training on the haematological status of women field hockey and soccer players. *J. Sports Med. Phys. Fitness* **29**, 179–183.

Ekblom B. (1986) Applied physiology of soccer. *Sports Med.* **3**, 50–60.

Evangelista M., Pandolfi O., Fanton F. & Faina M. (1991) Functional model of female soccer players: analysis of functional characteristics of female soccer players. *Abstract from the 2nd World Congress on Science and Football.* Conference Agency Limburg, Maastricht.

Jacobs I., Westlin N., Karlsson J., Rasmusson M. & Houghton B. (1982) Muscle glycogen and diet in élite soccer players. *Eur. J. Appl. Physiol.* **48**, 297–302.

Jensen K. & Larsson B. (1992) Variations in physical capacity among the Danish national soccer team for women during a period of supplemented training (abstract). *J. Sports Sci.* **10**, 144.

Knapik J.J., Bauman C.L., Jones B.H., Harris J.M. & Vaughan L. (1991) Pre-season strength and flexibility imbalances associated with athletic injuries in female collegiate athletes. *Am. J. Sports Med.* **19**(1), 76–81.

Møller-Neilson J. & Hammar M. (1989) Women's soccer injuries in relation to the menstrual cycle and oral contraception use. *Med. Sci. Sports Exerc.* **21**(2), 126–129.

Reilly T. & Thomas V. (1976) A motion analysis of work rate in different positional roles in professional football match play. *J. Hum. Movement Studies* **2**, 87–97.

Rhodes E.C. & Mosher R.E. (1992) Aerobic and anaerobic characteristics of élite female university soccer players (abstract). *J. Sports Sci.* **10**, 143–144.

Watts E. (1989) Athletes' anaemia. *Br. J. Sports Med.* **23**, 81–83.

Withers R.T., Whittingham N.O., Norton K.I., La Forgia J., Ellis M.W. & Crockett A. (1987) Relative body fat and anthropometric prediction of body density of female athletes. *Eur. J. Appl. Physiol.* **56**, 169–180.

Chapter 8

The referee

The referee is the umpire with special knowledge of the rules and regulation in football. He or she leads the game and whose decisions are final at the moment of the incident (Fig. 8.1). These decisions cannot be disputed and corrected afterwards. This protects the referee and supports his or her authority on the pitch. Also a so-called "wrong decision" by the referee is a decision of fact.

Adherence to the rules must be guaranteed by the referee, as these are determined by the official procedure of matches at national and international level. These rules are compiled in a rule book and have existed in the present form with few exceptions since 1938, edited by La Federation Internationale de Football Associations (FIFA) and the International Football Association Board (IFAB). The Board was founded in London in 1886 when an international referee and rule commission was set up for the purpose of consultation and decision-making in case of changes of rules and regulations.

The Board consists of four delegates from each of five organizations:

1 The Football Association (England).
2 The Scottish Football Association.
3 The Irish Football Association (Northern Ireland).
4 The Football Association of Wales.
5 FIFA (since 1913).

In votations, the four British associations have one vote each. FIFA as the representative of more than 150 member associations has four votes. Changes in the rules can only be made at the annual general meeting of the Board in June and must have at least 75% of the votes of the members present. The decisions of the Board are binding for all national associations and members of FIFA. The national associations are not allowed to make any changes of the rules without a prior decision by the Board.

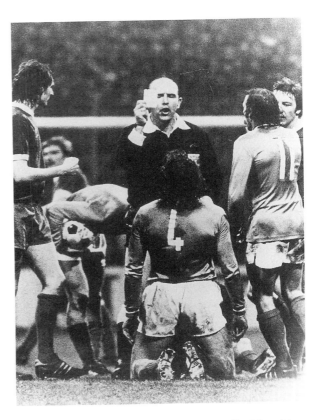

Fig. 8.1 The referee in the center of action. © IOC archives (photo by C. Champinot).

The physical and psychological demands on referees have increased enormously in the 1980s. Apart from ordinary health checks fitness tests are regarded as essential for evaluating the referee's physical performance capacity and, thus, his or her ability to make positive contributions to the game. The fitness tests are settled by FIFA for referees qualifying for the international list and aim to evaluate two main physiological factors, namely speed and endurance.

Minimum standards for performance have been adopted for referees (Table 8.1). A referee in male football runs between 7—8 and 11—12 km per game, including periods of high-intensity running interspersed with periods of standing still, walking, or jogging. Training for referees is therefore essentially the same as for the players, which includes both long-distance and medium-distance running, as well as speed training, strength training, and stretching. The training must be regular — at least 3—4 times a week —

Table 8.1 Minimum standards for referees

Speed tests	Maximal time (s)	
	Male	Female*
Test 1, running 50 m Rest time 15 min	7.5	9.0
Test 2, running 200 m Rest time 15 min	32.0	42.0
Test 3, running 50 m	7.5	9.0
Test 4, running 200 m Rest time 15 min	32.0	42.0

Endurance test	Minimum distance (m)	
	Male	Female*
The 12-min run (Cooper test)	2700	2000

* New standards are being discussed in FIFA, with the aim to fix higher standards.

and the referee has to prepare before a game in the same was as a player, i.e. with proper nutrition.

The referee also has an important role in the medical supervision of the game. The referee has to make quick and reliable decisions when a player is injured. Therefore, the referee has to have some basic medical education and knowledge of causes and symptoms of the most frequent football injuries, namely:
1 Head injuries with or without unconsciousness.
2 Chest and stomach/abdominal injuries.
3 Injuries to the joints.
4 Fractures.

Apart from the medical evaluation the referee has to make an observation of the nature of the accident such as:
1 Foul play.
2 Attack by an opponent.
3 Ball contact.
4 Falling on goal-post, net hooks, corner flag posts, stone edges, or advertising hoardings.

Finally, the referee has to make strict observations of the reactions of the injured player and the rest of the team. In cases of serious injury, the player concerned usually raises an arm to give a sign to the reserve bench, or other players make gestures for assistance, especially if the game is not interrupted. In the case of minor injuries, simulations, and intentional time delays, these reactions are more rarely seen.

According to the laws of the game, team assistants (trainers, masseurs, or physicians) are only allowed to enter the field of play when the referee is convinced that a player has genuinely been seriously injured. As a rule, only two assistants may come onto the pitch when the referee signals them to do so. The medical evaluation of injured players is done as quickly as possible. All major treatments must be done outside the playing area. Treatment on the pitch should be limited to serious injuries and especially in the case of unconsciousness, shock of various degrees, and bleeding. In any case the referee has to demand that the injured player leaves the pitch. The decision "to continue or be substituted" has to be made outside the pitch in such cases. When players suffer from open bleeding cuts, they are not allowed to take further part in the game until the bleeding has stopped.

In international matches, the immediate removal from the field of play by first-aid assistants by the shortest route is organized. Intentional simulation of a serious injury is regarded as unfair behavior which must be followed by a caution (yellow card). Players must bear in mind the basic idea of fair play. Any simulation of serious injury may cause incorrect decisions to be taken if actual serious injury occurs. Coaches and players should be especially aware of this.

Chapter 9

Evaluation of

physical performance

During a football match it is difficult to isolate and evaluate objectively physical performance. However, the most important physical factors which influence a player's match-play performance can be evaluated outside of a game situation using football-specific testing programs. The ultimate aim of using a physical performance test or where applicable an advanced laboratory test is to obtain information which can be used to improve a player's overall match-play performance. For example, information gained from a program of well-chosen tests can be used to design optimal individual training strategies and/or used to monitor the effectiveness of a specific training program. There are also many peripheral benefits which can be gained by implementing a testing program. For instance, test objectives should always be defined to the players and the theoretical background concerning each test clearly explained. This serves as a good educational process. Also testing on a regular basis can motivate players to work harder during the training.

There are many practical factors which must be considered when testing sessions are to be incorporated into the regular training program; in addition to the fact that there are normally 16 or more players who need to be evaluated, considerations must be made for the amount of allocated training time, the availability of testing equipment, and facilities where the tests can be carried out. As testing programs often displace at least part of a normal training session, it is important that time is used effectively and that there is a justifiable reason for testing. A test should never be used without a purpose.

To be beneficial to the coach and player, a testing program must include more than the administration of the test itself: test objectives need to be clearly defined; an appropriate test (which is valid and reliable) must be selected; it is necessary to plan when it is

most effective to carry out the test; the administration of the test should be well organized; test results should be analyzed as soon as possible after a test has been performed; and direct feedback given to the players, preferably on an individual basis. These factors, together with general principles of testing, are discussed in more detail in the following sections.

Principles of testing

Reasons for testing

Before using any test, the reason for testing should be clearly defined. As previously mentioned, a test should never be used without a purpose. A summary of the main reasons for testing football players is presented below.

To develop an individual physical profile. The aim of developing a physical profile is to identify a player's physical strengths and weaknesses. This can be achieved through the administration of a series of football-specific tests. The information gained from these tests can then be used to set up short- and long-term goals and optimize individual training strategies. In the event of a long-term injury, chronic sickness, or planned rest period, a player's predetermined physical profile will also provide data which can be used for comparison purposes.

To evaluate objectively the effect of a specific training program. The aim of a training program is to improve performance. To quantify changes in performance that have occurred as a result of the training, baseline data is needed. Baseline data is collected before the start of a training program using a test (pre-test) which must be specific to the type of training that is to be performed. The same test is then repeated (post-test) usually after 6 or more weeks of training. Thereafter, the subsequent progress of players should be periodically monitored through repeated tests.

To monitor progress during rehabilitation. During a rehabilitation program it is important to monitor how well an injured player is responding to treatment and to know when the player is ready to return to competitive football. Players who return prematurely to competitive football can have a higher risk of a recurring injury (Ekstrand 1982). In Fig. 9.1 the results from a football-specific endurance test (Ekblom 1989), administered repeatedly throughout the season, illustrate the progress of an injured player back to pre-injury status.

To monitor the health status of a player. The general health status of a player can be monitored by checking heart rate and other physiological responses to standardized submaximal exercise. Early signs of over-training may be detected by regularly monitoring a player's physical performance capacity. Heart rate response to standardized exercise can also be used to evaluate how well players adapt to new, unaccustomed surroundings, e.g. professional and national teams when competing in a foreign country.

Scientific research. To understand more about the physical limitations of performance during match-play, sport scientists need to test football players. In Fig. 9.2 a subject is shown breathing expired air into a Douglas bag to help quantify the aerobic energy demand of a training exercise.

Selecting a test

Once the reason for testing has been clearly defined, an appropriate test must be selected. Factors to be considered when selecting a test are discussed below.

Specificity for football. Information gained from a test will be of no benefit to the coach or player unless the recorded measurement can be applied to football.

Reliability. Test−retest reliability refers to how reproducible a test result is from trial to trial, or day to day. Factors which affect reliability can be classified into biological or experimental (Sale 1991). The former refers to the relative consistency with which a subject can perform, while the latter concerns variations in the way the test is administered (see "Test administration" below). For repeated testing, it is necessary to determine whether any difference in two test results, for a given player, can be attributed to a change in the physical status of the player or whether the difference is within the expected measurement variation for the test. Test−retest reliability is usually reported in the form of a correlation coefficient (r); the closer this coefficient is to 1 the more reliable the test is.

Feasibility. When selecting a test, considerations must be made for such factors as the playing status of the team and availability of facilities and appropriate equipment, as well as for the amount of time required to carry out the test and analyze the test results. For example, with a team which train twice a week it is not feasible to use time-consuming tests. Time can also be a problem for the coach of a national team where the squad of players are only together for short

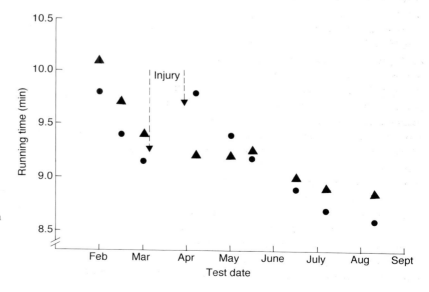

Fig. 9.1 Running times for a football-specific endurance test (Ekblom 1989) repeated regularly during the season in Sweden: (▲) indicates mean times for the team, while (●) represents the performance of a player who was injured after the third test.

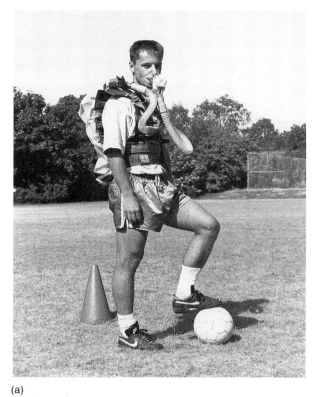
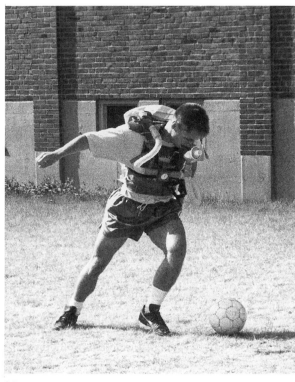

(a)

(b)

Fig. 9.2 To quantify the aerobic demands of a training drill, the player's expired air is collected in a Douglas bag and then analyzed for oxygen and carbon dioxide concentration. Courtesy of Styrbjörn Bergelt.

periods of time. Furthermore, a "select" squad of players are usually assembled to prepare for a game, therefore exhaustive exercise tests are not recommended in this instance.

Test administration

When learning how to administer a test it is important to be aware of variables which can affect test results. The most common sources of error are identified below.

Standardization of test conditions and procedures

Conditions. Testing conditions, e.g. running surface, preparation of test areas, and calibration of measuring equipment, must be standardized each time a test is performed. While test conditions can usually be accurately reproduced for tests performed in a research or clinical setting, problems can arise with field tests,

e.g. if performed on a football pitch the type or condition of the surface can change throughout the year. Extreme variations in environmental conditions should be avoided.

Procedures. The standardization of testing procedures refers to the way in which the test is administered. For example, when a battery of tests are performed on the same day, the order in which each player performs the tests should be standardized. Where possible, exhaustive exercise tests should be performed last.

Test results should not generally be documented the first time a test is used due to the possibility of there being a "learning effect."

Pre-test condition of players

Players should be well rested before being tested. Usually, at least 24 h should be allowed after a competitive match. Where players have just recovered from an injury or an acute illness this should always be noted. With female players it is advisable to note any players experiencing detrimental side-effects caused by menstruation.

Players should always warm-up before the test. In addition to whole-body exercises, a standardized test-specific warm-up should also be performed. Not only will this help to minimize the risk of injury but it also optimizes the functioning of various physiological mechanisms which can affect performance (Asmussen & Boje 1945).

An often overlooked consideration when testing is clothing and footwear. Suitable clothing should be worn which will not interfere with performance, and in running or jumping tests the same type of shoes should be worn for repeated tests.

Instructions and test administration

It is essential that players clearly understand how each test should be performed. The test administrator must also ensure that the test functions smoothly. Players will lose confidence in testing programs if problems continually arise.

When using a test where it is not possible to test all the players in the team at the same time, other activities should be planned so that players are not "waiting around" for long periods. However, such activities must not be strenuous enough to affect test results.

Motivation

Performance tests where players are required to exercise to voluntary exhaustion or to exert a maximal effort are both physically and mentally very demanding. Such tests can be greatly affected by motivation. It is therefore very important that players are well motivated and mentally prepared for the type of exercise that is to be performed.

When to administer a test

It is not possible to define exactly when and how often it is most effective to administer a test. Some general guidelines are:
1 When the objective of testing is to evaluate the effect of a training program, sufficient time should be

allowed for the desired adaptation to take place, a period of 6 weeks between tests is usually the minimum time advisable.
2 It is useful to test players just before they are released at the end of each season and again when training resumes.
3 Data for physical profiles should be collected toward the end of the pre-season period when players reach their peak performance levels.

Interpretation of test results

An integral part of any testing program is to interpret the test results and give direct feedback to each player. In the following section some recommendations for analyzing, interpreting, and presenting test results are described.

Analysis of data. Test results should be rapidly processed and analyzed so that feedback can be given to the players, if possible on an individual basis. From a pedagogic viewpoint the ranking of test results is not advisable. Alternative methods include expressing a result as a percentage change from a previous test or the attained percentage of an individual goal.

There are many tests which involve multiple trials, e.g. a sprint test, where the recorded test result can be either the best time or the mean of the best two or three trials. There is no single rule which covers all possibilities, but it is important to be consistent. It should also be noted that a test result can sometimes be presented in different units of measurement, e.g. to account for the effect of body weight.

Mean scores and recommended values. Comparing test results with "recommended" values or reported mean scores of selected squads of players is not often a good idea as different testing conditions and procedures can greatly affect a test result. For example, a 15-m sprint time can be affected by the running surface, timing equipment, the method used to start the sprint, environmental conditions, and so on. It is more important that the coach is able to interpret each player's test result in direct relation to how it affects overall football performance.

Individual differences. Players will respond differently to the same training program due to variables such as heredity, current training status, and motivation. However, a plausible explanation should be sought for players who fail to show an expected improvement after a set period of time. Also, "target" performances for a given test should be individualized.

Tests for football players

When designing a testing program for football players, tests should be selected to provide as much information as possible in the context of football, while remaining logistically feasible for the caliber of players to be tested. Tests which do not meet these guidelines should be avoided. For example, data on handgrip strength exists for football players, however this test has no relevance for the physical demands of football.

For the tests described in the following section, where necessary, readers are referred to original manuscripts or suitable references to compliment the description of methodologic procedures. At the end of the section a simple testing model is presented which can be used to evaluate the physical performance profile of all football players.

The next section is aimed at both male and female outfield players. Special considerations should be made for goalkeepers.

Football-specific endurance

Playing football is a form of intermittent exercise consisting of repeated short bouts of high-intensity exercise interspersed with periods of running at different speeds, walking, and standing still. Although each player only performs high-intensity exercise for a relatively small percentage of the total game time, such periods are instrumental in determining the path of the ball and thus the eventual outcome of the game.

Only small (non-significant) differences from game to game are found in the distance a player covers by high-speed running (Bangsbo 1992a). Thus, although the amount of high-speed running during a game can be influenced by factors such as tactical strategies and motivation, it has been suggested that the amount of this type of exercise performed during a match is influenced most by a player's football-specific endurance capacity (Bangsbo & Lindqvist 1992).

A preliminary evaluation of a player's football-specific endurance capacity can be made from a measurement of performance using an exercise protocol which includes the type of exercise performed during match-play. A significant relationship has been found between the distance covered by high-speed running during a game and performance during a prolonged intermittent exercise test with alternating short bouts of high- and low-intensity exercise (Bangsbo & Lindqvist 1992). However, this test is time consuming (> 95 min per player) which is not practical for general testing purposes.

Three types of football-specific endurance field tests which can be performed on a football field are presented below. Each test is based on a different performance principle: (a) the time taken to cover a set distance; (b) the time to fatigue during an exercise protocol with a progressively increasing running speed; and (c) performance during repeated sprints. These are discussed in detail below. Due to the strenuous nature of these tests it is recommended that such tests are not performed within 48 h of a competitive match.

Time taken to cover a set distance

A field test for football players (after Ekblom 1989). This test includes forward, backward, sideways, and "slalom" running, turning, and jumping. The aim of the test is to complete four test circuits in the shortest possible time.
1 Test circuit (Fig. 9.3). The test circuit is constructed within the perimeter of a football field. Although the design of the test circuit can be varied, it is important that the same layout is used when the test is repeated.
2 Performing the test. Players start at 15-s intervals and are instructed to complete four laps of the test circuit in the shortest possible time. Up to eight players can be tested together.
3 Test result. The test result is the time taken to cover four laps of the test circuit. For the test circuit illustrated in Fig. 9.3, Ekblom (1989) reported that for a Swedish semi-professional team ($n = 11$) the time to complete four laps decreased from (mean $\pm$ SD) 10 min 21 ± 43 s early in the pre-season to 8 min 49 ± 24 s during the competitive season (see Fig. 9.1).

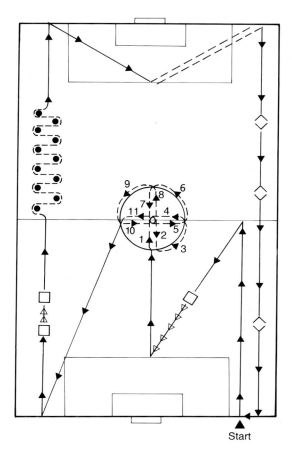

Fig. 9.3 This figure illustrates a field test which includes four laps of forward (▶), backward (▷) and sideward (═) running, turning (□) and jumping (◊). Any part of the test circuit may be modified but should be the same for repeated tests (after Ekblom 1989). ●, cone.

*Time to fatigue during exercise
with a progressive increase in running speed*

Continuous multistage fitness test (MFT) (after Brewer *et al.* 1988). The MFT consists of repeated 20-m shuttle runs with a progressively increasing running speed. The aim of the test is to complete as many shuttles as possible.

1 Test circuit. Two straight parallel lines marked on the ground exactly 20 m apart.
2 Performing the test. Players run back and forth between the two lines at a running speed which

increases every minute. This is controlled by a series of "bleeps" pre-recorded on an audio-cassette* in that players must always have reached the appropriate line at the sound of a "bleep." Players are required to stop running when they drop behind the required pace. The average running speed at the start of the test corresponds to a slow jog ($9\,km\cdot h^{-1}$) but is increased every minute, i.e. the time between the "bleeps" becomes shorter. A change of running speed corresponds to a new "running level" (first min, level 1; second min, level 2; etc.). A whole squad of players can be tested at the same time.

3 Test results. The test score is presented as the number of completed running levels plus the number of additional completed shuttles performed at the last running level, e.g. a test score of 12 + 5 means the player stopped after five shuttles at level 12. There are nine shuttles at the first running level. Mean test scores for a variety of players are presented in Table 9.1.

Intermittent yo-yo endurance test (after Bangsbo 1994). The yo-yo test is based on the same principle as the previously described multistage fitness test, however, a 5-s recovery period is included after every pair of 20-m shuttles[†]. The reason for this is to more closely simulate the intermittent exercise pattern of football match-play. As before the aim of the test is to complete as many shuttles as possible while keeping up with the required pace.

1 Test circuit. Two markers are placed on the ground exactly 20 m apart (two lines can also be used) and a third marker is placed 2.5 m behind the start marker.

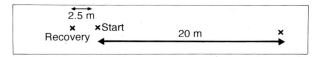

2 Performing the test. Test procedures are similar to those previously described for the multistage fitness test. However, on returning to the start cone (i.e. after completing two 20-m shuttles) there is a 5-s recovery

* Audio-cassette available from the National Coaching Foundation, 4 College Close, Beckett Park, Leeds LS6 3QH, UK.
† Audio-cassette available from DIF, Brøndby Stadion 20, 2605 Brøndby, Denmark.

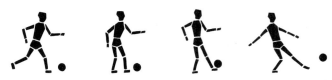

Table 9.1 Results of multistage fitness test. A score $X + Y$ means that Y levels were completed at level X

n	Players	Test result	Reference
Male			
135	English professionals	13 + 12	Davis *et al.* (1992)
16	English national team	13 + 13	J. Brewer (personal communication)
15	U16 Swedish top-class	12 + 8	P.D. Balsom (unpublished data)
23	U16 Swedish national squad	12 + 10	P.D. Balsom (unpublished data)
20	U18 Swedish top-class	13 + 5	P.D. Balsom (unpublished data)
17	Senior Swedish First Division	14 + 1	P.D. Balsom (unpublished data)
Female			
20	Australian national squad	10 + 4	Tumilty & Darby (1991)
18	English national squad	11 + 7	Davis & Brewer (1992)
19	Senior Swedish top-class	11 + 5	P.D. Balsom (unpublished data)
24	Swedish national squad	12 + 0	P.D. Balsom (unpublished data)

period during which the player jogs around the recovery cone and back to the start ready to perform the next two shuttles.

3 Test result. See "Continuous MFT" above. The mean score recorded for a group of top-class Danish male football players was 17 + 2.

Performance decrement during repeated sprints

Two tests are presented which involve repeated sprints interspersed with active recovery periods.

Test A (after Balsom 1990). This test consists of 20 repeated $10 \times 10 \times 10$ m sprints interspersed with 42 s active recovery periods. The aim of the test is to perform each sprint circuit in the shortest possible time.

1 Test circuit (Fig. 9.4). The test circuit consists of a 10-m sided equilateral triangle (sprint circuit) and a recovery circuit which has the same dimensions as the perimeter of the penalty area.

2 Performing the test. Each player is instructed to complete the sprint circuit ABCA (Fig. 9.4) in the

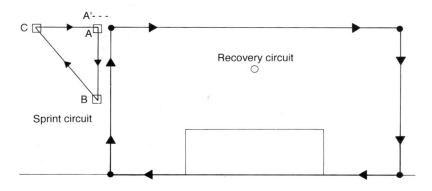

Fig. 9.4 The dimensions of the field test. The perimeter of the penalty area is used as the recovery circuit (after Balsom 1990).

shortest possible time, starting at A′ on a line 1 m behind A, and sprinting in straight lines from A to B, B to C, and C back to A. Each sprint should be timed using a suitable electronic timing device. After completing the sprint circuit the player has 42 s to complete the recovery circuit and return to the start ready for the next sprint. A stopwatch should be used to time the recovery period which begins as soon as the player finishes each sprint. The player should be verbally guided back to the start by shouting out the times "10, 20, 30, 40, 41" (s), followed by the command "Go" at 42 s. This procedure is repeated until 20 sprint circuits have been completed.

3 Test results (modified from original test). Three components of performance can be presented: (a) fastest sprint time; (b) sum of 20 sprint times; or (c) fatigue index (the difference between the mean of the first two and the mean of the last two sprint times).

Test B (after Bangsbo 1994). This test consists of seven 34-m sprints interspersed with 25 s active recovery periods. The aim of the test is to complete each sprint in the shortest possible time.

1 Test circuit (Fig. 9.5). The sprint circuit goes from A to B and the recovery circuit back to C.

2 Performing the test. A lap consists of a sprint from A through the markers, which should be posts higher than 160 cm, to B and a jog back to C. The jog back to C must be completed in 25 s. The test consists of seven sprints and six recovery jogs.

3 Test results. The seven sprint times for each player can be divided into three different test results: (a) the fastest sprint time; (b) the mean time of the seven sprints. (If a player falls or stumbles the time of this trial is omitted. The mean of the previous and next trial is used instead.) (c) Fatigue index: the fastest sprint time (of the first two sprints) is subtracted from the slowest sprint time (of the last two sprints).

Mean test scores (Bangsbo 1994) for top-class Danish males (*n* = 11) were (a) fastest time: 6.80 s (range 6.53–7.01 s); (b) mean time: 7.10 s (range 6.83–7.31 s); and (c) fatigue index: 0.64 s (range 0.15–0.92 s).

Laboratory tests

While a coach can gain useful information from a football-specific endurance field test, the exercise physiologist can compliment this data by evaluating

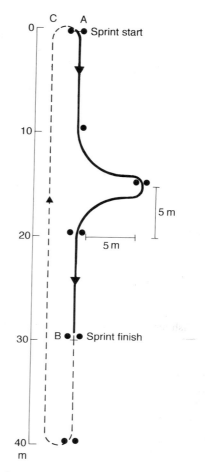

Fig. 9.5 The sprint and recovery circuit (after Bangsbo 1994).

the basic physiological functions which influence a player's ability to perform repeated bouts of high-intensity exercise. However, more work is needed to better determine the relationship between football-specific endurance and the conventional aerobic and anaerobic parameters measured in the exercise laboratory. Below, conventional tests of maximal aerobic power, anaerobic threshold and anaerobic capacity are presented.

Maximal aerobic power tests. Maximal aerobic power is the maximal energy output that can be produced by aerobic processes within the limitation of the functional capacity of the circulatory system (Åstrand & Rodahl 1986). It is assessed by determining maximal oxygen uptake, i.e. the highest amount of oxygen that the body can use during exhaustive exercise while breathing air at sea-level. There is evidence to suggest that recovery between repeated short duration bouts of high-intensity exercise is dependent on oxidative processes and may be enhanced if maximal aerobic power is increased (Balsom et al. 1994). Furthermore, players with a higher maximal oxygen uptake will utilize a higher percentage of fat as fuel during exercise thus sparing muscle glycogen which may help to delay the type of fatigue often observed towards the end of a game (Jacobs et al. 1982).

The average maximal oxygen uptake of top-class male ($55-65$ ml·kg^{-1}·min^{-1}) and female ($50-60$ ml·kg^{-1}·min^{-1}) football players is well above the mean value of a normal population (Swedish male, around 45 ml·kg^{-1}·min^{-1}; female, around 40 ml·kg^{-1}·min^{-1}) but lower than that of top-class endurance-trained athletes (male, $70-75$ ml·kg^{-1}·min^{-1}; female, > 60 ml·kg^{-1}·min^{-1}).

Maximal oxygen uptake can be accurately measured by a direct method, only gross estimations can be made from indirect measurements.

1 Direct measurements. Maximal oxygen uptake can be measured using a progressive exercise protocol to exhaustion, preferably performed on a motor-driven treadmill for football players. The player's ventilation during the last minutes of exercise is measured and the oxygen and carbon dioxide fraction of expired air analyzed. This methodology is explained in detail by Åstrand and Rodahl (1986, pp. 360–363). As test results are extremely reproducible (± 3 ml·kg^{-1}·min^{-1}), small training-induced changes can be accurately detected. However, this method is time-consuming and involves equipment which must be operated by skilled technicians.

2 Indirect measurements. Only gross estimations ($\pm 15\%$) of maximal oxygen uptake can be made based on heart rate measurements during submaximal exercise on a cycle ergometer (Åstrand & Ryhming 1954). However, under standardized conditions, heart rate response for a standardized submaximal exercise intensity performed on a cycle ergometer is reproducible to within ± 5 beats·min^{-1}. Thus, with repeated tests, for a given player, a decrease of greater than 5 beats·min^{-1} in heart rate can be indicative of an increase in maximal aerobic power. It should be noted, however, that in addition to extrinsic factors there are several intrinsic factors such as emotional stress and acute illness which can elevate heart rate at a sub-

maximal work-rate but which are not related to changes in maximal aerobic power.

It is also possible to predict a player's maximal oxygen uptake by using a field test. Such tests include continuous exercise protocols where players run a set distance, e.g. $2-5$ km, in as short a time as possible, or have a set time to run as far as possible, as in the 12-min Cooper test (Cooper 1968). However, again only a gross estimation can be obtained.

Anaerobic threshold test. There is much controversy surrounding the concept of anaerobic threshold but in general terms it can be defined as the point during gradually increasing submaximal exercise above which global energy production is supplemented by anaerobic mechanisms (Wasserman 1984). For endurance athletes it is desirable to be able to produce energy primarily via aerobic pathways at as high an exercise intensity as possible. However, the concept of the anaerobic threshold for football players is less clear due to the intermittent exercise pattern of match-play. Many different approaches have been used to evaluate anaerobic threshold. The simplest and most straightforward of which is the onset of blood lactate accumulation (OBLA) test. A typical exercise protocol for a treadmill test which can be used to evaluate OBLA includes four or five 4-min bouts of submaximal running with incremental exercise intensities. The initial exercise intensity is always relatively low and selected based on the training status of the subject. Blood lactate concentration, and oxygen uptake are measured during the last 60 s of each 4-min interval. Heart rate is continuously monitored throughout the test. The data obtained from this test can then be used to identify the running speed, oxygen uptake and heart rate which results in a blood lactate concentration of 4 mmol·l^{-1} (although a 2 mmol·l^{-1} limit is sometimes used). For a more detailed description see Thoden (1991).

Anaerobic capacity tests. Anaerobic capacity refers to the highest anaerobic energy yield that can be attained during a short duration bout of high-intensity exercise (Bouchard et al. 1991). Although it is clear that anaerobic energy yield is important for a football player, less is known about the relationship between the so-called anaerobic capacity and football-specific endurance. However, a significant relationship has been found between performance during an anaerobic capacity test and performance during a football-specific high-intensity intermittent exercise test (Balsom 1988).

Tests which claim to measure anaerobic capacity can be divided into those which measure oxygen deficit during supramaximal exercise and those which record a parameter of performance during a 30 s or greater period of exercise. However, unlike the testing of aerobic power, there is currently no single test which can accurately measure maximum anaerobic energy yield.

In recent years there has been a renewed interest in the evaluation of anaerobic capacity by calculating oxygen deficit during a bout of supramaximal exercise (Medbo *et al.* 1988). However, the accuracy to which the energy demand of supramaximal exercise can be predicted is questionable (Bangsbo 1992b) and the source of error for this method can be large. The oxygen deficit of top-class players during supramaximal exercise has been reported by Ekblom (1988).

A considerable amount of performance data has been reported for football players performing cycle ergo-meter tests of varying duration, e.g. the 30-s Wingate test (see Bar-Or 1987), and the Cunningham and Faulkner treadmill test (Cunningham & Faulkner 1969). Due to the fact that these tests can be performed in controlled laboratory conditions, they may be useful in certain circumstances, e.g. to collect baseline data for comparison purposes during rehabilitation or to detect early signs of overtraining.

1 Wingate test. The test is performed on a friction loaded (Wingate) cycle ergometer. The resistance is usually standardized to 7.5% of the subject's body mass. Subjects are instructed to pedal as fast as possible, from a flying start, for 30 s. Power output is most accurately measured by instantaneously recording the angular velocity of the flywheel. The following three measures of performance can be calculated: (a) peak 5 s power output; (b) mean power output; and (c) fatigue index, i.e. the difference between the peak and lowest 5 s power output divided by the peak 5 s power output. Peak power for "explosively" trained athletes often exceeds 1000 W. Test−retest reliability coefficients are high, between 0.90 to 0.98.

2 Cunningham and Faulkner treadmill test. With this test the time to voluntary exhaustion for running on a motorized treadmill with a speed of 12.8 km·h^{-1} and a 20% slope is recorded. Subjects "hop" on to the moving treadmill belt and continue running until exhaustion. Test−retest reliability is between 0.76 and 0.91.

A mean running time of 92 s has been reported for the Canadian Olympic football team (Rhodes *et al.* 1986) and 60 s for an American NCAA second Division team (Balsom 1988). For a comprehensive review of anaerobic tests see Vandewalle *et al.* (1987) and Bouchard *et al.* (1991).

Sprinting

During match-play the average sprint performed by a player is around 15 m with an upper distance of around 40 m. The ability to accelerate rapidly is important in football as this action most often denotes a form of urgency where a player is attempting to gain possession of the ball or preventing an opponent from doing so. Professional players have been shown to be faster than non-professional players over distances from 5 to 40 m (Brewer & Davis 1992, Kollath & Quade 1993). Thus, even though speed in football is determined by an integration of physical, perceptual, skill, and tactical factors, i.e. it is more intricate than simply running between two points in the shortest possible time, it appears that "pure" sprinting ability is an important factor.

With football players, it is most specific to record sprint times over distances between 5 and 40 m. However, with such distances, inter-player variations, especially of top-class players, will be very small. For example, the range of 15-m sprint times, measured on grass with photoelectric cells, for the Swedish National team ($n = 16$) was 2.32−2.48 s. Therefore, when recording sprint times it is necessary to use accurate electronic timing equipment, e.g. photoelectric cells, and ensure that test procedures and conditions are carefully standardized between tests. Factors such as starting procedures, the type of running surface and the positioning of the time measuring instruments can all significantly affect test results.

The unacceptably high measurement error that can be incurred when using a stop-watch is illustrated by the results of an experiment where 15-m sprint times (on indoor tartan track) were recorded for a group of players ($n = 28$) simultaneously with a stop-watch and two photoelectric cells (Clausen AB, Laholm, Sweden). While the range of sprint times recorded with the photoelectric cells for the whole group was 0.19 s (range 2.35−2.54 s), when photoelectric cell times were compared to those recorded by the stop-watch, individual discrepancies greater than 0.2 s were found. The type of running surface has also been shown to influence sprint times significantly. Although it is most natural for football players to run on grass, considerations must be made for the condition of the surface which can frequently change.

When using photoelectric cells to record sprint times, starting procedures must be standardized as differences in the way time recording is initiated can influence the test result. When a photoelectric cell is used to trigger the time recording, a flying start, e.g. of 1 m, is recommended to avoid false starts. With this procedure, starting is self-determined which eliminates reaction times.

Test protocols

When recording sprint times the following components can be tested.

Acceleration. When evaluating a player's ability to accelerate, a distance of between 5 and 15 m, from a standing start, is recommended.

Maximum or peak running speed. A player will reach maximal speed between 30 and 50 m. This component can be evaluated by using a flying start with photoelectric cells placed at 5 or 10 m intervals between 30 and 50 m. Mean running velocity (m·s^{-1}) between two photoelectric cells is then calculated.

Kinematic analysis. In addition to recording sprint times, technical aspects of sprint performance can be analyzed with the use of high-speed cinematography in conjunction with computer modeling and simulation techniques.

Electromyography (EMG) analysis. EMG measurements can be used to evaluate co-ordination. By recording EMG activity from active muscle groups during sprinting, patterns of activation can be identified which, for example, can be compared before and after a training program.

Agility tests. Agility may be defined as the ability to shift quickly the direction of movement and is dependent on a combination of factors such as speed, strength, balance, and co-ordination (Wilmore 1982). During a match, players are frequently required to

make rapid changes of direction. Two examples of a test circuit which can be adapted into an agility test for football players have been previously described in the section "Football-specific endurance" (Balsom 1990, Bangsbo 1994). Another test of agility for football players is shown in Fig. 9.6.

In a research study by Ekblom *et al.* (1982) a force platform was used to obtain information on a player's ability to change direction rapidly. To evaluate the effect of an 8-week eccentric strength-training program, a force platform was used to measure contact time and force during foot plant when changing direction. The test circuit is shown in Fig. 9.7. This study found that following the training period contact time on the plat-

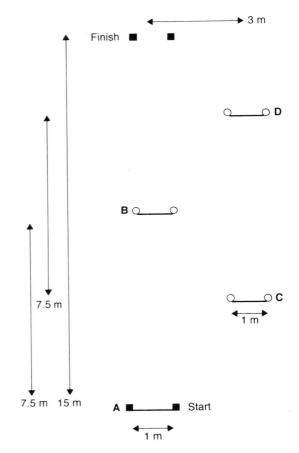

Fig. 9.6 Test circuit for the agility test. The player runs from A (the start) to B, back to A, from A through the cones (at C) to D, from D back to C, then through the cones at B to the finish.

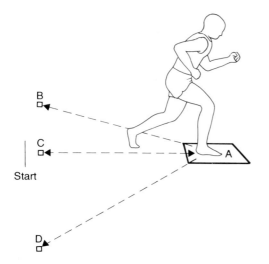

Fig. 9.7 Test circuit used by Ekblom *et al.* (1982) to study the effect of eccentric training on ability to change direction, i.e. run from C to A and back to B, C and D.

form decreased when changing direction and it was concluded that agility performance could be improved through eccentric strength training.

Anaerobic power tests

Anaerobic power tests with different technical demands than running may also be performed in the laboratory to compliment sprint times. Anaerobic power may be defined as the maximal rate of anaerobic energy production during short duration high-intensity exercise. Anaerobic power tests usually last up to 15 s and maximal work output is recorded, during different types of exercise, e.g. staircase stepping (Margaria stair-climbing test; Margaria *et al.* 1966), repeated jumps (Bosco *et al.* 1983), and all-out cycle ergometer tests. While performance during the cycle test reflects the ability of the active muscles to convert chemical energy to mechanical power, with the jump and stair-climbing tests an elastic energy component is also evaluated (Bosco *et al.* 1983).

Cycle ergometer tests. Short duration cycle ergometer tests lasting between 5 and 10 s can be used to measure peak power output. These tests are performed on a Wingate cycle ergometer with a resistance of around 7.5% of the player's body mass.

Margaria stair-climbing test. This test calculates power output during stair climbing. Subjects are required to ascend 12 stairs (each approximately 17.5-cm high), two at a time, as fast as possible. The test measurement, recorded using two "switch" mats or photoelectric cells, is the time taken to travel from the fourth to eighth stair. Power is then calculated using the formula:

$$\text{power} = (W \cdot 9.8 \cdot d)/t$$

where W = subject's body mass (kg); d = vertical distance between the two timing devices (cm); and t = time taken from fourth to eighth stair (s). The test–retest coefficient of this test is between 0.85 and 0.90.

Bosco 15-s jump test. During this test subjects perform a series of repeated jumps for 15 s on a force platform or contact mat. From the recorded data, i.e. total number of jumps, flight time, and contact time, several performance parameters can be calculated; for example, the average jump height, average work performed, and the average generated power. Test–retest reliability coefficient is about 0.95.

For a comprehensive review of these and other anaerobic power tests see Vandewalle *et al.* (1987) and Bouchard *et al.* (1991).

Jumping ability

When jumping, vertical displacement is determined by the vertical velocity of the body's center of gravity at take-off which in turn is a measure of the ability of the activated muscles to produce kinetic energy (power). In football, apart from the obvious benefits of being able to out-jump an opponent in an aerial duel, power is also important for acceleration, quick stop and start movements, and rapid changes of direction which occur frequently during match-play. For example, it has been demonstrated that there is a significant relationship between jumping ability and 15-m sprint times (Fig. 9.8).

A crude assessment of jumping ability can be made using a Sargent jump test where a player jumps with an outstretched arm and makes a fingertip chalk mark as high as possible on a wall. However, when evaluating jumping ability there are parameters other than jump height that can be analyzed. A more specific

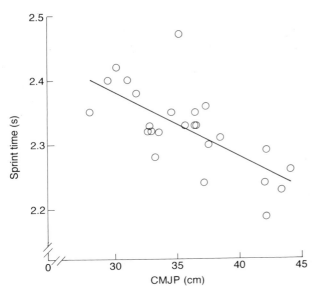

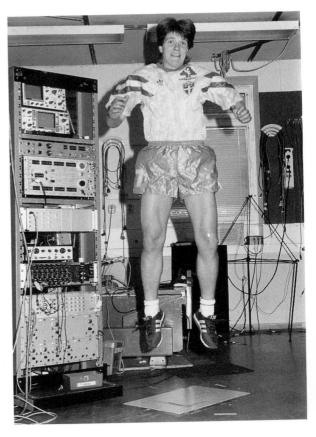

Fig. 9.8 Relationship between counter movement jump height with arm swing (CMJP) and 15-m sprint times. $n = 25$ players in Swedish U16 national squad; $r = 0.70$.

Fig. 9.9 A force platform being used to record data on jumping ability. Courtesy of Styrbjörn Bergett.

method of evaluating jumping performance is with a "contact mat" or force platform (Fig. 9.9) where the flight time recorded during a jump is used to calculate jump height using the equation

$$h = 1.226 \cdot t^2$$

where h = jump height and t = flight time (Bosco *et al.* 1983). In addition to flight time, contact time on the mat during repetitive jumps can also be recorded. In scientific laboratories a force plate can be used to provide additional information about take-off forces and other biomechanical parameters of interest, e.g. power and work output. For field tests, a contact mat is an excellent tool which can provide sufficient information for a comprehensive analysis of jumping ability.

When using a contact mat or force platform, flight time is used to calculate the vertical displacement of the body's center of gravity. For this measurement to be valid the take-off and landing posture of the body must be the same, i.e. the center of gravity of the body should be the same distance from the ground at take-off and landing. Any difference in the position of the body between the instant of take-off and landing can falsify the calculation of jumping height. The most

common deviations in body position between take-off and landing are differences in the degree of knee flexion, ankle extension, and the position of the arms.

Jumping ability is associated with such factors as muscle strength, power production and co-ordination (Oddsson & Westing 1991). Therefore, jumping ability is best evaluated using a protocol which includes different forms of jumping to evaluate as many of these factors as possible. The information gained from a battery of four to five different types of jump can be used to develop individualized training programs. The test program presented below, consisting of four different kinds of jumps, was introduced by Oddsson and Westing (1991). This test has been applied to a large group of international top-class athletes of different sports (Oddsson & Thorstensson 1992; Table 9.2). As only short rest periods are necessary between jumps

Table 9.2 Mean jumping performance
of élite competitors in different sports
(± SD in brackets) (after Oddsson &
Thorstensson 1992)

	n	CMJ	CMJP	BJ	RJ	BJ–RJ*	BJf–BJc†	CMJ–CMJP‡
Volleyball	12	0.44 (0.03)	0.51 (0.05)	0.36 (0.06)	0.38 (0.04)	0.95	3.04	1.16
Olympic diving	7	0.37 (0.07)	0.42 (0.08)	0.33 (0.04)	0.31 (0.06)	1.06	3.13	1.14
Football (male)	16	0.37 (0.04)	0.42 (0.03)	0.33 (0.04)	0.35 (0.04)	0.94	2.90	1.14
Football (female)	15	0.27 (0.03)	0.32 (0.03)	0.27 (0.03)	0.25 (0.05)	1.08	2.54	1.19
Table tennis	10	0.38 (0.04)	0.40 (0.05)	0.30 (0.04)	0.31 (0.06)	0.97	2.70	1.05
Karate	8	0.35 (0.04)	0.43 (0.05)	0.28 (0.03)	0.34 (0.05)	0.82	2.70	1.23
Badminton	6	0.42 (0.06)	0.44 (0.08)	0.32 (0.03)	0.37 (0.07)	0.86	2.77	1.05
Biathletes	5	0.33 (0.06)	0.37 (0.06)	0.26 (0.05)	0.28 (0.05)	0.93	2.45	1.12

BJ, bounce jump; CMJ, counter movement jump without arm swing; CMJP, counter movement jump with arm swing; RJ, rocket jump.
* Bounce jump to rocket jump ratio.
† Bounce jump flight time to contact time ratio.
‡ CMJ to CMJP ratio.

a whole squad of players can be tested in a relatively short period of time.

Test procedures

Counter movement jumps — with arm swing (CMJP) or without arm swing (CMJ). These are maximal jumps performed starting from an upright standing position, with an initial counter movement action where the body's center of gravity is lowered before being propelled vertically up. During this movement extensor muscles can store and utilize elastic energy by first contracting eccentrically and then immediately concentrically (Cavagna *et al.* 1968). This type of muscle activation has been termed the stretch shortening cycle (Komi 1984). Counter movement jumps should be performed both with and without an arm swing. When no arm swing is permitted the hands are held on the hips.

Rocket jump (RJ). This jump is initiated from a static position with no counter movement. The subject sits in a fully crouched position with the trunk vertical and is instructed to jump vertically upward using only the legs for propulsion. This starting position prevents the subjects from using a counter movement. The jump gives an estimation of dynamic concentric work produced mainly by the hip, knee, and ankle extensors. During this jump hands are held on the hips. It should be noted that it is essential to perform this jump with the correct technique as small deviations, e.g. if there is an initial counter movement, can markedly affect test results.

Bounce jumping (BJ). BJ involves a series of repeated jumps where subjects are instructed to jump as high as possible (with hands on hips) with a minimal contact time on the ground. Both contact and flight time are recorded. This test gives an evaluation of maximal power production during jumping.

Football-specific jumping. When jumping to head a ball in football it is most natural to include a run up with a couple of steps followed by a one-foot take-off. An extra dimension of co-ordination is now involved. Thus, a more football-specific jumping test is a jump to head a suspended ball. To calculate jump height the player's standing height is subtracted from the highest height of the ball above the ground where contact can be made.

Performance parameters. Figure 9.10 shows the relationship (*n* = 37) between CMJP height and the height jumped to head a suspended ball. From this graph it can be suggested that some players (e.g. player 1) should focus on improving physical components of jumping performance while others (e.g. player 2) should focus on more functional training as player 2 is not able to fully utilize his jumping ability to head the ball.

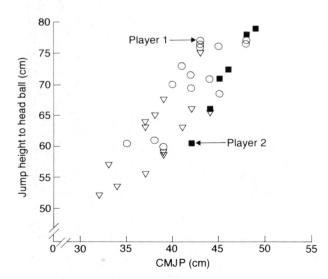

Fig. 9.10 Relationship between counter movement jump height with arm swing (CMJP) and the height jumped to head a suspended ball. All players (*n* = 37) are from a Swedish First Division club. ▽, U16; ○, U18; ■, A-team.

The vertical displacement achieved when jumping can be greatly influenced by the arm swing before take-off. Good jumpers are able to co-ordinate their arm swing to help drive the body upward. By testing jumping performance using a counter movement jump both with and without arm swing, an indication of the effectiveness of the arm swing can be made using the ratio CMJP−CMJ. The mean CMJP−CMJ ratio for the Swedish national male team was found to be 1.14 (range 1.03−1.29) (see Table 9.2) indicating that players increase their vertical jump height by on average 14% with the arm swing. However, for three players the increase was less than 5% suggesting that these players could improve their jumping ability by a more co-ordinated arm swing.

During BJ the ratio between flight and ground contact time is another interesting parameter. The ratio for 'powerful' jumpers is larger than 3 (see Table 9.2) indicating that they stay three times longer in the air than on the ground. The highest value to date (4.0) was found in an élite volleyball player (L. Oddsson personal communication). For football players with a low "flight−contact" ratio, training should focus more on the power component of the jump.

Using the results in Table 9.2 it can be seen that top-class volleyball players have a RJ height of 38 cm and a BJ height of around 36 cm. The ratio BJ−RJ can be used as an initial indicator of whether the player should focus on slow high resistance strength training (i.e. if the ratio is much higher than 1) or fast "explosive" training (i.e. if the ratio is much lower than 1).

Strength

Strength, defined as the ability to develop force in a single muscle contraction (Atha 1981), is specific to the type of muscle action, i.e. concentric or eccentric, and the speed and pattern of movement. Lower extremity muscle strength is influential in such football-specific movements as sprinting, jumping, tackling, changing direction, and kicking, whereas during heading and tackling, trunk and upper body strength is also utilized. Although it has been found that the leg strength of top-class players is greater than players of a lower caliber (Öberg 1989), it is difficult to quantify the relative importance of strength in football. Even within a team considerations must be made for each player's style of play.

Some studies have investigated the relationship between strength of certain muscle groups, e.g. knee extensor and hip flexors, and kicking performance (e.g. Narici *et al.* 1988). However, due to the complex interaction of different muscle groups involved in kicking and the high speed of muscle action ($> 700°\cdot s^{-1}$) many other factors must also be considered.

Strength can be expressed and tested in a variety of ways. The reason for testing strength should ultimately determine the type of test to be used. The most efficient method of monitoring adaptation to strength training is to use the same exercise for both training and testing (Sale & MacDougall 1981). Laboratory tests can underestimate training progress where movement patterns differ from those performed during the training. Thus, to evaluate the effect of a strength training program, where conventional weight training machines or free weights are used, progress can be monitored by recording the maximum weight that can be lifted for either 1 or 5 repetitions of movement (RM). Although a 5 RM measurement is harder to obtain, it is often considered a safer alternative, especially during the early stages of a training program when players are still learning correct lifting techniques. However, during these exercises, muscles are not contracting maximally throughout the entire range of motion and the maximum weight that can be lifted is limited by the weakest point in the range of motion.

During an isokinetic movement where force is applied at a constant velocity, a muscle can contract maximally throughout the range of motion. Using an isokinetic dynamometer, the torque produced during a constant velocity concentric, and in some cases eccentric, muscle action can be recorded at different speeds of movement for a full range of motion (Fig. 9.11). Isometric torques can also be recorded at a fixed joint angle. Differentiating features of commercially available isokinetic dynamometers have been reviewed by Sale (1991). In Fig. 9.12 knee extensor torque is being measured on the SPARK system (Seger *et al.* 1988).

Strength testing can be used to identify gross muscle weaknesses or functional imbalances, between legs and between agonistic and antagonistic muscle groups of the same leg, e.g. between knee flexor (hamstring) and knee extensor (quadriceps) muscle groups. Developing a strength profile of both legs is useful for comparison purposes in cases of long-term injury,

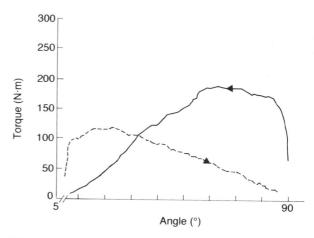

Fig. 9.11 A concentric torque displacement curve ($n = 1$) for the quadriceps and hamstring muscles. (——), knee extension; (– – – –), knee flexion.

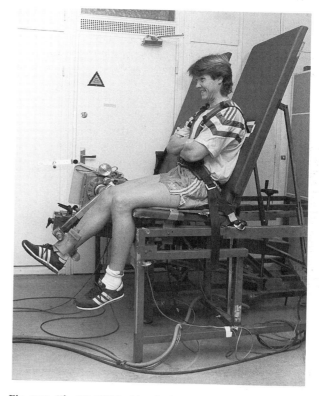

Fig. 9.12 The SPARK isokinetic dynamometer being used to measure knee extensor torque. Courtesy of Styrbjörn Bergelt.

especially following knee surgery with post-operative joint immobilization (cf. Halkjaer-Kristensen & Ingemann-Hansen 1985). It has been shown that following immobilization, gross discrepancies can exist in bilateral leg strength without players being aware of any functional impairment (Grimby et al. 1980). In a study where a group of athletes who had returned to competitive sport following knee surgery were tested 5–10 years post-operation, bilateral strength differences of up to 20% were found (Arvidsson et al. 1981). Therefore, regular testing during rehabilitation programs should be used to monitor progress and ensure that muscle strength is restored close to pre-injury status before the player fully resumes normal training and playing competitive matches.

The day-to-day variation of isokinetic strength measurements has been reported to be around 10% (Westing et al. 1988). This variation can be affected by such factors as the degree of central nervous system stimulation and activation of antagonistic muscles (Narici et al. 1992).

Strength testing protocol for football players

When recording strength measurements using an isokinetic dynamometer it is particularly important that players are familiarized with the equipment before a test value is recorded.

While in principle, extension and flexion torques around the ankle, knee, and hip are of some interest, such an extensive testing protocol for a large group of football players can be impractical due to time restraints. A more feasible testing protocol includes the measurement of concentric knee flexor and extensor torque at two different speeds of motion (Poulmedis 1985, Öberg et al. 1986, Rochcongar et al. 1988). The slower speed being either 30 or $60°\cdot s^{-1}$ with a faster speed of c. $180°\cdot s^{-1}$.

In addition to bilateral comparisons of peak and angle-specific torques, and between angle-specific torques produced by agonistic and antagonistic muscle groups, i.e. hamstring to quadriceps (ham–quad) ratio, torques produced by a given muscle group at fast and slow speeds of movement (fast–slow speed ratio) may also be compared.

Generally, in studies where comparisons have been made between the strength of players' dominant and non-dominant legs no significant bilateral difference

has been found. It is recommended that for individual players, bilateral strength differences should not exceed 10–15% (Goslin & Charteis 1979). It has been suggested that for a given speed of movement the peak ham–quad ratio should be within a range of 0.3–0.8 (Grimby et al. 1980), however, more research is needed here, especially as the comparison of angle-specific torques may be of more value (Westing & Seger 1989). A fast–slow ($30–180°\cdot s^{-1}$) speed ratio of 0.65 has been reported for Swedish national players; this was higher than that reported for First (0.58) and Fourth (0.58) Division players (Öberg et al. 1986). It would appear that the capability of producing torque at high movement speeds is greater for top-class players.

Torques should be corrected for the effect of gravity, i.e. gravity effect torques (GET), especially if comparisons are to be made with data from other studies and when ham–quad ratios are calculated (Filyaw et al. 1986).

Flexibility

Flexibility describes the range of motion at a skeletal joint. It is unique to each joint and is limited by many factors. The aim of evaluating range of motion is to evaluate the degree to which movement about a joint is limited by the musculotendinous unit. In football, flexibility testing can be used to identify lower extremity muscle tightness which uncharacteristically restricts joint motion (Ekstrand et al. 1982). In addition to possibly hindering performance muscle tightness may make a player more prone to injury (for a review see Knapik et al. 1992). A suitable range of motion for a given joint should allow a player to perform sport-specific skills while placing minimal stress on the surrounding soft tissue (Hubley-Kozey 1991). In a study where lower extremity flexibility of 180 Swedish football players was evaluated, muscle tightness was diagnosed in 113 (67%) of the players, which was significantly greater than a control group (Ekstrand 1982).

Flexibility can be tested in a two-step approach. Initially, a battery of tests can be used as a screening process for a preliminary evaluation of flexibility in the lower extremities. A "non-pass" test result in the screening process, i.e. restricted range of motion about a joint, can be followed up with an objective measure of angular displacement using a goniometer.

Screening process

The purpose of the screening process is to use a series of simple field tests to identify subjectively where range of motion may be uncharacteristically restricted by muscle tightness. These tests are presented and described in Fig. 9.13. The aim of these tests is to identify those players who are unable to attain the marked position in the figure. Players who fail to reach this position should be selected for further tests. Unfortunately, these tests do not allow for the assessment of too much flexibility, but this is extremely rare, at least among male football players. It is important to emphasize that players who pass the screening tests still need to stretch regularly before and after training and matches.

Goniometric measurements

Goniometric measurements of range of motion allow for an objective measurement which can be documented and used for comparison purposes, e.g. after a training program or period of rehabilitation. The methodology concerning these measurements is described in more detail by Ekstrand *et al.* (1982).

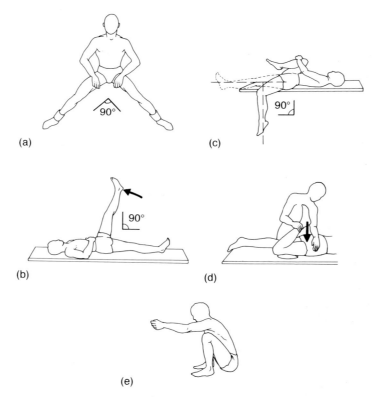

Fig. 9.13 Flexibility measurements. (a) Hip abduction (tests hip adductors). In an upright seated position, with straight legs, the legs are opened as wide apart as possible (fail: < 90°). (b) Hip flexion (tests hamstrings). With the player in the supine position, the straight leg is passively pushed back (hip flexion). Upward movement at the hip should be prevented (fail: < 90°). (c) Gaenslen's test for (i) psoas, and (ii) quadriceps. Player lays on a table and holds the flexed knee of the non-tested leg. The opposite leg is extended and lowered over the side of the table. Thigh should not lie above the horizontal (fail: knee flexion from horizontal > 90°). (d) Knee flexion which tests quadriceps (rectus femoris). The leg is passively flexed toward the thigh, hips must not rise up (fail: foot does not touch buttocks). (e) Dorsiflexion (tests soleus). In a squatted position with feet at shoulder width apart the player attempts to hold the heels of the feet on the ground (fail: both heels are not touching the ground). Courtesy of Niclas Carlson, Scandinavia Chiropractor School, Stockholm.

Other measures of flexibility

The "sit and reach" test is commonly used to evaluate the flexibility of football players. To perform this test players sit with straight legs and, by flexing at the hip, reach forward as far as possible with straight arms (hands together) in the horizontal plane. A major limitation of this test, however, is that it involves rotational movement around more than one joint and thus it is difficult to make a clear diagnosis from the test result (Hubley-Kozey 1991). Furthermore, a player with long arms and short legs can record a "false high" test value, likewise a player with short arms and long legs can record a "false low" test value.

A testing model for football

A testing model to evaluate players at all levels of the game has been designed. The model is based on an initial screening process where players are tested on three basic physical performance components, namely, football-specific endurance, sprinting, and jumping (Fig. 9.14). The information gained from the screening process is then used to identify those players who would benefit the most from a specific physical

training program designed to improve performance in an identified area of weakness. This may be in the form of a general training program based solely on the test results from the screening process or in the form of a more individualized training program that is based on the results from a series of more advanced laboratory tests where component factors of the basic performance are evaluated (Fig. 9.15). Thus, the model represents an organized testing structure which can be used to develop effective individualized training programs. Furthermore, by identifying "good" test results individual training can focus on other aspects of the game.

The screening process is not time consuming and the tests require only basic equipment which means that, at least in some form, they can be administered by all coaches. Furthermore, the results obtained from these tests are easy to process and analyze which means that direct feedback can be given almost immediately to the players. The test results are analyzed to identify those players who would benefit the most from a specific physical training program. However, those players with "good" test results should still be retested at regular intervals to ensure that this level of performance is maintained. Unfortunately, it is not possible to

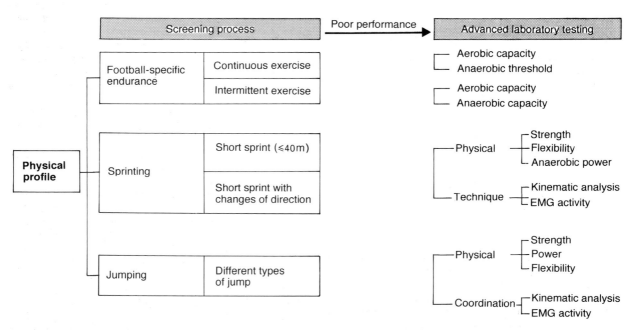

Fig. 9.14 A testing model for football.

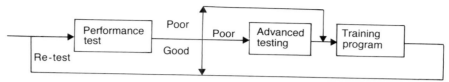

Fig. 9.15 Priniciple of using a screening process.

present absolute test results to define "good" or "poor" performance as, in addition to the many methodological factors which can influence a test score, other factors such as the team's playing status and the age and sex of the players must be considered. Even within a team different performance levels can be defined based on the positional roles. As a general guideline, the mean test score in the team can often be used as a reference point.

Where possible, the players who perform poorly on the tests used in the screening process should be tested further using more advanced laboratory tests. This will enable a more specific training program to be developed which will make the training as efficient and effective as possible.

Conclusion

Information gained from performance testing should be used to improve overall match-play performance. Before testing, objectives should be clearly defined, during the test administration conditions and procedures should be standardized, and after the test feedback should be given to the players as soon as possible. Testing should only include tests which are football-specific, these may be in the form of simple performance tests where the whole team is tested together or more advanced laboratory tests where players are tested individually.

References

Arvidsson I., Erikson E., Häggmark T. & Johnson R.J. (1981) Isokinetic thigh muscle strength after ligament reconstructions in the knee joint. Results from a 5−10 year follow-up after reconstruction of the anterior cruciate ligament in the knee joint. *Int. J. Sports Med.* **2**, 7−11.

Asmussen E. & Boje O. (1945) Body temperature and capacity for work. *Acta Physiol. Scand.* **10**, 1−22.

Åstrand P.O. & Ryhming I. (1954) A nomogram for calcu-lation of aerobic capacity (physical fitness) from pulse rate during submaximal work. *J. Appl. Physiol.* **7**, 218.

Åstrand P.O. & Rodahl K. (1986) *Textbook of Work Physiology*, 2nd edn. McGraw-Hill, New York.

Atha J. (1981) Strengthening muscle. In D.I. Miller (ed.) *Exercise and Sport Science Reviews*, pp. 1−73. American College of Sports Medicine Series.

Balsom P.D. (1988) *Physiological variables and performance decrementation for soccer players*. Graduate thesis, Springfield College, Massachusetts.

Balsom P.D. (1990) A field test to evaluate physical performance capacity of association football players. *Sci. Football* **3**, 9−11.

Balsom P.D., Sjödin B. & Ekblom B. (1994) Enhanced oxygen availability during high intensity intermittent exercise decreases anaerobic metabolite concentrations in blood. *Acta Physiol. Scand.* in press.

Bangsbo J. (1992a) Time motion characteristics of competitive soccer. *Sci. Football* **6**, 34−40.

Bangsbo J. (1992) Is the oxygen deficit an accurate quantitative measure of the anaerobic energy production during intense exercise? *J. Appl. Physiol.* **73**, 1207−1208.

Bangsbo J. (1994) *Fitness Training for Football: A Scientific Approach.* HO + Storm, Bagsværd, Copenhagen, Denmark.

Bangsbo J. & Lindqvist F. (1992) Comparison of various exercise tests with endurance performance during soccer in professional players. *Int. J. Sports Med.* **13**, 125−132.

Bar-Or O. (1987) The Wingate anaerobic test: An update on methodology, reliability and validity. *Sports Med.* **4**, 381−394.

Bosco C., Luhtanen P. & Komi P.V. (1983) A simple method for measurement of mechanical power in jumping. *Eur. J. Appl. Physiol.* **50**, 273−282.

Bouchard C., Taylor A.W., Simoneau J.-A. & Dulac S. (1991) Testing anaerobic power and capacity. In McDougall J.D., Wenger H.A. & Green H.J. (eds) *Physiological Testing of the High-Performance Athlete*, pp. 175−221. Human Kinetics, Champaign, Illinois.

Brewer J. & Davis J.A. (1992) A physiological comparison of English professional and semi-professional soccer players. *J. Sport Sci.* **10**(2), 146−147.

Brewer J., Ramsbottom R. & Williams C. (1988) *Multistage Fitness Test.* National Coaching Foundation, Leeds, UK.

Cavagna G.A., Dusman B. & Margaria R. (1968) Positive work

done by the previously stretched muscle. *J. Appl. Physiol.* **24**, 21–32.

Cooper K.H. (1968) A means of assessing maximal oxygen intake: correlation between field and treadmill testing. *J. Am. Med. Assoc.* **162**, 1139–1149.

Cunningham D.A. & Faulkner J.A. (1969) The effect of training on aerobic and anaerobic metabolism during a short exhaustive run. *Med. Sci. Sports Exerc.* **1**, 65–69.

Davis J.A. & Brewer J. (1992) Physiological characteristics of an international female squad. *J. Sport Sci.* **10**, 142–143.

Davis J.A., Brewer J. & Atkin D. (1992) Pre-season physiological characteristics of English First and Second Division football players. *J. Sport Sci.* **10**, 541–547.

Ekblom B. (1988) Fysiologiska aspekter på fotbollsspel (Physiological aspects of football match-play). In Forsberg A. & Saltin B (eds). *Konditionsträning.* Swedish Sports Research Council, Farsta, Sweden.

Ekblom B. (1989) A field test for soccer players. *Sci. Football* **1**, 13–15.

Ekblom B., Andersson G., Malm S. & Nilsson R. (1982) *En studie av excentriskt muskelarbete i handboll* (A study of eccentric muscle function in handball). Undergraduate thesis, Specialarbete, Gymnastik och Idrotts Högskolan, Stockholm.

Ekstrand J. (1982) *Soccer injuries and their prevention.* Medical dissertation No. 130, Linköping University, Sweden.

Ekstrand J., Wiktorsson M., Öberg B. & Gillquist J. (1982) Lower extremity goniometric measurements: a study to determine their reliability. *Arch. Phys. Med. Rehab.* **63**, 171–175.

Filyaw M., Bevins T. & Fernandez L. (1986) Importance of correcting isokinetic peak torque for the effect of gravity when calculating knee flexor to extensor ratios. *Phys. Ther.* **66**, 23–32.

Goslin B.R. & Charteis J. (1979) Isokinetic dynamometry: normative data for clinical use in lower extremity (knee) cases. *Scand. J. Rehab. Med.* **11**, 105–109.

Grimby G., Gustafsson E., Peterson L. & Renström P. (1980) Quadriceps function and training after knee ligament surgery. *Med. Sci. Sports Exerc.* **12**(1), 70–75.

Halkjaer-Kristensen J. & Ingemann-Hansen T. (1985) Wasting and training of the human quadriceps muscle during the treatment of knee ligament injuries. *Scand. J. Rehab. Med.* Suppl. 13.

Hubley-Kozey C.L. (1991) Testing flexibility. In McDougall J.D., Wenger H.A. & Green H.J. (eds) *Physiological Testing of the High-Performance Athlete*, pp. 309–359. Human Kinetics, Champaign, Illinois.

Jacobs I., Westlin N., Karlson J., Rasmussin M. & Houghton B. (1982) Muscle glycogen and diet in élite soccer players. *Eur. J. Appl. Physiol.* **48**, 297–302.

Knapik J.J., Jones B.H., Bauman C.L. & Harris J. (1992) Strength, flexibility and athletic injuries. *Sports Med.* **14**(5), 277–288.

Kollath E. & Quade K. (1993) Experimental measurement of the professional and amateur soccer player's sprinting speed. In Reilly T., Clarys J. & Stibbe A. (eds) *Science and Football II*, pp. 31–36. E. & F.N. Spon, London.

Komi P.V. (1984) Physiological and biomechanical correlates of muscle function. Effects of muscle structure and stretch shortening cycle on force and speed. In Terjung R.L. (ed.) *Exercise Reviews*, Vol. 12, pp. 81–121. Collamore Press, Lexington.

Margaria R., Aghemo P. & Rovelli E. (1966) Measurement of muscular power (anaerobic) in man. *J. Physiol.* **21**, 1662–1664.

Medbo J.I., Mohn A.C., Tabata I., Bahr R., Vaage O. & Sejersted O.M. (1988) Anaerobic capacity determined by maximal accumulated O_2 deficit. *J. Appl. Physiol.* **64**, 50–60.

Narici M.V., Sirtori M.D. & Mognoni P. (1988) Maximal ball velocity and peak torques of hip flexor and knee extensor muscles. In Reilly T., Lees A., Davids K. & Murphy W.J. (eds) *Science and Football*, pp. 429–433. E. & F.N. Spon, London.

Narici M.V., Sirtori M.D. & Mognoni P. (1992) Isokinetic torques and cross sectional area ratios of knee flexor and extensor muscles. *J. Sport Sci.* **10**(2), 171–172.

Öberg B. (1989) *Lower extremity muscle strength in soccer players.* Medical dissertation No. 190, Linköping University, Sweden.

Öberg B., Möller M., Gillquist J. & Ekstrand J. (1986) Isokinetic torque levels for knee extensors and knee flexors. *Int. J. Sports Med.* **7**, 50–53.

Oddsson L. & Thorstensson A. (1992) Jumping performance in élite athletes — application of a test predicting vertical jumping ability. *Med. Sci. Sports Exerc.* **24**(5), S104.

Oddsson L.I.E. & Westing S.H. (1991) Jumping height can be accurately predicated from selected measurements of muscle strength and biomechanical parameters. In *Proceedings of the 9th International Symposium on Biomechanics in Sports*, pp. 29–33. Iowa, USA.

Poulmedis P. (1985) Isokinetic maximal torque power of Greek élite soccer players. *J. Orthop. Sport Phys. Ther.* **6**(5), 293–295.

Rhodes E.C., Mosher R.E., McKenzie D.C., Franks I.M. & Potts J.E. (1986) Physiological profiles of the Canadian Olympic soccer team. *Can. J. Appl. Sport Sci.* **11**(1), 31–36.

Rochcongar P., Morvan R., Jan J., Dassonville J. & Beillot J. (1988) Isokinetic investigation of knee extensors and knee flexors in young French soccer players. *Int. J. Sports Med.* **9**, 448–450.

Sale D. (1991) Testing strength and power. In McDougall J.D., Wenger H.A. & Green H.J. (eds) *Physiological Testing of the High-Performance Athlete*, pp. 21–106. Human Kinetics, Champaign, Illinois.

Sale D. & MacDougall J.D. (1981) Specificity in strength training: A review for the coach and athlete. *Can. J. Appl. Sport Sci.* **6**, 87–92.

Sargent D.A. (1921) The physical test of a man. *Am. Phys. Educ. Rev.* **26**, 188−194.

Seger J., Westing S.H., Hanson M., Karlson E. & Ekblom B. (1988) A new dynamometer measuring concentric and eccentric muscle strength in accelerated, decelerated, or isokinetic movements. *Eur. J. Appl. Physiol.* **57**, 526−530.

Thoden J.S. (1991) Testing aerobic power. In McDougall J.D., Wenger H.A. & Green H.J. (eds) *Physiological Testing of the High-Performance Athlete*, pp. 107−174. Human Kinetics, Champaign, Illinois.

Tumilty D.McA. & Darby S. (1991) Physiological characteristics of Australian female soccer players. *J. Sports Sci.* **10**(2), 145.

Vandewalle H., Peres G. & Monod H. (1987) Standard anaerobic exercise tests. *Sports Med.* **4**, 268−289.

Wasserman K. (1984) The anaerobic threshold measurement to evaluate exercise performance. *Am. Rev. Respir. Dis.* Suppl. 129, S35−S40.

Westing S.H. & Seger J. (1989) Eccentric and concentric torque−velocity characteristics, torque output comparisons, and gravity effect torque corrections for the quadriceps and hamstring muscles in females. *Int. J. Sports Med.* **10**, 175−180.

Westing S.H., Seger J., Karlson E. & Ekblom B. (1988) Eccentric and concentric torque−velocity characteristics of the quadriceps femoris in man. *Eur. J. Appl. Physiol.* **58**, 100−104.

Wilmore J.H. (1982) *Training for Sport and Activity: The Physiological Basis of the Conditioning Process*. Allyn & Bacon, Boston.

Chapter 10

Physical conditioning

Training in football has to cover the many different aspects of performance during match-play (see Chapters 3 and 4). The training can be divided into four main areas: technical, tactical, psychological/social, and fitness training. The various components of training should be combined in a way that accommodates the needs of a group of players.

The aim of fitness training in football is to enable a player to cope with the physical demands of football and to ensure that a player's technical abilities can be utilized throughout a match.

Training methods

A major part of fitness training in football should be performed with a ball as such training has several advantages. Firstly, the specific muscle groups used in football are trained. Secondly, the players develop technical and tactical skills under conditions similar

to those encountered during a match. Thirdly, this form of training provides greater motivation for the players compared to training without the ball. However, when training with a ball the players may not work hard enough, as many factors, such as tactical limitations, can lower the exercise intensity. To increase the demands of a training game new rules may be introduced. As an example, Fig. 10.1 shows how the heart rate (HR) of a player increased when the playing field in a four against four game was extended from one-third to one-half of a football field.

Under some circumstances it might be necessary to train without a ball. In this case the training should mainly be on grass, with the players wearing football boots and performing movements that resemble those during match-play.

Individual fitness training

In football, the physiological demands of a player during a match are influenced by several factors such as the player's tactical role and technical standard. Therefore, players in a team have different training needs. A part of the fitness training may, therefore, be performed on an individual basis, when the training can be focused on either improving a player's strong or weak abilities. It is important to be aware that due to hereditary differences there will always be differences in the physical capacity of players irrespective of training programs. However, players who are physi-

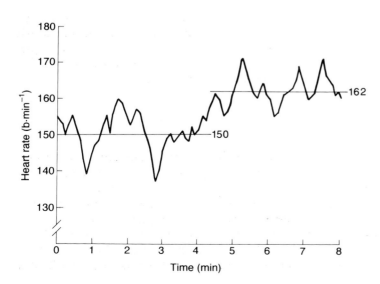

Fig. 10.1 Heart rate for a player during a four against four game on one-third of a football field (left) and on one-half of a football field (right). Mean heart rate for the two periods of the game is represented by the horizontal lines.

cally weaker may be able to compensate through superior qualities in other aspects of football. This type of player is also needed in a team, and it is important for the coach to choose a playing system and style which fits the strength of the available players.

Training of youth players

There is evidence to suggest that training of youth players does not need to be focused on improving physical performance. Often young players get a sufficient physical training effect by regular drills and games. The time saved by excluding fitness training should be spent on training to improve technical skills. The players will greatly benefit from this type of training when they become seniors. Figure 10.2 shows exercises which can be used to improve the technical level of young players.

When training youths one should be aware that there is a large difference in maturation status within a given age group. The adolescent growth spurt may start as early as 10 years of age or it may not start until the age of 16. On average, girls mature about 2 years earlier than boys. As maturation status can have a profound effect on physical performance, care should be taken not to underestimate genuine football talents due to physical immaturity in comparison with the other players in the same age group. Another important aspect of youth training is the training dose. The coach should carefully observe how the individual players respond to training, as young players can easily be given too much training.

Training of female players

The overall exercise intensity in female football is not as high as in the male game due to the lower physical capacity of female players (see Chapter 7). On the other hand, the activity profile of female football is very similar to that of male football, and there is little difference in the training potential of men and women, i.e. the response to training from a baseline level is similar. Therefore, male and female players should train in the same way and the training advice given in this chapter can be used for both genders.

With the rapid development of female football, the overall intensity of the female game has been elevated, and it is, therefore, important to emphasize training

at a high intensity. On the other hand, sudden large increases in the amount of training and intensity within a short period of time should be avoided, as alterations in the menstrual cycle may occur when the training becomes too demanding. This condition is generally reversible after several days to weeks of rest or much reduced training.

Components of fitness training

Fitness training in football can be divided into a number of components based on the different types of physical performance required during a match (Fig. 10.3). The terms aerobic and anaerobic training are based on the energy pathway that dominates during the exercise periods of the training. Aerobic and anaerobic training represent exercise intensities below and above the maximum oxygen uptake, respectively. However, during a game, the exercise intensity varies continuously. Figure 10.4 shows examples of exercise intensities during games and drills within aerobic and anaerobic training. Some overlapping exists between the categories of training, e.g. the exercise intensity during aerobic high intensity (aerobic$_{HI}$) training may in short periods become as high as during speed endurance training.

The separate components within fitness training are briefly described below.

Aerobic training

Aerobic training will improve a player's potential to maintain a high overall work-rate throughout a match and it may also minimize a decrease in technical performance and lapses in concentration induced by fatigue towards the end of a game.

Specific aims of aerobic training for football players

1 To improve the capacity of the cardiovascular system to transport oxygen. Thus, a larger percentage of the energy required for intense exercise can be supplied aerobically allowing a player to work at a higher exercise intensity for prolonged periods.
2 To improve the capacity of muscles specifically used in football to utilize oxygen and to oxidize fat during prolonged periods of exercise. Thus, the limited

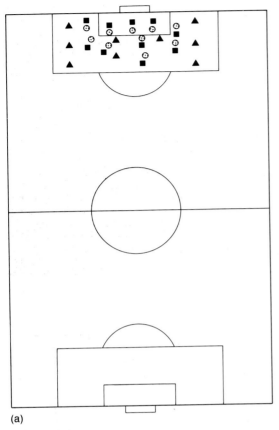

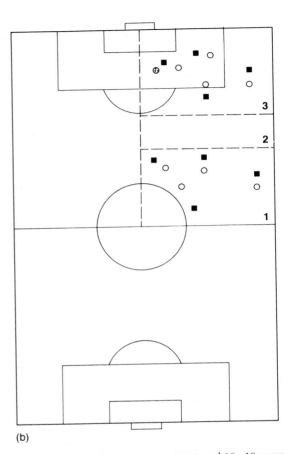

(a)   (b)

Fig. 10.2 A drill (a) and a game (b) which can be used to improve the technical ability of youth players 6—12 and 12—16 years of age, respectively.

(a) *Area of field*: penalty area. *Number of players*: 10. *Organization*: nine cones are placed in the penalty area. Each player has a ball. *Description*: the players are dribbling in the penalty area and on a given sound or hand signal the players have to bring the ball to a cone and touch the cone. Each cone may only be touched by one player. *Rules*: the players are not allowed to kick the ball to the cone, it has to be dribbled. The aim of the drill is to train the players to dribble and to maintain a good sense of orientation while handling the ball. It is important to allow all of the players to be successful in touching the cones which can be achieved by timing the signal.

(b) *Area of field*: one-fourth of a football field divided into three zones — two outer zones (1 and 3) and one middle zone (2). *Number of players*: 16 — eight against eight. *Organization*: four players from each team start in the two outer-zones. *Rules*: no player is allowed to touch the ball in the middle zone. *Scoring*: a team scores a point, if the ball is played from one of the outer-zones to the other three times in a row, without the other team capturing it. The main aim of the game is to improve the ability of the players to perform long passes.

⊙, ball; ▲, cone; ■, players on one team; ○, players on the other team.

stores of muscle glycogen are spared and a player can exercise at a higher intensity towards the end of a game.

3 To improve the ability to recover after a period of high-intensity exercise. Thus, a player requires less time to recover before being able to perform in a subsequent period of high-intensity exercise.

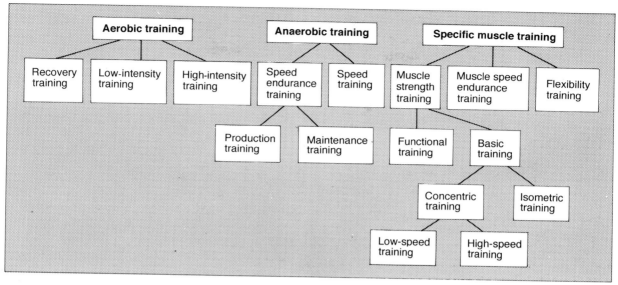

Fig. 10.3 Components of fitness training in football.

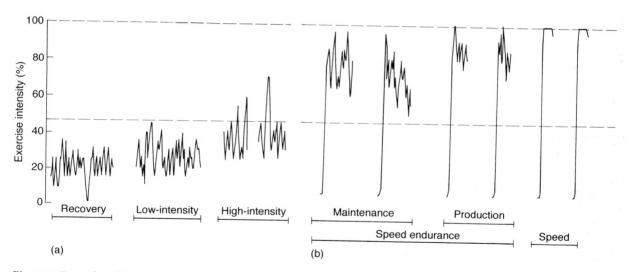

Fig. 10.4 Examples of the exercise intensities of a player within (a) aerobic; and (b) anaerobic training, expressed in relation to maximal intensity (100%). The exercise intensity eliciting the maximum oxygen uptake and the maximal exercise intensity of the player are represented by the lower and the higher horizontal lines, respectively.

Components of aerobic training

Aerobic training can be divided into three overlapping components: (a) recovery training; (b) aerobic low-intensity training (aerobic$_{LI}$); and (c) aerobic high-intensity training (aerobic$_{HI}$) (Fig. 10.3).

As aerobic training should be mainly performed with a ball, the definition of the three categories of aerobic training take into account that the HR of a player will alternate continuously during the training. Table 10.1 illustrates the principles behind the various categories of aerobic training. It is misleading to quan-

Table 10.1 Principles of aerobic training

	HR (% of $HR_{max.}$)		HR (beats·min^{-1})	
	Mean	Range	Mean*	Range*
Recovery training	65	40–80	130	80–160
Low-intensity training	80	65–90	160	130–180
High-intensity training	90	80–100	180	160–200

HR, heart rate.
* If $HR_{max.}$ is 200 beats·min^{-1}.

tify training by the total exercise time. Any activity, if it lasts for 15 or 90 min, can have a favorable effect on a player's aerobic work capacity.

The separate components within aerobic training are briefly described below.

Recovery training. During recovery training the players perform light physical activities, such as jogging and low-intensity games, in which the mean HR is around 130 beats·min^{-1} (see Table 10.1). This type of training may be carried out the day after a match or the day after a hard training session to help a player return to a normal physical state. Recovery training may also be used in periods involving frequent training sessions and competitive matches, in order to avoid the players becoming overtrained.

Aerobic low-intensity (aerobic$_{LI}$) training. A football player should be able to maintain the same level of physical and technical performance throughout a match. Therefore, part of the fitness training should aim at improving the ability to exercise for long periods of time (endurance) at varying running speeds. Endurance capacity can be elevated with aerobic$_{LI}$ training in which a player exercises either continuously or intermittently with a mean HR around 160 beats·min^{-1} (see Table 10.1). During an intermittent aerobic$_{LI}$ training session the work periods should be longer than 5 min. If the training is performed without a ball it is recommended that continuous exercise at varying intensities is used, e.g. alternating between exercise

intensities corresponding to 70, 80, and 90% of maximal HR ($HR_{max.}$) each third minute.

Figure 10.5 shows an aerobic low-intensity training game and the alterations in HR for a player during the game.

Aerobic high-intensity (aerobic$_{HI}$) training. It has been demonstrated that the distance covered by high-intensity running during a match is related to the standard of football, i.e. top-class players cover the most distance. Thus, it is important that players are capable of repeatedly exercising at high intensities for prolonged periods of time during a match. The basis for this capacity is a high maximum oxygen uptake, which can be elevated by aerobic$_{HI}$ training. During this type of training a player exercises intermittently with an average HR around 180 beats·min^{-1} (see Table 10.1). In addition to the intermittent exercise inherent to a game of football, different intermittent training models can be used in the aerobic$_{HI}$ training. Three of these training forms are described here.

1 *Fixed time intervals.* In fixed time interval training, the duration of the exercise and rest periods is determined in advance, e.g. alternating between 2 min of exercise and 1 min of rest. If the exercise periods are longer than 1 min the rest periods should be shorter than each exercise bout, otherwise the overall intensity will be too low. The shorter the exercise periods, the higher the exercise intensity should be, according to the principles given for this type of training. Rest periods should include some form of recovery exercise, such as jogging. The above principles are valid for training both with and without a ball.

2 *Alteration of the rules.* By changing the rules during a training game the exercise intensity may be varied, e.g. alternating between using and not using the rule of exactly two touches each time a player is in contact with the ball. Set times can be implemented where the rules are changed to either increase or decrease the exercise intensity.

3 *Natural variations.* Training games can be structured so that the exercise intensity changes in a natural way during a game. Figure 10.6 shows an example of an aerobic$_{HI}$ training game where limitations of the players' actions within an area of the field result in an elevated exercise intensity during periods of the game. This is illustrated by the fluctuations in HR of a player during the game shown in Fig. 10.6.

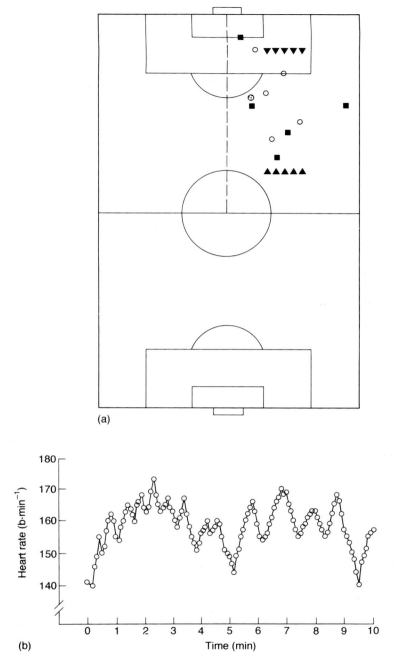

(a)

(b)

Fig. 10.5 Aerobic low-intensity game. (a) The playing field; and (b) the heart rate of one player performing the game. *Area of field*: one-quarter of a football field divided into two halves. *Number of players*: 10 — five against five. *Organization*: each team defends a row of cones (five or more) positioned at least 1 m apart in a straight line on each half of the playing field. *Description*: the teams try to knock over the cones of the opposing team with the ball. When a team succeeds, they place the cone on their own line. The game immediately continues after a scoring. Play is allowed both in front of and behind the line of cones. *Rules*: ordinary football play. *Scoring*: the game is won by the team which has the most cones on their line at the end of the game. If the exercise intensity level is too low a rule may be introduced so that a cone may only be knocked down when all the players from the attacking team are in the opponent's half of the field. If one player from the defending team is not within the defending half when a cone is knocked down then the attacking team takes two cones to their defending line. Symbols as on Fig. 10.2.

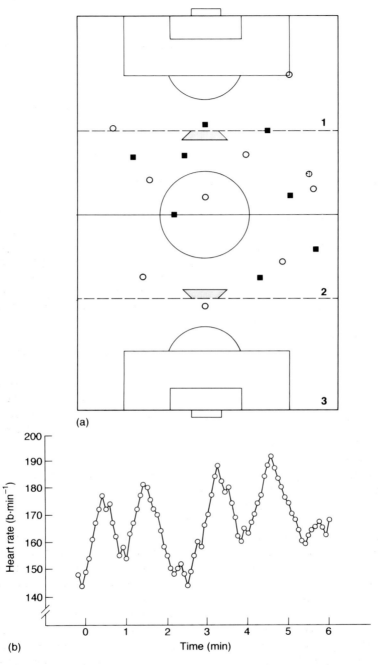

Fig. 10.6 Aerobic high-intensity game. (a) The playing field; (b) the heart rate of one player performing the game. *Area of field*: a football field divided into three zones (1–3). Two goals are placed back-to-back in the middle of each half. *Number of players*: 16 — seven against seven plus two goalkeepers. *Rules*: in zone 2 the number of ball touches per player is limited to a maximum of two and a team is only allowed six passes. The goalkeepers may use their hands inside a certain area. *Scoring*: ordinary scoring, i.e. scoring from behind. The demands are greatest when the players are inside the zone between the two goals. The length of the middle zone will influence the exercise intensity of the players, i.e. the longer the zone, the higher the intensity. If the exercise intensity level is too low a rule may be introduced so that a goal can only be scored when all the players from the attacking team are in the attacking zone (1 or 3). If one player from the defending team is not within the defending zone (3 or 1) when a goal is scored then the score counts as two. Symbols as on Fig. 10.2.

Anaerobic training

Anaerobic training can increase a player's potential to perform high-intensity exercise during a game.

Specific aims of anaerobic training for football players

1 To improve the ability to act quickly and to produce power rapidly during high-intensity exercise. Thus, a player reduces the time required to react and elevates performance of a sprint during a game.
2 To improve the capacity to produce power and energy continuously via the anaerobic energy-producing pathways. Thus, a player elevates the ability to perform high-intensity exercise for longer periods of time during a game.
3 To improve the ability to recover after a period of high-intensity exercise. Thus, a player requires less time before being able to perform maximally in a subsequent period of exercise and is therefore able to perform high-intensity exercise more frequently during a game.

Components of anaerobic training

Anaerobic training can be divided into (a) speed training; and (b) speed endurance training (see Fig. 10.3). The aim of speed training is to improve a player's ability to perceive, evaluate, and act quickly in situations where speed is essential. Speed endurance training can be separated into two distinct categories: (a) production training; and (b) maintenance training. The purpose of production training is to improve the ability to perform maximally for a relatively short period of time, whereas the aim of maintenance training is to increase the ability to sustain exercise at a high intensity.

Anaerobic training must be performed according to an interval principle. During speed training the players should perform maximally for a short period of time (<10 s). The periods between the exercise bouts should be long enough for the muscles to recover to near resting conditions, so to enable a player to perform maximally in a subsequent exercise bout. During the speed endurance training the exercise intensity should be almost maximal. In the production training the duration of the exercise bouts should be relatively

short (20−40 s), and the rest periods in between the exercise bouts should be comparatively long (2−4 min) in order to maintain a very high intensity throughout an interval training session. In the maintenance training the exercise periods should be 30−120 s and the duration of the rest periods should approximately equal the exercise periods, as the players should become progressively fatigued. Table 10.2 illustrates the principles of the various categories of anaerobic training.

The two types of anaerobic training are briefly described below.

Speed training. When playing football a player performs many activities that require rapid development of force such as sprinting or quickly changing in direction. As a player's speed during match-play may influence the outcome of a game, speed training is very important. In football, speed is not merely a physical problem, it also involves rapid decision-making which must then be translated into quick movements. Therefore, speed training should mainly be performed with a ball.

Speed training should be performed at an early stage in a training session, when the players are not tired. However, it is very important that the players have warmed up thoroughly. Figure 10.7 shows a speed training drill.

Speed endurance training. High blood lactate concentrations measured from top-class players during match-play indicate that the lactate-producing energy pathway is highly stimulated in football and should be specifically trained (see Chapter 4). This can be achieved through speed endurance training, which improves the capacity to perform high-intensity exercise repeatedly. Speed endurance training is very demanding both physically and mentally for players. Therefore, it is recommended that this type of training is only used with top-class players. When there is a limited amount of time available for training, time can be better utilized on other forms of training.

The adaptations caused by speed endurance training are mostly localized to the exercising muscles. Thus, it is very important that a player performs movements in a manner similar to that during match-play. This can be obtained with high-intensity games or drills with a ball. Figure 10.8 illustrates a game within the maintenance category of speed endurance training

Table 10.2 Principles of anaerobic training

		Duration		Intensity	Number of repetitions
		Exercise (s)	Rest		
Speed training		2–10	> 5 times exercise duration	Maximal	2–10
Speed endurance training	Production	20–40	> 5 times exercise duration	Almost maximal	2–10
	Maintenance	30–90	As exercise duration	Almost maximal	2–10

and it also shows HR and blood lactate values for a player during the game.

Maintenance training should be placed at the very end of a training session, as the players will be physically affected for a long period after this training. It is, however, important that the players perform some type of light exercise after the training to allow for rapid recovery.

Specific muscle training

Specific muscle training involves training of muscles in isolated movements. The aim of this type of training is to increase performance of a muscle to a higher level than can be attained just by playing football. Specific muscle training can be divided into (a) muscle strength; (b) muscle speed endurance; and (c) flexibility training (see Fig. 10.3). The effect of this form of training is specific for the muscle groups that are trained, and the adaptation in the muscle is limited to the kind of training performed.

Below, muscle strength and muscle endurance training is briefly described. For an overview of flexibility training for football players see Bangsbo (1994).

Muscle strength training

A player's ability to produce force during a football match is not solely dependent on the strength of the muscles involved in the movement. The power output is also influenced by the player's ability to co-ordinate the action of the muscles at the right time (timing). Thus, a high level of basic strength cannot be effectively utilized during match-play if a player is not able to co-ordinate the activation of the different muscle groups during a movement. In a similar way, the ability to co-ordinate muscle involvement is of limited use if a player does not have a good sense of timing in a game situation. Smaller players who possess a well-developed ability to co-ordinate and time movements, are often able to compete, e.g. in a heading situation, with players who are taller and have higher basic strength levels. When planning a muscle strength training program it is therefore important to recognize that the ability to utilize strength during a game depends on several factors.

The specific aims of muscle strength training for football players are:
1 To increase muscle power output during explosive activities in a football match such as tackling, jumping, and accelerating.
2 To prevent injuries.
3 To regain strength after an injury.

Components of strength training. Strength training can be divided into (a) functional strength training;

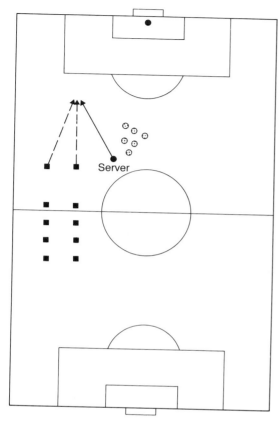

Fig. 10.7 Speed training drill. *Area of field*: half a football field with one full-size goal. *Number of players*: 10 plus one goalkeeper. *Organization*: the players work in pairs. The drill may start from different positions on the field. *Description*: two players stand in front of a server. The server kicks the ball toward the goal. The players start to sprint immediately after the ball has been served. The player who reaches the ball first tries to score, i.e. becomes the attacker, while the other player becomes the defender. *Scoring*: ordinary scoring. It is important that the players try hard to get to the ball first. The player who gains possession of the ball should be encouraged to make a direct run towards the goal and shoot. By varying the position of the serve, the players will need to concentrate throughout the exercise. Symbols as on Fig. 10.2.

and (b) basic strength training (see Fig. 10.3). Common for the two types of training is that the exercise should be performed with a maximum effort. After each repetition, a player should rest a few seconds to allow for a higher force production in the subsequent muscle contraction. The number of repetitions in a set should

not exceed 15. During each training session a muscle group should perform two to four sets, and rest periods between sets should be longer than 1 min. During this time the players can exercise with other muscle groups. Before a strength training session the players should be thoroughly warmed up. The two types of strength training are briefly described below (Table 10.3).

In *functional strength training*, movements related to football are used. The training can consist of games where typical football movements are performed under conditions that are physically more stressful than normal. Alternatively, the training can take the form of maximal force development in isolated movements relevant for football, e.g. jump training. Figure 10.9 shows an exercise of the latter type of functional strength training.

During *basic strength training* muscle groups are trained in isolated movements. For this training different types of conventional strength training machines and free weights can be used, but the body weight may also be used as the resistive load. When planning a strength training program, it is important to take into consideration the way that the muscles function when playing football. A muscle can contract under different conditions. Based on the separate muscle actions the basic strength training can be divided into isometric, concentric, and eccentric muscle strength training. In an isometric muscle contraction the length of the muscle does not change during force production; in a concentric action the muscle length shortens when the muscle contracts; and in an eccentric muscle action the length of the muscle increases as it is contracted.

During isometric strength training a weight load of 85–100% of maximum force is held at a given joint angle for 5–15 s (see Table 10.3). The rest period between each repetition should approximately equal the work time. When performing isometric strength training it is important to train the muscles at joint angles that are relevant for football.

Eccentric muscle strength training is difficult to perform with machines and free weights because eccentric muscle strength exceeds concentric muscle strength. Since large weight loads are needed, a player will have difficulties in returning the weights to the starting position after each repetition.

Maximal force development during a concentric contraction is decreased with increasing speed of

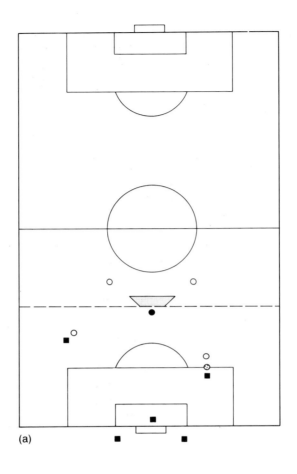

(a)

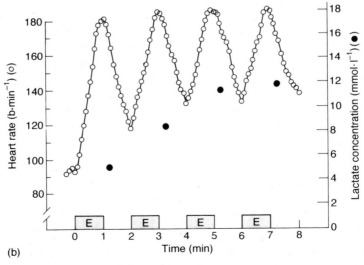

(b)

Table 10.3 Principles of specific muscle training

(a) Basic muscle strength training

	Work load	Number of repetitions	Rest between repetitions (s)	Number of sets
Concentric				
Low speed	5 RM	5	2−5	2−4
High speed	50% of 5 RM	15	1−3	2−4
Isometric	85−100% of max. sustained for 5−15 s	5−10	5−15	2−4

RM, repetition maximum.

(b) Muscle speed endurance training

		Duration		Number of sets
	Work load	Exercise (s)	Rest	
Concentric	Constant frequency (20−60·min^{-1})	15−60	As exercise time	2−4
Isometric	50−80% of maximal force	15−60	As exercise time	2−4

contraction. It has been observed that performing concentric strength training with high loads and low velocities can have a beneficial effect on maximal force development at slow contracting speeds, e.g. during a tackle in football. On the other hand, strength training at slow speeds only to a minor extent improves strength during fast movements. Similarly, training with light loads at moderate velocities will mainly increase force developments at these speeds and only result in a small improvement in strength at slow speeds. Therefore, it is advisable to divide the concentric strength training into slow-speed and high-speed training. Generally, in football the leg muscles should be trained at both slow and high speeds while the muscles of the upper body should be trained mainly at slow speeds. Figure 10.10 shows an exercise which

Fig. 10.8 (*Opposite*) Speed endurance game (maintenance training). (a) The playing field; and (b) the heart rate (○) and blood lactate concentration (●) of one player performing the game. E, exercise. *Area of field*: one-third of a football field with two full-size goals. *Number of players*: 10 − four against four plus two goalkeepers. *Organization*: two players in each team take turns to play. The teams perform player-to-player marking. *Description*: the teams have to attack one and defend one goal. *Scoring*: ordinary scoring. *Intervals*: exercise periods of 1 min and rest periods of 1 min. The players should be motivated to continuously exercise at a high intensity. If one player cannot cope with the marking of an opponent the intensity of the other players can be affected. Therefore, it is important to have players of equal ability marking each others. In order to avoid delays extra balls should be placed in the goals. Symbols as on Fig. 10.2.

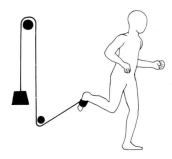

Fig. 10.9 Functional strength training — kicking exercise. A player performs kicking movements with added resistance. The resistance should be relatively low in order for the speed of the kick to be high.

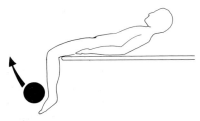

Fig. 10.10 Exercise for basic strength training of the thigh muscles (quadriceps). The player kicks forwards and upwards. The upper body should be kept still. For isometric strength training the load should be held in a given position.

can be used to improve isometric and concentric strength of the thigh muscles (quadriceps).

During the first part of a strength training period a player should train with rather low loads a couple of times per week. Before starting the more extensive strength training, baseline measurements of muscle strength should be obtained. A useful measure is the maximum load of a given movement, that can be executed for five consecutive repetitions of the movement (5 RM).

Several principles can be used in concentric strength training. Table 10.3 illustrates a principle which is based on the 5 RM determinations and which allows for muscle groups to be trained at both slow and high speeds. During an intensive strength training period new 5 RM determinations should be made about every third week so that training loads can be suitably adjusted. This is necessary in order to achieve further improvements in strength.

To utilize improvements effectively in basic muscle strength during match-play, it is important that a player, either during or after an intensive basic strength training period, frequently performs a significant amount of training with a ball.

Muscle speed endurance training

Regular football training can develop a high level of muscle speed endurance, especially for the leg muscles. For the muscles of the upper body, however, it may be beneficial to develop a higher level of anaerobic endurance. This can be obtained by speed endurance training.

The specific aims of muscle speed endurance training for football players are:
1 To improve a muscle's capacity to sustain intense exercise.
2 To improve the recovery of a muscle after intensive exercise. Thus, the muscle can perform high-intensity contractions more frequently during a game.

Principles of muscle speed endurance training. Several principles can be used for muscle speed endurance training. The exercise can be performed for a given time, e.g. 20 s, either at a fixed joint angle (isometric) or as a concentric movement at a constant frequency. The exercise should be repeated 2–4 times for each muscle group separated by rest periods of equal duration as the exercise periods. Table 10.3 shows the principle of muscle speed endurance training and Fig. 10.11 illustrates an exercise which can be used to improve the speed endurance of the oblique muscles.

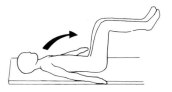

Fig. 10.11 Exercise for speed endurance training of the oblique muscles. The legs are held still in the air with the knees bent. The upper body moves upwards and turns alternatively to the left and right.

Planning of fitness training

Football players need a high level of fitness to cope with the physical demands of a game (see Chapters 3 and 4) and to allow for their technical skills to be utilized throughout a match. Therefore, fitness training is an important part of the overall training program. However, the amount of emphasis placed on fitness training depends on several factors, such as the players, competency in other areas of the game and the exercise intensity during training sessions which are not specifically designed to develop fitness.

When planning fitness training the phases of the playing season should be taken into account. A year may be divided into an off-season, a season, and a mid-season break. Table 10.4 shows how the different types of fitness training can be structured through the various periods of a year. The higher the number given, the more important is the form of training. However, it should be emphasized that there may be major deviations in the prioritization of the various aspects of fitness training due to specific demands of

a team. The structure of fitness training during the various periods of a year is briefly discussed below.

Off-season

The off-season term covers the period between the last match of one season and the first match of the next. At an élite level the duration of this period varies from 2 to 7 months, out of which 5–16 weeks may be used for preparation in the club for the following season.

After a playing season the players should regularly perform aerobic$_{LI}$ (Table 10.4). In order to help the players to relax mentally from football, parts of the training can consist of other ball games, e.g. hockey, basketball, or badminton. By maintaining a certain amount of endurance training after the end of the season, the decrease in fitness, which always occurs on cessation of normal training and competition, will be minimized. This will allow for a slow rebuilding of the players' physical capacity when training starts again in the club, and time can be spent on improving other performance characteristics in football, e.g.

Table 10.4 Prioritizing of fitness training throughout the year

	Off-season			Season			Mid-season break		Season			
Aerobic training												
Low-intensity	3344	4445	5555	4433	4343	4343	4334	4445	4343	4343	4343	4343
High-intensity	2223	3234	4445	4555	5555	5555	5443	3345	5555	5555	5555	5444
Anaerobic training												
Speed endurance	1111	1111	2234	4555	3453	4534	5431	1135	4453	4534	5345	3453
Speed	1111	1111	2234	4555	5555	5555	5552	2245	5555	5555	5555	5554
Muscle strength training												
Basic	3334	5555	5543	2222	2222	2222	2222	2222	2222	2222	2222	2222
Functional	2222	3333	3344	4343	4343	4343	4342	2234	4343	4343	4343	4322
Muscle speed training	1111	1112	3333	3333	3333	3333	3332	2233	3333	3333	3333	3333
Flexibility training	3232	3434	4444	4444	4444	4444	4443	3344	4444	4444	4444	4444

1, very low priority; 2, low priority; 3, moderate priority; 4, high priority; 5, very high priority.

technical skills. Sustaining a relatively high fitness level during the off-season will also help the players reach peak physical performance at the beginning of the season, even with a short preparation period in the club (5–6 weeks). In addition, a gradual transition between individual training out of the club and the training at the club keeps the risk of injuries low.

During the last part of the off-season it is important to play matches regularly at a high competitive level. Such matches should be supplemented by frequent sessions of aerobic$_{HI}$ training, speed training and, for élite players, speed endurance training as well.

In the first part of the off-season it is feasible to emphasize basic strength training, since the adaptations can be easily maintained. As the start of the season approaches, the amount of basic strength training should be reduced and more time should be allocated to functional strength training and playing football.

Season

Aerobic$_{HI}$ training should be given a high priority during a season (see Table 10.4). Speed training, and for top-class players, speed endurance training, should also be performed regularly. Endurance capacity may be maintained by frequently including prolonged training sessions with only short rest periods. The extent of strength training during the season should be determined by the total training time available.

Mid-season break

In some countries the season is divided into two halves. During the first part of the mid-season break when the players are not training at the club, it is important to prioritize aerobic$_{LI}$ training (see Table 10.4). By performing this type of training the players will be able to return to their previous level of endurance during the subsequent period of training at the club. The aerobic$_{LI}$ training will also facilitate the transition between the two periods and at the same time reduce the risk of injuries. Toward the start of the second half of the season high-intensity training should be emphasized.

Conclusion

The performance potential of a player can be improved by fitness training, which can be divided into aerobic training, anaerobic training, and specific muscle training. Common to all types of fitness training is the fact that the exercise performed during the training should be as similar as possible to playing football. This is one of the main reasons as to why the majority of fitness training in football should be performed with a ball. As a supplement to the general fitness training, exercises may also be designed to satisfy the individual needs of the players. Fitness training for both males and females should follow the same principles. Training for young players, prior to and during early puberty, should not be focused on the physical aspect, but should mainly emphasize technical training. For further discussion of the practical aspects of fitness training in football and additional suggestions on activities which can be used in football see Bangsbo (1994).

Reference

Bangsbo J. (1994) *Fitness Training for Football: A Scientific Approach.* HO + Storm, Bagsværd, Copenhagen, Denmark.

Chapter 11
Nutritional aspects

Nutrition is, all too often, low on the long list of priorities facing coaches and team physicians preparing players for competition. It is assumed that players have enough nutritional knowledge to eat well-balanced diets and to adjust their food and fluid intakes to cope successfully with the demands of training and playing under varying climatic conditions. For example, the long European season presents players with the challenge of training and competing under conditions which threaten them with dehydration in summer and with hypothermia in winter. Furthermore, some games are played in the afternoons while others have to be played at night.

When players are unable to complete heavy training sessions or keep up with the rest of the team then their failure is usually blamed on "lack of commitment" or in the case of professional players on "too many late nights." Rarely is the cause of underachieving linked with inadequate nutritional preparation for training. It is assumed that players know enough about the links between nutrition and sports performance not to neglect their diets. Unfortunately, for too many, the interest in nutrition is limited only to what foods can be eaten just before a game in order to gain a competitive advantage. It does not extend, however, to how ordinary foods can be used as part of nutritional strategies to prepare for and to recover quickly from competition and training. Usually the interest in nutrition increases when (a) players have a weight problem; (b) they question changes in the composition of pre-game meals; or (c) they are encouraged to eat a new "wonder food" which has been adopted by a team, usually in return for sponsorship.

Unfortunately, the information available on the influence of food and nutrition on the performance of football players, is sparse compared with the encyclopedic literature on nutrition and endurance sports

(Coggan & Coyle 1991). This may be the main reason why the role of nutrition in football has not had a high profile. Nevertheless, there are lessons we can learn from other sports on the links between foods, nutrition, and sports performance. Soccer is a running sport which demands endurance and the ability to sprint frequently with very little recovery. Therefore, the literature on the influences of nutrition on endurance and sprint sports provides a starting point for the development of a knowledge based on the contribution of nutrition to improving the performance of football players.

The aim of this chapter is, therefore, to provide the reader with enough nutritional information to understand the reasons for the dietary advice offered in the following pages and to be able to assess critically the claims for new performance-enhancing foods (ergogenic foods) which will inevitably become available to players in the future.

Food intake

Food, in all its infinite varieties, is described by nutritional science in terms of its content of macro- and micronutrients. Macronutrients are carbohydrates, fats, and proteins, whereas the micronutrients are vitamins and minerals. Water is an essential ingredient in our diets even though it is not a nutrient. Carbohydrates and fats provide fuels for energy metabolism in the form of glucose and fatty acids. Protein provides the biologic building blocks for growth and repair of all the tissues of the body. In this chapter nutrients rather than foods will be the focus of attention. To translate nutrients into foods familiar to all football players would be an impossible task because it would require relevant examples of foods from almost every country in the world. Nevertheless, it is essential that these nutritional principles are translated into foods which are familiar to players. Ideally, a dietitian should be consulted to help players choose local foods which are consistent with the nutritional strategies known to improve performance. Or at least, reference should be made to one or more of the increasing number of recipe books for sportsmen and sportswomen (e.g. Clark 1990).

Carbohydrates

Foods containing large amounts of carbohydrates include bread, potatoes, pasta, rice, and cereals. Carbohydrate is stored in skeletal muscles and liver as glycogen, a polymer of glucose. They are described in terms of the amount of glucose released during analyses namely, as millimoles (mmol) of glucosyl units per kilogram of muscle. For example, human skeletal muscle has a glycogen concentration in the range $60-150$ mmol glucosyl units$\cdot$kg^{-1} wet weight (w.w.) samples or $258-645$ mmol glucosyl units$\cdot$kg^{-1} dry weight (d.w.) samples. The size of the liver glycogen store depends on whether the person is fed or fasted. When fed, an adult man, with a liver weighing about 1.8 kg, has a liver glycogen concentration of approximately 550 mmol glucosyl units (w.w.), whereas after an overnight fast the concentration of glycogen falls to about 200 mmol. After a number of days on a high-carbohydrate diet the liver glycogen concentration can increase to as much as 1000 mmol (w.w.) (Nilsson & Hultman 1973). Interestingly, however, an overnight fast does not appear to lower muscle glycogen concentration as it does with liver glycogen (Maughan & Williams 1981). Liver glycogen is the reservoir which maintains blood glucose concentrations at optimum levels. The brain and central nervous system use approximately 120 g of blood glucose a day as their main fuel for energy production. A reduction in blood glucose concentrations to very low levels is called hypoglycemia and this condition may cause dizziness and headaches. The uptake of glucose by the liver, following the digestion and absorption of carbohydrate foods, is not under hormonal control. But the hormone insulin controls the entry of glucose into fat and muscle cells.

The recommended daily carbohydrate intake for sportsmen in training, is $60-70\%$ of their daily energy intake (Devlin & Williams 1991). However, it is worth re-examining the terms in which these recommendations are expressed. For example, the recommendation that our daily carbohydrate intake should be $500-600$ g (Costill & Miller 1980) is applicable for men but not for women. It is inappropriate for women because it is equivalent to the whole of their daily energy intake. Therefore, a more useful way of prescribing daily carbohydrate intake is one based on body weight, i.e. an amount of carbohydrate per kilogram of body weight. This approach leads to less confusion and is more precise than the general guidance offered to the population as a whole. As an illustration of this point, in Table 11.1, the carbohydrate intake of professional football players, reported by Jacobs *et al.* (1982), is equivalent to 47% of their daily energy intakes, whereas the values for distance runners is 53% of their daily energy intakes. When the carbohydrate intake of the two groups are expressed in terms of their body weights, then the value for the professional football players is equivalent to 8 g$\cdot$kg^{-1} body weight$\cdot$day^{-1}, whereas, the value for the endurance runners is equivalent to 6 g$\cdot$kg^{-1} body weight$\cdot$day^{-1}. And, of course, the replenishment of glycogen stores after exercise is related to the absolute amount of carbohydrate consumed rather than the percentage of energy intake it represents for any individual.

Fat

Our main source of fat intake is from dairy products such as butter, cheese, and milk. But fat in foods is difficult to avoid because it is present in many fresh foods and an ingredient in almost all processed and pre-prepared foods.

Fat is stored in the body in fat cells of which there are two types, namely white adipose tissue (WAT) and brown adipose tissue (BAT) cells. In these cells, fat is stored as triglycerides. The triglycerides are made up of free fatty acids (FFAs) and glycerol and are found in muscle as well as in adipose tissue cells. WAT cells are the long-term storage sites for fat and it is from these cells that fatty acids are mobilized for use as metabolic fuels for energy metabolism. BAT, on the other hand, is believed to be important only for very young children under conditions which stimulate cold-induced thermogenesis. It has no real physiological significance in adults because the amount of brown fat is almost insignificant in relation to the abundance of white fat.

Hydrolysis or splitting up triglycerides releases FFAs and glycerol in a ratio of three FFAs to one glycerol molecule. The FFAs are transported to other tissues, such as skeletal muscle, in loose combination with a plasma protein called albumin. The amount of FFAs taken up by working muscles is dictated by their plasma concentration and the blood flow to the tissue (Gollnick 1977). However, the FFAs are not necess-

Table 11.1 Energy, protein, fat, and carbohydrate (CHO) intakes of endurance runners and football players

Group	Season	Energy (kcal) (kJ)	Protein (g) (%)	Fat (g) (%)	CHO (g) (%)	Reference
Distance runners ($n = 50$)	In-season	3170 (13 314)	114 (14)	116 (33)	417 (53)	L. Piearce & C. Williams (unpublished data)
Football players ($n = 8$)	In-season	4952 (20 798)	170 (14)	217 (39)	596 (47)	Jacobs *et al.* (1982)
Football players ($n = 18$)	Pre-season	4492 (18 866)	159 (14)	168 (34)	586 (52)	Hickson *et al.* (1986)
Football players ($n = 18$)	In-season	3346 (14 053)	201 (17)	138 (37)	389 (46)	Hickson *et al.* (1986)
Football players ($n = 8$)	In-season	3392 (14 246)	127 (16)	127 (35)	400 (49)	L. Piearce & C. Williams (unpublished data)

arily used immediately they are taken up by active muscles because their oxidation is controlled by the oxidative capacity of the muscles (Gollnick 1977). The oxidative capacity of a muscle is dictated by the number of mitochondria they have available to use the FFAs offered to them (see Chapter 4). Those FFAs which are not immediately oxidized in the mitochondria are stored as triglycerides in the muscle. These pools of triglycerides increase with training and decrease during prolonged exercise (Jansson & Kaijser 1987). While there is a greater amount of energy produced from aerobic metabolism of FFAs than from the aerobic metabolism of an equal amount of carbohydrate, the rate of production is slower from FFAs than from glycogen (McGilvery 1975). It is important to remember that the limitation to fat metabolism is not its mobilization or transport nor, during submaximal exercise, the supply of oxygen, but the limited number of mitochondria in skeletal muscles available to oxidize this high energy fuel (Golnick 1977).

In addition to it's role as a fuel, fat is also important as a storage site for the fat soluble vitamins A, D, E,

and K. It also provides padding to protect internal organs of the body. There are essential fatty acids (EFA) which must be part of our diets, if we are to maintain good health. The EFA linoleic acid and linolenic acid are essential constituents of cell membranes, especially nerve tissue. About 1−2% of our total energy intake should come from EFA.

The average man has about 15% of his body weight as fat whereas, the equivalent value for a lean woman is about 20%. Professional football players have a lower than average body fat content (Davis *et al.* 1992). Midfield players have values of 10% whereas, goalkeepers are heavier and have about 13% of their body weight as fat (Davis *et al.* 1992). A relatively large proportion of this stored fat is available as a fuel both during rest and during exercise. Weight for weight, fat provides twice the energy we obtain from carbohydrate oxidation (see "Energy balance" below).

Protein

Meats, fish, and eggs are the main contributors of

protein to our diets but we also derive some protein from foods containing cereals and vegetables. Proteins, unlike carbohydrates and fat, are not designed to be fuels for energy production because proteins are part of the structure of every cell in the body. They are also part of hormones and enzymes which contribute to the regulation of energy production and the general health of the individual.

All proteins are made up from an infinite combination of only 20 amino acids. They are the building blocks of the body and, as such, far too valuable to be used as fuels for energy production. Nevertheless, there are occasions when amino acids have to be used in this uneconomic way. When the body's carbohydrate stores are low, amino acids are oxidized in skeletal muscle as a contribution to adenosine triphosphate (ATP) resynthesis.

Of the 20 amino acids, eight are essential or indispensable. They cannot be manufactured by the body and so they must be part of our diets (Table 11.2). Proteins in meat, eggs, and fish, contain all the essential amino acids and so these foods have "high biological value." Cereals and vegetables contain proteins with only a few of the essential amino acids and so individually they are of low biological value, however, they still contribute to our protein intake, even though it is less than meals containing either meat, eggs, or fish. Combining several foods of low biological value is a method of obtaining all the essential amino acids in one meal and is a dietary strategy used by vegetarians.

Many sportsmen and sportswomen share the same beliefs as the first Olympians about the beneficial values of high protein diets. There is a long held, but misguided, belief that athletes who want to develop strength must consume large quantities of meat. Although protein is an essential part of our diet it should only contribute about 15% or less to our daily

energy intake. Even sedentary people eat enough meat, eggs, and fish to cover their daily protein requirements. The World Health Organization (WHO 1985) recommends a daily protein intake of 1 g of protein per kilogram of body weight. The daily protein intakes of even female endurance athletes, who are not normally preoccupied with gaining strength, is about 1.5 g per kilogram of body weight and so well above the WHO recommendations. The WHO recommendations are, however, too low for athletes who are involved in prolonged heavy training (Lemon 1991). Their daily intake should be the equivalent of 1.2–1.7 g of protein per kilogram of body weight. One of the consequences of eating more meat, however, is that it can increase fat intake, especially some red meats. Most sportspeople, including football players, try to avoid gaining excess body fat. Therefore, choosing lean meats, such as white meat, reduces the daily fat intake and so helps avoid gaining body fat. In addition, eating less fat has the added advantage that it allows us to eat more carbohydrate at each meal.

Vitamins

The micronutrients, namely vitamins and minerals, are only needed in very small quantities. They are not fuels for energy metabolism, but their presence enables the body's many complex biochemical reactions to occur smoothly to sustain healthy and active tissues. Eating a wide variety of foods, especially fresh fruit and vegetables, ensures that we have a sufficient supply of vitamins to cover the needs of all cellular activities. The vitamins are classified as either fat soluble or water soluble and a summary of their roles and the foods in which they are found are shown in Tables 11.3 and 11.4. In the Western world, vitamin deficiency is rare in people who eat a varied diet containing plenty of fresh foods. The people at risk of nutrient deficiency are those who follow fad diets which have a low nutrient and energy content.

Minerals

Minerals are also essential for healthy and active lives and are described as either major or trace minerals (trace elements) according to their contribution to our long-term health. A summary of their contributions to normal functions of the body, along with examples of

Table 11.2 The essential amino acids

Isoleucine	Phenylalanine
Leucine	Threonine
Lysine	Tryptophan
(Histidine for children)	Valine
Methionine	

Table 11.3 Fat soluble vitamins, their main functions, and foods which are good sources of these vitamins

Vitamin	Main function	Sources
A	Essential for vision in dim light; necessary for skin and growth, also for maintenance of mucous membranes	Milk, butter, cheese, fortified margarine, egg yolk, liver, and fatty fish, as retinol; carrots, dark green vegetables, tomatoes, as carotenes
D	Promotes the absorption of calcium and phosphate from food and is therefore essential for bones and teeth	Sunshine on skin, fortified margarine, oily fish, egg yolk, fortified breakfast cereals
E	An anti-oxidant, protects cell membranes from damage by the products of oxidation	Vegetable oils, nuts, vegetables, cereals
K	Essential for the formation of proteins involved in blood clotting, especially prothrombin	It is synthesized by bacteria in the gastrointestinal tract; dark green leafy vegetables: cabbage, sprouts, spinach, cauliflower

the types of foods in which they are found, are shown in Tables 11.5 and 11.6. The minerals not shown in these tables, but which are also essential parts of a healthy diet are chloride, molybdenum, manganese, boron, nickel, lithium, aluminium, lead, and antimony. The precise nature of the role of these trace elements are not so well known as are the contributions of the major minerals to human metabolism.

There are no good reasons to recommend vitamin and mineral supplements for football players who eat a wide range of foods in sufficient quantity to cover their energy expenditures. Neither is there any good evidence to suggest that vitamin (Van de Beek 1991) and mineral (Clarkson 1991) supplements improve exercise capacity. There are, however, some people who may be at risk. Sportswomen may have inadequate iron and calcium intakes, especially when they are trying to lose body weight by reducing their daily energy intakes. Furthermore, women of child-bearing age must ensure that they have an increased intake of folic acid, one of the B vitamins. An inadequate intake of this particular vitamin is linked with neural tube defects in children, such as spina bifida. Many breakfast cereals and some breads have folate and folic acid; as well as other vitamins and minerals added to them. Therefore, even if the diet is low on fresh fruit and

vegetables for short periods of time the vitamins and minerals in many fortified foods can help cover the shortfall in intake of these essential ingredients of a healthy diet. If our energy intake is too low, then even a well-balanced diet, made up of a wide range of foods, will not provide enough of the essential nutrients to sustain healthy recovery, growth, and repair of tissues. Therefore, there is a danger that missing meals, because of the demands of a busy life style and heavy training, can lead to undernourished, underachieving football players.

Energy balance

One of the most frequently asked questions in nutrition is "How much should I eat to stay fit and healthy?" Of course, the prescription for good health is the same for everyone whether or not they participate in sport. A healthy diet is one in which over half of the daily energy intake is provided by carbohydrate-containing foods, less than a third from fat, and the remainder of our food intake should come from proteins. The amount of food we eat each day should be sufficient to match our energy expenditure. Ideally, we should be in energy balance, but the amount we should eat

Table 11.4 Water soluble vitamins, their main functions, and foods which are good sources of these vitamins

Vitamin	Main function	Sources
C	Aids wound healing and iron absorption; involved in the formation of collagen which is a protein used in the structure of connective tissues and bone	Fresh fruits especially citrus fruits and green vegetables; it is also found in potatoes
Thiamin (B_1)	Involved in energy production from carbohydrates; important for central nervous system which uses glucose for energy metabolism	Cereals, nuts, pulses are good sources; green vegetables, roots, pork, fruits, fortified breakfast cereals
Riboflavin	Involved in the release of energy, especially from fat and protein	Good sources are found in liver, milk, cheese, yoghurt, eggs, green vegetables, yeast extract, fortified breakfast cereals
Niacin	Involved in the release of energy from carbohydrates and fats	Good sources are found in liver, beef, pork, mutton, meat, fish, yeast extracts; also found in fortified breakfast cereals and instant coffee
B_{12}	Necessary for the formation of blood cells and nerve fibres	Good sources are offal and meat, eggs, milk; almost no plant foods contain B_{12}; also found in fortified breakfast cereals
Folate	Involved in the formation of red blood cells and essential substances such as the genetic material DNA	Liver, dark green vegetables, e.g. broccoli, spinach; nuts, wholemeal bread, oranges, rice, fortified breakfast cereals

depends on several factors, not only the amount of exercise we take each day. Therefore, it is helpful to consider more fully the concept of energy balance because it will provide the basis for a sound understanding of the essential elements in the formulae for weight loss and weight gain.

Energy intake and energy expenditure are expressed in terms of kilocalories (kcal), or more correctly, kilojoules (kJ). These are units of heat (1 kcal = 4.2 kJ) because the laboratory methods used to assess the energy contents of foods involve measuring the heat released during their complete combustion (Jequier & Schutz 1983). Therefore, food intake and energy expenditure are commonly described in terms of kilocalories. For example, the complete oxidation of 1 g of fat yields 9 kcal (37.6 kJ) whereas the oxidative metabolism of 1 g of carbohydrate (glucose) yields only 4.0 kcal (17 kJ).

When the amount of food we eat provides sufficient energy to match our energy expenditure, then we should neither gain nor lose weight because we are in energy balance. This is often described in terms of the following simple equation:

energy intake = energy expenditure ± energy stored.

One of the mistaken assumptions of many people, especially adolescents, is that they will gain weight (i.e. fat) whenever they eat and are not active. This assumption often leads to an inappropriate reduction in food intake, a reduction in body weight but more importantly a decrease in the capacity to train hard. What is often overlooked is that energy expenditure is made up of three components:

1 Basal metabolic rate (BMR).
2 The thermic effect of food intake (TEF), which is the energy expended on digestion, absorption, and storage

Table 11.5 Major minerals, their main functions, and foods which are good sources of these minerals

Mineral	Main function	Sources
Calcium	Formation and maintenance of bones, teeth; involved in blood clotting, nerve function and contraction of muscles	Milk, cheese, yoghurt, canned fish are rich sources; also in dark green leafy vegetables, white flour, bread
Sodium	Involved in the nerve function and in the regulation of fluid balance	Salt, either added to food during preparation or added to the meal at the table
Potassium	A constituent of all cells and involved in all neural activity in the body	In all foods except sugars, fats, oils; raw foods have more potassium than processed foods
Magnesium	Involved in the release of energy in cells, in activity of enzymes and contractile activity of muscles	In most foods, whole-grain cereals, nuts, spinach are particularly good sources
Phosphorous	Present in bone and in teeth and an essential component of all cells of the body	Good sources are milk, cheese, eggs, meat, fish

Table 11.6 Trace minerals, their main functions, and foods which are good sources of these minerals

Mineral	Main function	Sources
Zinc	Essential for growth and repair of tissue cells, sexual maturation, involved in enzyme activity, taste, perception	Milk, cheese, eggs, meat, fish, whole-grain cereals, pulses
Iodine	Involved in the formation of thyroid hormones	Milk, seafood, seaweed; iodine-fortified foods such as salt
Fluoride	Increases the resistance of teeth to decay	Tea, fish, fluoridated water, toothpaste
Selenium	An anti-oxidant, protects cell membranes against damage by free radicals	Cereals, meat, fish offal, cheese, eggs
Copper	Intrinsic part of many enzyme systems also enables the body to use iron effectively	Good sources include fish, green vegetables, liver
Chromium	Involved in the action of insulin and so the control of carbohydrate and fat metabolism	Good sources include nuts, prunes, dark green vegetables, green peas, vegetable oils, corn, orange juice
Iron	Present in hemoglobin in red blood cells; involved in enzyme activity and energy production in mitochondria	Red meat and offal are good sources of iron; bread, cereals, flour and vegetables contain some iron; some breakfast cereals are fortified with iron

of foods and it amounts to about 10% of the daily energy intake.

3 The energy (thermic) cost of exercise (TEE), which includes the daily round of normal activities as well as the cost of training or playing football.

The basal metabolic rate demands about two-thirds of our daily energy intake to cover all the domestic activities of the body. Therefore, it accounts for the largest part of our daily energy expenditure. The BMR for people in the age range 18−30 years can be estimated from the following equations (WHO 1985):

males: BMR (kcal/24 h) = 17.5 W + 651
$\quad$ BMR (kJ/24 h) $\quad$ = 73.5 W + 2734;

females: BMR (kcal/24 h) = 14.7 W + 496
$\quad$ BMR (kJ/24 h) $\quad$ = 61.8 W + 2083

where W is body weight in kilograms.

Using these equations, along with a few assumptions about levels of physical activity, the daily energy expenditure of players can be estimated. This information is useful in providing advice about the amount of food players should eat to cover their energy expenditures. Ideally, the time spent in different activities, throughout the day, should be recorded for each player for several days. Then their calculated BMR values are multiplied by the appropriate physical activity levels (PAL).

PAL, as multiples of BMR, have been calculated for different types of activity. Football has a PAL value of 7.5. The PAL value for someone who has very little activity is 1.3 and so their daily energy expenditure and intake would be 1.3 × BMR. This is, however, equivalent to the minimum amount of food we need for survival and provides enough energy for only essential movements (WHO 1985). Men who have a moderate level of activity would have a PAL value of 1.7 whereas, the equivalent value for women would be 1.6 (HMSO 1991). For most people, participating in football, whether as professionals or as recreational players, is the most exercise they get in a day. Therefore, when they are not playing or training they probably have life styles which have only moderate amounts of additional activity. Thus the amount of time spent expending large amounts of energy are probably small when averaged out over the whole day. A physical activity factor of about 1.6−1.7 can be used, as a guide to assessing the daily energy expenditures and intakes

of men. For example, a male 70 kg midfield player would have a BMR of 1876 kcal·day^{-1} (7879 kJ·day^{-1}) (17.5 times body weight plus 651) (WHO 1985). Assuming an average daily activity level equivalent to 1.7, then his energy expenditure would be approximately 3189 kcal (13 394 kJ) (plus 10% for TEF), i.e. approximately 3500 kcal·day^{-1} (14 700 kJ·day^{-1}). Therefore, in order to maintain a constant body weight and cover his energy expenditure he should eat about 3500 kcal (14 700 kJ) a day. Equivalent activity values for female football players would be between 1.5 and 1.6, from which their energy expenditures and intakes can be calculated in a similar manner.

A simpler approach to assessing whether or not a player is achieving energy balance is to record body weight on a weekly basis. The stability of the body weight of a player is a useful guide to the adequacy of food intake, especially in an environment were food is freely available. However, body weight alone is a poor indicator of body composition. Players can, for example, gain body weight without becoming fatter because their muscle mass has increased. Similarly, players can lose body weight while increasing their body fat content because their loss of lean mass is greater than the gain in fat mass. Therefore, some routine assessment of body composition, such as skinfold measurements, along with dietary assessment are helpful as additional methods of monitoring the total fitness of players (Davis et al. 1992).

The ideal way of assessing the average daily energy intake of players is for them to weigh and record all the food and drink they consume for a week. Dietary analysis of these records provide a good description of the players energy intakes which includes not only information about the daily consumption of macronutrients, carbohydrates, fats, and proteins, but also details about the vitamin and mineral intakes. This procedure is, however, tedious and only highly motivated people will persist with accurate record keeping for several days. Therefore, many studies have used information gathered from 3 or 4 days of dietary records where, in many instances the food intake was estimated rather than weighed. Useful as this information is, it can only provide a snapshot of the energy intake and the composition of the diet over the period of observation. Nevertheless, without dietary records of food intake, it is virtually impossible to assess whether or not individuals involved in sport are eating the quality and quantity of foods necessary to support their active and healthy life styles. Therefore, even a simple dietary record covering no more than 3 days is a helpful screening method to ensure that players are not following fad diets or routinely skipping meals.

There are, unfortunately, too few studies on the energy intakes of football players and so it is difficult to generalize about their nutritional status. But those that are available show that although their energy intakes are larger than those of the general population, they are not as large as they are imagined to be. For example, the energy intakes of Dutch professional football players has been reported to be 3373 kcal·day^{-1} (14 099 kJ·day^{-1}) (van Erp-Baart *et al.* 1989), which is similar to values reported for English and American players (see Table 11.1). But these values are less than the energy intakes of 4952 kcal (20 699 kJ) reported for a group of Swedish professional football players (Jacobs *et al.* 1982). By way of comparison, recent nutritional surveys show that British men consume each day the equivalent of 2450 kcal (10 241 kJ) (Gregory *et al.* 1990). Whereas, the daily value for American men is 2667 kcal (11 148 kJ) (Grandjean 1989).

The amount of food players eat is also a function of the environment in which they live and train. In training camps, for example, regular meals are provided for players and so their food intake may be greater than when they have to prepare their own meals. Some evidence for this change in the energy intakes of football players was provided by Hickson *et al.* (1989).

They showed that there was a marked reduction in the energy intakes of college football players during the competitive season when they were living on their own and faced with the task of providing their own meals (see Table 11.1). Whether or not this decrease in energy intake during the season is a common phenomenon, remains to be established.

It is important to recognize how much of our energy intake we obtain from foods eaten between meals, i.e. snacks. For example, the distribution of energy intake throughout the day for a group of young amateur football players is shown in Fig. 11.1 — the snacks account for 22% of their daily energy intakes. This pattern of eating is a useful strategy for achieving energy balance. During periods of heavy training players may not be able to tolerate large meals before or immediately after training and so eating small snacks, made from high-carbohydrate foods, or ingesting carbohydrate-containing drinks throughout the day is one way of ensuring that neither energy intake nor training capacity suffers.

For most people, there are only rare occasions when energy intake must match energy expenditure on a daily basis. Energy balance is necessary, however, for those sportspeople who have to compete, or train hard, on a daily basis for several days at a time. Professional cyclists, such as those who compete in the Tour de France, need to restore their energy reserves on a daily basis for 2–3 weeks. They are able to achieve energy balance, averaged over a few days by supplementing their meals with high-carbohydrate drinks and snacks between meals (Brouns *et al.* 1989).

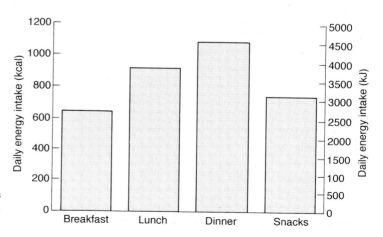

Fig. 11.1 Daily energy intakes of football players from meals and snacks (L. Piearce & C. Williams unpublished data).

Weight loss

When players try to lose body weight quickly by reducing their food intake, especially at the beginning of the competitive season, they encounter several problems. It is the time of the year when training is prolonged and most intense. Therefore, failure to achieve the appropriate energy and fluid intake leads to a gradual reduction in the player's capacity to train hard. This, in turn, casts doubt on the suitability of the individual for team selection. Players with weight problems should decrease their fat intake by paying particular attention to the composition of the foods they eat in order to avoid the consumption of too much fat. Fat is not only present in obviously fatty foods such as dairy products and fatty types of meat but it is also a hidden ingredient in many foods which first appear to be high in carbohydrate such as cakes, doughnuts, and chocolates; furthermore fat, in the form of cooking oil, is used worldwide for cooking even fresh foods low in fat. Decreasing the daily amount of fat eaten also enables players to eat more carbohydrate before they feel full and so they should be able to continue to train hard, while at the same time reducing their body fat content. Changing the composition of the diet is the key to successful weight loss for those who are training hard. It is in the selection of the appropriate foods to replace high-fat foods that players can benefit from the help of a sports dietitian. Using a menu of "food exchanges" players can be guided in their choice of foods so that they eat less of the high fat containing foods and still achieve the right energy intake to match their energy expenditure.

In practice a weight loss of no more than $1\,kg \cdot week^{-1}$ is generally recommended by health professionals. To achieve this loss of fat there are a couple of options open to players. One is to reduce daily energy intake by 1000 kcal (4180 kJ) a day for a week. Another is to increase energy expenditure by a 1000 kcal (4180 kJ) a day while keeping energy intake constant. A third option is to increase energy expenditure by about 500 kcal (2090 kJ) and decrease energy intake by about the same amount. Of course, a weight loss of less than 1 kg a week is an easier goal to achieve but a program which can become part of the life style of the individual is the preferable way of reducing body fat. One of the responsibilities of coaches and team doctors, which is too frequently overlooked, is the education of players about the consequences of energy imbalance when their playing days are over. Players who continue to eat more or less the same amounts of food when they no longer train hard, or even play football as a recreational sport, will inevitably increase their body fat and decrease their muscle mass. Therefore, they should be told about the health risks associated with increases in body fat.

Carbohydrate intake and performance

The early laboratory studies of Christensen and Hansen (1939) over half a century ago established the link between a high-carbohydrate diet and improvements in exercise capacity. They showed that their subject's cycling time to exhaustion was twice as long after they had consumed a high-carbohydrate diet for 3–4 days than when they exercised to exhaustion after a period on their normal mixed diets. Building on these early studies, Bergström and Hultman (1966) showed how a high-carbohydrate diet immediately after exercise increased muscle glycogen stores to values that are higher than those recorded before exercise. They were the first to make direct measurements of glycogen concentrations in skeletal muscles, using a needle biopsy technique, before and after exercise and confirmed the central role of this carbohydrate store as a fuel for energy production during prolonged exercise (Hultman 1967).

There are now abundant laboratory-based studies showing that endurance capacity during cycling is improved following dietary carbohydrate loading (Coggan & Coyle 1991) and although the evidence for improvements in running performance is not as extensive, it is nevertheless just as convincing. There are also several field studies directly or indirectly relevant to football which support the recommendations from laboratory studies that increasing the carbohydrate content of the diet improves performance. It is now clear, for example, that football players who start a game with low muscle glycogen concentrations perform less well than those who have normal stores of carbohydrate before competition. Saltin (1973) showed, using film analysis of an exhibition match, that a group of players with low muscle glycogen concentrations before the game ran less and had lower average speeds than a control group of players. The physical demands of football cause significant reductions in the muscle glycogen stores of players (Jacobs *et al.* 1982). Therefore, there is clearly a need to ensure that muscle glycogen stores are restocked before competition if fatigue during the second half of a game is to be delayed.

Bangsbo *et al.* (1992) examined this nutritional advice by using a field test that simulated the activity pattern of football players, for 45 min, and then monitored their ability to complete multiple sprints on a laboratory treadmill after carbohydrate loading. The professional football players ran 0.9 km further (16.2 vs. 17.1 km) during the multiple sprint test, after carbohydrate loading, than when they performed the test after consuming their normal mixed diets.

An increase in carbohydrate intake can also be achieved, to good effect, by supplementing food intake with glucose drinks. Muckle (1973) reported an increase in the number of goals scored when players had their normal diets supplemented with a glucose syrup solution (46%) during the day before the game and again 30 min before competition. The glucose syrup supplementation was provided for a team of professional players for 20 matches while the remaining 20 matches of the season were used as control. The number of goals scored in the second half of each game increased and there was a reduction in the number of goals conceded. Contact time with the ball also increased during the period when the team were receiving the glucose syrup.

Evidence that the ingestion of a glucose polymer solution improves players' work-rates during a football match has also been provided by Kirkendall *et al.* (1988). They filmed a game in which a group of players consumed a concentrated carbohydrate solution (*c.* 15.5%) before the game and at half-time. The players who consumed the carbohydrate solution covered more ground during the second half of the game than those players who consumed a sweet placebo solution. Indirectly the results of this study confirm the benefits of consuming additional carbohydrate before a game, reported by Muckle (1973) 15 years earlier.

Some clue to the mechanism(s) responsible for the improvements in performance after consuming additional carbohydrate was reported in a recent study. When players consumed 0.5 l of a 7% glucose solution 10 min before a match and at half-time, the decreases in their muscle glycogen concentrations were less than those in a control group of players who consumed only water (Leatt & Jacobs 1989). This glycogen sparing effect would be a distinct advantage because players could run longer before reduced muscle glycogen contents forced them to reduce their work-rates.

Recovery

Recovery from training and competition is particularly important during football tournaments, especially when there are only a few days between games. Not only is the amount of carbohydrate consumed by football players important, but the type and timing of carbohydrate intake must also be considered as part of a nutritional strategy to improve the rate of recovery from exercise (Coyle 1991). Appropriate nutritional intervention can help optimize the recovery process by ensuring that glycogen stores are restocked as soon as possible.

The results of the Bergström and Hultman study (1966) and others have been used as the bases of methods for carbohydrate or glycogen loading prior to prolonged exercise (Åstrand 1967). The recommendations offered by these early studies are that skeletal muscle glycogen concentrations should first be depleted by prolonged exercise. For the next 3 days the muscle's glycogen stores should be kept low by avoiding eating carbohydrate-containing foods. This means increasing the consumption of protein and fats in order not to decrease overall energy intake. This period is then followed by 3 days on a high-carbohydrate diet (Åstrand 1967). Glycogen supercompensation is achieved by this exercise and dietary manipulation, however, the 3 days on a low-carbohydrate diet is not a pleasant experience and most people feel less than "fit" during this period. As more studies have been carried out on the glycogen loading procedures it has become clear that the original recommendations are now unnecessary. The more recent studies recommend simply tapering training during the week before competition and increasing the carbohydrate intake during the 3 days before the event (Sherman *et al.* 1981). Of course, players who are training frequently should have a diet which is high in carbohydrate. A day or two of rest or light training and their normal high-carbohydrate diet should be sufficient for players to restock their glycogen stores.

The most rapid restocking of glycogen stores occurs

during the first few hours after exercise (Piehl 1974). During this early recovery period the membranes of muscle cells appear to be more permeable to glucose than before exercise. Therefore, to take advantage of these favorable conditions for glycogen resynthesis, it is obviously important to eat foods that will provide glucose quickly immediately after exercise (Robergs 1991).

Foods that increase blood glucose concentrations rapidly are not always the obvious ones. For example, bread is generally regarded as a complex carbohydrate and sugar as a simple carbohydrate, but the increases they produce in blood glucose concentrations are quite similar. A method has been developed for classifying foods in relation to the changes in blood glucose they produce called the glycemic index (GI), and the standard is 50 g of white bread, which has a GI reference value of 100 (Coyle 1991). Glucose has also been used as a standard but concern over whether or not all the glucose clears the stomach has favored the use of bread (Wolever *et al.* 1991).

Ivy (1991) showed that subjects who drank a carbohydrate solution which provided the equivalent of 2 g·kg^{-1} body weight of carbohydrate immediately after prolonged heavy exercise had a glycogen resynthesis rate 300% greater than normal values. However, when the post-exercise carbohydrate intake was delayed for 2 h then the rate of glycogen resynthesis was 47% slower. Blom *et al.* (1987) found that the maximum rate of glycogen resynthesis occurred when their subjects consumed 0.7 g·kg^{-1} body weight every 2 h, during the first 6 h of recovery. Therefore, the optimum amount of carbohydrate needed to maximize rapid restocking of muscle glycogen stores is about 1.0 g·kg^{-1} body weight (Robergs 1991). When this prescription is followed there is an improvement in performance. Runners who drank a carbohydrate–electrolyte solution to provide the equivalent 1.0 g·kg^{-1} body weight of carbohydrate immediately after completing a 90-min treadmill run, at 70% $V_{O_{2max.}}$, were able to run a further 62 min after 4 h of recovery. In contrast, a control group, who drank an equivalent volume of sweetened water during the 4-h recovery period could only complete 40 min of treadmill running (J. Fallowfield & C. Williams unpublished data). Therefore, carbohydrate ingestion immediately after exercise does improve recovery. All published studies to date, on rapidly replacing glycogen stores after

exercise, have used carbohydrate-containing solutions rather than solid foods. Fluids have the advantage of not only providing glucose rapidly but they also help replace the water lost as sweat during exercise. Furthermore, carbohydrate-containing fluids are often more acceptable than solid foods, after exercise, because they are more palatable and more easily accessible.

Increasing the carbohydrate content of the diet of players is absolutely essential if they need to fully recover in 24 h. If they are left to decide how much food they need during this recovery period, then experience shows that they will not eat enough carbohydrate. Even if they eat exactly the same amount of foods during the recovery period as they would normally consume, this is still not enough to restore their exercise capacity in 24 h. Fallowfield and Williams (1993) showed that runners were unable to reproduce a 90-min training run when they consumed their normal daily amount of carbohydrate, plus extra energy in the form of protein and fat. But the runners who increased their carbohydrate intakes from their normal intake values of 6 to 9 g·kg^{-1} body weight were able to complete the standard 90 min training run. The type of carbohydrate used to supplement a normal mixed diet does not seem to matter. Brewer *et al.* (1988) showed that runners who supplemented their normal diets with either simple or complex carbohydrates improved their endurance capacity by 25% after only a 3-day recovery period. The simple carbohydrates used to supplement the runner's diets were chocolate bars, whereas the complex carbohydrate supplements were extra bread, pasta, potatoes, and rice. Therefore, for relatively short recovery periods foods containing predominantly simple or complex carbohydrates are equally effective in improving endurance capacity.

There are some studies on the changes in muscle glycogen concentrations of players after competition but very few which have also studied changes in performance. Jacobs *et al.* (1982) reported changes in muscle glycogen concentrations of professional football players during the 24-h after a league game. Their study showed that the lower the muscle glycogen concentrations were at the end of the game, the greater the amount of glycogen replaced in 24 h (Fig. 11.2) confirming the predictions of the early laboratory studies (Bergström & Hultman 1966). There were,

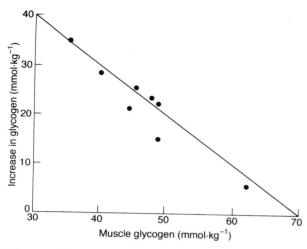

Fig. 11.2 Changes in muscle glycogen concentrations, during 24-h recovery after a football match, in relation to post-match muscle glycogen concentrations of professional players (after Jacobs *et al.* 1982).

however, only modest increases in muscle glycogen concentrations after the 24 h recovery period, even though the players increased their carbohydrate intakes. This may have been the consequence of a delay in consuming the additional carbohydrate intake or the result of other factors known to delay glycogen resynthesis. Muscle fibers that experience some damage as a result of direct injury or an excessive amount of unaccustomed exercise, or simply unusually hard training, do not restock their glycogen stores as quickly as expected (Costill *et al.* 1990). In contrast, even though each gram of glycogen is stored with about 3 g of water (Olsson & Saltin 1970), dehydration does not appear to inhibit glycogen resynthesis (Neufer *et al.* 1991).

Nutritional recommendations for training and competition

It is important to remember that the most effective contribution of nutrition to improved performance is not, as often believed, the pre-match meal but the long-term nutritional support of training. Training improves performance when it includes exercise of the appropriate mixture of intensity, duration, and frequency. Heavy training of long duration causes dehydration and lowers the body's carbohydrate

stores. Failure to recover from heavy training means that the essential contribution of frequency of training, to the process of adaptation, is lost. Therefore, to sustain high-quality training every day for several days, players must eat enough carbohydrate to restock muscle and liver glycogen stores and drink sufficient fluids to ensure rehydration. In order to put this recommendation into practice the social habits of players may have to be modified because they may be contributing to their own dehydration.

Ideally, training programs should include days of light training, as active recovery, after days of heavy training. This type of preparation allows players to recover from minor injuries and to replenish their carbohydrate stores without unnecessary intrusion into their normal eating habits. When daily recovery is essential then the food and fluid intake of players should be prescribed and monitored to ensure that the nutritional preparation is effective in achieving recovery and avoiding the effects of residual fatigue.

Recovery in 24 h will occur if players eat foods which provide them with the equivalent of about $10\,g\cdot kg^{-1}$ body weight of carbohydrate. In order to achieve this target and to make the most of the rapid rate of glycogen replacement after exercise, players should drink carbohydrate-containing solutions immediately they return to the changing rooms and even before they shower. Their carbohydrate intake should be at least $1\,g\cdot kg^{-1}$ body weight every 2 h until their next meal. Because the bulkiness of many carbohydrate-containing foods may prevent players eating the amount prescribed, then high-density carbohydrate foods and beverages can be used to meet the dietary recommendations for recovery. Small snacks of high-carbohydrate foods can be eaten throughout the recovery period and this helps avoid the abdominal discomfort which can occur when large meals are consumed. Under normal circumstances, snacks contribute a significant amount to the daily carbohydrate intake. By way of illustration, Fig. 11.3 shows the amount of carbohydrate consumed during the three main meals and snacks of a group of eight football players. Snacks consumed between meals provided 22% of their daily carbohydrate intake. There is, of course, no reason why snacks should not contribute more to our daily energy intake, especially if they are in the form of high-carbohydrate, low-fat foods.

Drinking concentrated glucose solutions less than

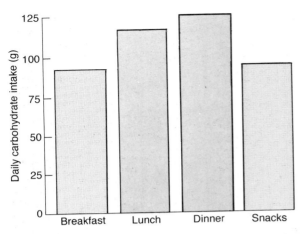

Fig. 11.3 Daily carbohydrate intakes of football players from meals and snacks (L. Piearce & C. Williams unpublished data).

an hour before training or competition has been discouraged because of evidence which appeared to show that this practice reduces endurance capacity (Foster *et al.* 1979). When you drink a concentrated glucose solution it first produces a large increase in blood glucose which is followed by an increase in insulin. Insulin is the hormone which controls the entry of glucose into fat and muscle cells. Therefore, the large increase in this anabolic hormone is followed by a rapid fall in blood glucose concentration, often to such low concentrations that they are classified as hypoglycemic. One of the other consequences of the rise in insulin concentrations is that it decreases the release of FFAs from fat cells. It has been suggested that this will decrease the availability of FFAs for energy production and so lead to an increase in glycogen degradation as compensation (Foster *et al.* 1979). A greater rate of glycogen utilization will, of course, lead to an earlier loss of this fuel and to a more rapid onset of fatigue.

More recent studies show that endurance running capacity is unaffected by consuming a concentrated glucose solution 30 min before exercise to exhaustion (Coyle 1991). Furthermore, when blood glucose concentrations fall briefly, during the early part of prolonged exercise, they are not detected by the runners nor is exercise regarded as being harder compared to conditions in which blood glucose concentrations are

normal. Therefore, the predicted detrimental effects, on exercise capacity, of the "insulin overshoot" as it has been called, does not occur. Nevertheless, drinking concentrated glucose solutions within the hour before exercise is not the best way to obtain rapid absorption and assimilation of carbohydrates. Dilute solutions are emptied from the stomach more quickly and assimilated more rapidly than concentrated carbohydrate solutions (Noakes *et al.* 1991). Drinking dilute carbohydrate beverages immediately before and during endurance races improves performance times by maintaining blood glucose concentrations and supplementing the limited glycogen stores in skeletal muscles (Tsintzas *et al.* 1993).

Pre-competition diets

When there are several days to prepare for competition, players should taper their training and then 2–3 days before the match increase their carbohydrate intake to the equivalent of $10\,g\cdot kg^{-1}$ body weight (Sherman *et al.* 1981). The carbohydrate restocking process can continue up to a few hours before training or competition and still make a significant contribution to performance (Wright & Sherman 1989). Therefore, meals taken 2–3 h before training or competition should consist of easily digestible high-carbohydrate foods (Fig. 11.4). But nutritional advice must be flexible enough to take into consideration what is the normal custom and practice of a team. Not only has the dietary advice to be translated into acceptable foods but it must also respect the cultural values associated with the eating habits of players. Therefore, a dietitian should be consulted to help advise players about the range of foods they can eat during their preparation for competition and during recovery. Nutritional preparation must also be flexible enough to cope with the demands of different environments such as competition in hot and humid climates or at altitude. In northern Europe, for example, professional football players have to survive long seasons which involves playing in a wide range of weather conditions. They play in extremely hot weather in late summer and then play in the cold, wet, and often snowy winters before emerging in the spring to finish the season playing in warm weather again. Therefore, the type and timing of meals must reflect the conditions as well as the energy needs of the players.

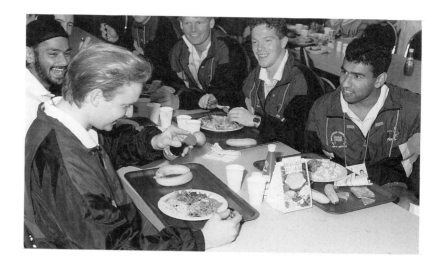

Fig. 11.4 A high carbohydrate diet is essential preparation for training and competition.

Fluid intake

Dehydration will probably have a more immediate impact on performance while playing and training in hot humid environments than will the gradual reduction in muscle glycogen. The opposite is true when playing and training in cooler climates of northern Europe. Fluid replacement is extremely important and so strategies have to be developed to ensure that players do not become so dehydrated that their performances suffer (Ekblom 1986) (Fig. 11.5). Weighing players before and after training and competition is a commendable practice which, even though it is time-consuming, pays dividends in terms of monitoring the functional fitness of a team. Drinking carbohydrate solutions and commercially available beverages have been shown to aid rehydration and improve performance (Maughan 1991). However, a carbohydrate solution should be chosen according to environmental conditions. Under hot and humid conditions, rehydration is more important than providing additional fuel (Fig. 11.6). When the weather is cool and the training is heavy and prolonged, then more concentrated carbohydrate solutions can be consumed to the

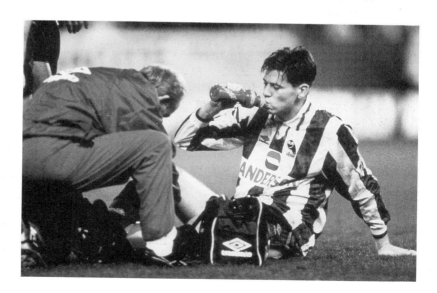

Fig. 11.5 Every opportunity should be taken to take in fluid and prevent dehydration.

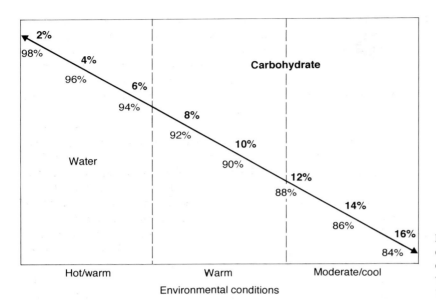

Fig. 11.6 Guidelines for composition of carbohydrate solutions in relation to environmental conditions (hot > 28°C; warm > 22°C cool < 22°C) (after Brouns 1991).

benefit of players (Brouns 1991). Although the concentrated carbohydrate beverages take longer to clear the gut, they will provide a larger glucose load (Noakes *et al.* 1991). However, dehydration still presents a real threat to players even when they train in temperate climates or even during the winter. Players training hard, while wearing layers of clothing in winter, will lose as much sweat as during training in the summer when they are lightly clothed (Ekblom 1986). Therefore players, coaches and team doctors should pay attention to this aspect of nutritional preparation for competition.

Post-match alcohol intake should not be confused with rehydration. Strong alcoholic drinks are diuretics and so players will lose more fluid than the volume of alcoholic beverages they drink. Social drinking during the evening before a game, coupled with missing breakfast is a recipe for disaster because of its effects on blood glucose concentration. Normally, blood glucose concentrations are maintained by the liver which is, in turn, restocked after each meal. However, during periods of fasting and between meals, liver glycogen is restocked by a process called gluconeogenesis. Alcohol consumption inhibits gluconeogenesis and so contributes to and compounds the reduction in blood glucose concentration during fasting (Newsholme & Start 1973). Therefore, playing

under these conditions, when blood glucose concentrations can fall to low levels may lead to poor decision-making and will result in poor performances.

Supplements

Football players, in particular and sportspeople in general have a poor knowledge of nutrition and nutritional strategies. Therefore it is not surprising that they are vulnerable to advertisements for powders, pills, and all kinds of wonder foods. Although most of the supplements cause more financial than physical harm to the players, they do pose a potential health threat. This occurs when players ignore sound nutritional advice and believe that supplements can provide them with an easy route to a balanced diet.

Nevertheless, from time to time, sportspeople are recommended to try, what appears to be at first sight, performance-enhancing products which have some basis for their claims. Bicarbonate loading is one practice which appears to give athletes a distinct advantage during short-term high-intensity exercise such as racing over 400 and 800 m (Lamb & Williams 1991). The effective dose appears to be about $0.3\,\text{g·kg}^{-1}$ body weight, taken $2-3\,\text{h}$ before exercise, however, this amount of bicarbonate is not tolerated by everyone without some unpleasant side-effects. Gastrointestinal discomfort is the most common reaction to this treatment, and it is not unusual for people to experience diarrhea and vomiting. Furthermore, there is not sufficient evidence to show that bicarbonate loading improves performance during periods of maximal exercise with brief periods of recovery. All in all, it is not a dietary practice which should be given serious consideration by football players.

Caffeine ingestion, in the form of several cups of coffee, before exercise has been shown in some studies to improve endurance capacity during cycling but the evidence for running is less convincing (Lamb & Williams 1991). Caffeine stimulates the release of fatty acids from WAT cells. If the increased concentration of fatty acids are oxidized by working muscle then they will reduce the amount of glycogen used for energy production. This glycogen sparing contributes to the improvement in endurance capacity. However, drinking coffee before exercise to exhaustion in a laboratory experiment is one thing, following this same practice an hour before a football match is quite another, for at least two reasons. The first is that caffeine is a diuretic and so players would lose more fluid than they ingested, and what is more they would need to empty their bladders at times when it was not only inconvenient, but if it was during a game, tactically disastrous. The second reason is that caffeine in the amounts needed to achieve an improvement in performance is banned by the International Olympic Committee (IOC). This also applies to the consumption of caffeine-containing products which are often sold by health-food stores.

Creatine, which is found in meat and fish, contributes to the formation of a high-energy compound called creatine phosphate. This compound plays a central role in energy production (see Chapter 4). During brief periods of high-intensity exercise the concentration of creatine phosphate is reduced to very low levels. Sprints of short duration are supported by the regeneration of ATP from creatine phosphate and they cannot be repeated until a significant amount of the creatine phosphate store has been replaced. Recovery periods of at least 30 s are needed to restock the creatine phosphate to sufficient levels to be able to repeat a sprint of maximal intensity. Training does not appear to increase creatine phosphate concentrations in resting skeletal muscle to values significantly above those found in a moderately active person. In con-

trast, training tends to increase resting muscle glycogen concentrations above those found in moderately active people. This response suggests that training and changes to the habitual diets of formerly untrained individuals improves their nutritional status in a direction which prepares them to meet the challenge of exercise successfully.

Recently, creatine supplementation has been shown to increase the resting concentration of creatine phosphate in skeletal muscles (Harris *et al.* 1992). This would, in theory give a player an advantage when performing multiple sprints. However, the amount of creatine that players would have to consume to achieve measurable improvements in performance has yet to be established. Dosages of *c.* 24–30 g of creatine a day for 2 days increased creatine phosphate concentrations by about 50%, but much of the ingested creatine was lost in the urine. This amount of creatine monophosphate consumed in these experiments is equivalent to eating approximately 6 kg of beef over 2 days (Harris *et al.* 1992). Therefore, there is insufficient research information on this topic to offer advice about dosages or indeed if this nutritional supplement is generally effective. Nevertheless, it is not a nutritional practice to be encouraged because not only is it impractical to undertake a nutritional strategy involving an expensive supplement of limited availability, more importantly it would undermine the recommendations about good nutritional practices.

The recommendation that players should eat a well-balanced diet coupled with the appropriate training and preparation for competition is one that can be put into practice by everyone, whether they are professional or recreational football players. In addition, the nutritional strategies used in preparation for, and recovery from training and competition can be employed using foods which are part of the normal diets of players worldwide.

Conclusion

Increased attention to the nutritional needs of players as well as a knowledge of nutritional strategies for recovery from heavy training will contribute to improved performance. Nutritional support for players will ensure that body weight and composition is under control and appropriate for the level of energy expenditure. Nutritional strategies during the preparation for, the participation in, and recovery from training and competition will only work when the player's maintenance diets are of adequate quality and quantity. Thereafter, attention to the carbohydrate and fluid intakes before and after training and competition is the most successful way of using nutrition as an effective aid to performance.

References

Åstrand P.O. (1967) Diet and athletic performance. *Fed. Proc.* **26**, 1772–1777.

Bangsbo J., Norregaard L. & Thorsoe F. (1992) The effect of diet on intermittent exercise performance. *Int. J. Sports Med.* **13**, 152–157.

Bergström J. & Hultman E. (1966) Muscle glycogen synthesis after exercise: an enhancing factor localised to the muscle cells in man. *Nature* **210**, 309–310.

Blom P.C.S., Hostmark A.T., Vaage O, Kardel K.R. & Maehlum S. (1987) Effect of different post-exercise sugar diets on the rate of muscle glycogen synthesis. *Med. Sci. Sports Exerc.* **19**, 491–496.

Brewer J., Williams C. & Patton A. (1988) The influence of high carbohydrate diets on endurance running performance. *Eur. J. Appl. Physiol.* **57**, 698–706.

Brouns F. (1991) Dehydration–rehydration: a praxis oriented approach. *J. Sports Sci.* **9**, Suppl. 1, 143–152.

Brouns F., Saris W.H.M., Stroecken J. *et al.* (1989) Eating, drinking and cycling, a controlled Tour de France simulation study; Part I effect of diet manipulation. *Int. J. Sports Med.* **10**, Suppl. 1, S41–S48.

Christensen E.H. & Hansen O. (1939) Arbeitsfahigkeit und Ehrnahrung (Work performance and nutrition). *Scand. Arch. Physiol.* **81**, 160–175.

Clark N. (1990) *Nancy Clark's Sports Nutrition Guidebook.* Leisure Press, Champaign, Illinois.

Clarkson P. (1991) Minerals: exercise performance and supplementation in athletes. *J. Sports Sci.* **9**, 91–116.

Coggan A.R. & Coyle E.F. (1991) Carbohydrate ingestion during prolonged exercise: effects on metabolism and performance. *Exerc. Sports Sci. Rev.* **19**, 1–40.

Costill D.L. (1988) Carbohydrates for exercise: dietary demands for optimum performance. *Int. J. Sports Med.* **9**, 1–18.

Costill D.L. & Miller J. (1980) Nutrition for endurance sport: carbohydrate and fluid balance. *Int. J. Sports Med.* **1**, 2–14.

Costill D.L., Pascoe D.D., Fink W.J., Robergs R.A. & Barr S.I. (1990) Impaired muscle glycogen resynthesis after eccentric exercise. *J. Appl. Physiol.* **69**, 46–50.

Coyle E.F. (1991) Timing and method of increased carbohydrate intake to cope with heavy training, competition and recovery. *J. Sports Sci.* **9**, Suppl. 1, 29–52.

Davis J.A., Brewer J. & Atkin D. (1992) Pre-season physiological characteristics of English First and Second division soccer players. *J. Sports Sci.* **10**, 541–547.

Devlin J.T. & Williams C. (1991) Food, nutrition and sports performance. *J. Sports Sci.* **9**, Suppl. 1, iii.

Ekblom B. (1986) Applied physiology of soccer. *Sports Med.* **3**, 50–60.

Fallowfield J. & Williams C. (1993) Influence of nutrition on recovery from exercise. *Int. J. Sports Nutr.* **3**, 150–164.

Foster C., Costill D.L. & Fink W.J. (1979) Effect of pre-exercise feeding on endurance performance. *Med. Sci. Sports* **11**, 1–5.

Gollnick P.D. (1977) Free fatty acid turnover and the availability of substrates as a limiting factor in prolonged exercise. *Ann. N.Y. Acad. Sci.* **301**, 64–71.

Grandjean A.C. (1989) Macro-nutrients intake of US athletes compared with the general population and recommendations for athletes. *Am. J. Clin. Nutr.* **49**, 1070–1076.

Gregory J., Foster K., Tyler H. & Wiseman M. (1990) *The Dietary and Nutritional Survey of British Adults.* HMSO, London.

Harris R.C., Soderlund K. & Hultman E. (1992) Elevation of creatine in resting and exercise muscle of normal subjects by creatine supplementation. *Clin. Sci.* **83**, 367–374.

Hickson J.F., Schrader J.W., Pivarnik J.M. & Stockton J.E. (1986) Nutritional intake from food sources of soccer athletes during two stages of training. *Nutr. Rep. Int.* **34**, 85–91.

HMSO (1991) *Dietary Reference Values for Food Energy and Nutrients for the United Kingdom.* Report on Health and Social Subjects No. 41. HMSO, London.

Hultman E. (1967) Studies on muscle metabolism of glycogen and active phosphate in man with special reference to exercise and diet. *Scand. J. Clin. Invest.* **19**, Suppl. 94, 1–64.

Ivy J.L. (1991) Muscle glycogen synthesis before and after exercise. *Sports Med.* **11**, 6–19.

Jacobs I., Weslin N., Karlsson J., Rasmussen M. & Houghton B. (1982) Muscle glycogen concentration and élite soccer players. *Eur. J. Appl. Physiol.* **48**, 297–302.

Jansson E. & Kaijser L. (1987) Substrate utilisation and enzymes in skeletal muscle of extremely endurance trained men. *J. Appl. Physiol.* **62**, 999–1005.

Jequier E. & Schutz Y. (1983) Long term measurements of energy expenditure in humans using a respiration chamber. *Am. J. Clin. Nutr.* **38**, 989–998.

Kirkendall D.T., Foster C., Dean J.A., Grogan J. & Thompson N.N. (1988) Effect of glucose polymer supplementation on performance of soccer players. In Reilly T., Lees A., Davids K. & Murphy W.J. (eds) *Science and Football*, pp. 33–41. E. & F.N. Spon, London.

Lamb D.R. & Williams, M.H. (eds) (1991) *Perspectives in Exercise Science and Sports Medicine*, Vol. 4. *Ergogenics: Enhancement of Performance.* Brown & Benchmark Press, Indianapolis.

Leatt P.B. & Jacobs I. (1989) Effect of glucose polymer ingestion on glycogen depletion during a soccer match. *Can. J. Sport Sci.* **14**, 112−116.

Lemon P.W.R. (1991) Effect of exercise on protein requirements. *J. Sports Sci.* **9**, Suppl. 1, 53−90.

Maughan R.J. (1991) Fluid and electrolyte loss and replacement during exercise. *J. Sports Sci.* **9**, Suppl. 1, 117−142.

Maughan R.J. & Williams C. (1981). Differential effects of fasting on skeletal muscle glycogen content in man and on skeletal muscle in the rat. *Proc. Nutr. Soc.* **40**, 45A.

McGilvery R.W. (1975) The use of fuels for muscular work. In Howald H. & Poortmans J.R. (eds) *Metabolic Adaptation to Prolonged Physical Exercise*, pp. 12−30. Birkhauser Verlag, Basel.

Muckle D.S. (1973) Glucose syrup ingestion and team performance in soccer. *Br. J. Sports Med.* **7**, 340−343.

Newsholme E.A. & Start C. (1973) *Regulation in Metabolism.* Wiley-Interscience Publication, London.

Nilsson L.H. & Hultman E. (1973) Liver glycogen in man — the effect of total starvation or a carbohydrate-poor diet followed by carbohydrate refeeding. *Scand. J. Clin. Lab. Invest.* **32**, 325−330.

Noakes T.D., Rehrer N.J. & Maughan R.J. (1991) The importance of volume in regulating gastric emptying. *Med. Sci. Sports Exerc.* **23**, 307−313.

Nuefer D.P., Sawka M.N., Young A.J., Quigley M.D., Latzka W.A. & Levine L. (1991) Hypohydration does not impair skeletal muscle glycogen resynthesis after exercise. *J. Appl. Physiol.* **70**, 1490−1494.

Olsson K.E. & Saltin B. (1970) Variations in total body water with muscle glycogen changes in man after exercise. *Acta Physiol. Scand.* **80**, 11−18.

Piehl K. (1974) Time course for refilling of glycogen stores in human muscle fibres following exercise-induced glycogen depletion. *Acta Physiol. Scand.* **90**, 297−302.

Robergs R.A. (1991) Nutrition and exercise determinants of post-exercise glycogen synthesis. *Int. J. Sport Nutr.* **1**, 307−337.

Saltin B. (1973) Metabolic fundamentals in exercise. *Med. Sci. Sports* **15**, 366−369.

Sherman W.M., Costill D.L., Fink W. & Miller J. (1981) Effect of exercise−diet manipulation on muscle glycogen and its subsequent utilisation during performance. *Int. J. Sports Med.* **2**, 114−118.

Tsintzas K.O., Liu R., Williams C., Campbell I.G. & Gaitanos G. (1993) The effect of carbohydrate ingestion during exercise on performance during a 30 km race. *Int. J. Sports Nutr.* **3**, 127−139.

Van de Beek E.J. (1991) Vitamin supplementation and physical exercise performance. *J. Sports Sci.* **9**, Suppl., 77−90.

van Erp-Baart A.M.J., Saris W.H.M., Binkhorst R.A., Vos J.A. & Elvers J.W.H. (1989) Nation-wide survey on nutritional habits in élite athletes: Part I carbohydrate, protein and fat intake. *Int. J. Sports Med.* **10**, Suppl. 1, S3−S10.

WHO (1985) *Energy and Protein Requirements.* Technical Report Series No. 724. World Health Organization, Geneva.

Wolever T., Jenkins D.J.A., Jenkins L.A. & Josse R.G. (1991) The glycemic index: methodology and clinical implications. *Am. J. Clin. Nutr.* **54**, 846−854.

Wright D.A. & Sherman W.M. (1989) Carbohydrate feedings before, during or in combination improve cycling performance. *J. Appl. Physiol.* **71**, 1082−1088.

Chapter 12

The German experience of peak performance in football

In football, top-level performance is required by a player who is trying to reach international level or a personal best. Maximum potential needs to be achieved in aerobic capacity, anerobic alactacid power, aerobic regenerative capability, regenerative and repair mechanisms (immunological power), creativeness, anticipation, understanding of the game, intelligence and personality.

Insufficient performance capacity or weakness in one of these components leads inevitably to functional disturbances of the body with a higher susceptibility to injuries and infections. The psychological state of a player can also be damaged, for example lack of concentration, psychological instability, false technical–tactical behavior, and so on. Main causes may include insufficiently developed capacity; exercise-reduced regenerative capacity (correlated with aerobic metabolic capacity) which may cause imbalances in the psychological, neurological, endocrinological, and immunological regulation; physical and/or psychological overloads; or for instance lack of active substances such as vitamins, minerals, or trace elements.

A stable top-level performance is only possible in combination with a stable psychological, neurological, endocrinological, and immunological state of health (Liesen & Hollman 1981). This is an important prerequisite for success throughout the whole season or during a long international tournament such as the World Cup. In the following text, tips and recommendations for the development of such a stable performance capacity as well as findings and procedures for the diagnosis of disturbances and for their treatment during training and competition periods are presented. The basis of the chapter are experiments and practical experiences gained over the last 15 years with professional football players especially in international tournaments such as the World Cup (1986 and 1990),

the European Cup (1988), and the Olympic Games (1984 and 1988).

Development of a stable psychological and physical performance capacity

There are a large number of football players with special capabilities who have developed technical skills and have given these an individual hallmark. Some also possess a strongly marked instinctive sense which can be associated with creative anticipation. A lot is demanded from a football player e.g. creativeness, understanding of the game, game control, and a specific intelligence for the game.

The localization of personality traits in the brain is situated on that side which is the youngest, most complex, and most sensitive. Here, the distinctiveness rate for regulatory procedures is very high. This is combined with a great sensitivity for disturbance factors. Due to different stress situations and through intensive football training and competitions high activations are achieved, e.g. from stress hormones like adrenocorticotrophic hormone (ACTH), catecholamines, or neuropeptides (Weicker & Werle 1991). The blood lactic acid, the worldwide approved measurement for the intensity of work-load for energy metabolism, is only partly controlled by these hormones. Therefore, lactic acid can only give indirect and incomplete information about stress to the brain during training. This knowledge is essential for precise controlling and planning of training. The practical methods of controlling and training metabolic parameters such as lactic acid, urea, uric acid, muscle enzymes, etc. are limited. All these parameters do not on their own control the personal development of a player or the ability to overcome injuries. New data have shown that parameters of the immune system, especially examination of the T-cell subsets, and hormones of the immune system (the cytokines), can give information about the impact of stress on the central nervous system during sports and determine whether rest and injury-prevention techniques are sufficient (Liesen et al. 1989a, Northoff & Berg 1991, Pedersen 1991, Liesen & Uhlenbruck 1992).

The combination of intensive work-loads (e.g. training with the ball, maximum sprints, tackles, jumps, and sprints with changes of direction) and psychological stress can lead to immunological suppression (Liesen *et al.* 1989a, 1989c). This indicates that the phases of regeneration and regenerative activities between the intervals of training are not sufficient. This is as significant in young players as it is in older ones. Young players are probably less susceptible to injuries or infections, but their ability to train in co-ordination and technique and to maintain a balanced mental state is reduced under these conditions. The following conclusions can be drawn.

1 There should be as little psychological stress as possible during training, and, most importantly, during active regenerative periods. The players must enjoy and accept the training. The aim is to avoid central stimulations build up by high concentration and maximal power. As a result, learning effects become possible in the sense of training adaptions.

2 Players of any age should have an active regeneration period of 10−20 min after every competition or training, with exercises for relaxation (stretching, psychoregulatory, and aerobic elements such as jogging without intervals), in order to obtain maximum training adaptions.

3 Players of any age need a training program with regenerative elements, especially on the day after competition.

The regenerative capacity of a player's central nervous system from heavy work-loads seems to correlate well with the player's aerobic capacity of energy metabolism.

The aerobic capacity of young football players at national levels is comparable to the professional players. (There is also no difference in the aerobic capacity between young and adult amateur players.) Overloads in training result in a reduction of the development of metabolic aerobic capacity. Speed, strength, agility, and elasticity are the most important physical capabilities for football players (Reilly & Vaughan 1976, Pohl *et al.* 1981, Öberg *et al.* 1984, Ekblom 1986). Young players with a high capability for speed and strength therefore have a much larger ability, not only for self-control, but also to control the physically weaker player who may be technically and tactically more gifted. This means that in young players, physical capabilities may be trained too intensely. The necessity for a reduction in technical−tactical training and the development of the personality of young players has already been indicated.

Football training has to be designed so that the regeneration of creatine phosphate storage after speed and strength exercise results almost entirely through aerobic metabolism. The ability to reproduce creatine phosphate by aerobic metabolism not only limits the physical capacity in a football player, but, in cases of high concentrations of lactic acid ($> 6-8\,\text{mmol}\cdot\text{l}^{-1}$ in the blood) and a high distribution of stress hormones, central fatigue may also hinder the technical, tactical, and creative capabilities of a player (Hillman *et al.* 1982, Liesen 1983).

In several thousand examinations of professional and amateur players the authors found that:

1 The basic endurance capacity of a player does not always reveal sufficient regeneration of creatine phosphate storage for swiftness and elasticity stress, i.e. aerobic capacity is not "player-specific."

2 Dependent on the player, position, and tactical needs, a player needs a defined endurance capability to regenerate himself or herself from sprints, jumps, etc., without a higher production of lactic acid.

In order to analyze the capability of aerobic metabolic capacity to regenerate creatine phosphate, the authors developed a special test — a $5 \times 30\,\text{m}$ sprint test.

Regulation of health and recuperation in training and competition

A top-level performance of an athlete during a single performance is determined by an optimum latent vitality of the psychological, neurological, and endocrinological reactions. A prerequisite, however, is a state of fitness (of the energy metabolism and its regulation) gained through training adaptations over months and years. For several repetitions of an athletic top-level performance, e.g. in a tournament, a high stability of these control systems is required combined with a fast and complete recuperative capacity from the preceding work-load. According to recent knowledge, the immune system plays an important role in this context. The immune system develops from molecular adhesions of the brain cells. It receives information from the brain via neuropeptides and other specific brain hormones, for which the immunocytes have specific receptors. Conversely, "irritations" of the cells of the immune system are noticed by the brain due to the production of hormones by the immune system (cytokines) which are picked up by specific receptors on the brain cells. An athlete requires a well-trained immune system in order to produce repeated top-level performances. Moreover, a well-developed immune system is needed for the regulation of extreme activations at high mental and physical capacities. This is the basic requirement for a maximum athletic performance.

Figure 12.1 shows the importance of the psyche and the immune system for the development of top-level performances, health, or even illness. It is frequently observed that top athletes are susceptible to infections and injuries. Mackinnon and Tomasi (1986) point out, however, that training and sports can lead to a stabilization of the immune system, so that athletes are able to develop better protection against infections and injuries. It is well known that, depending on the intensity and extent of the work-load during training sessions and sports competitions, a generalized inflammatory reaction in the body can be activated (Haralambie 1969; Haralambie & Flaherty 1970; Liesen & Hollman 1981; Northoff & Berg 1991). An acute-phase reaction of glycoproteins points to such an inflammatory reaction against future physical distress. The interleucines seem to be of importance as a control system, particularly on a local level. They are connected with the nerve cells of the brain; the local inflammatory reac-

tion is also centrally controlled. Due to the work-loads in training sessions and competitions the catabolic metabolism process is mainly developed on a cellular basis. The immune system, its cells, and their products have to clear away the structures (enzymes, contractile proteins, etc.), which have been changed during the work-load.

During this process, the cells of the immune system play an important role. However, the number of immunocompetent cells is not decisive, but their functional ability is (Liesen *et al.* 1989b, Order *et al.* 1989, Pedersen *et al.* 1989, Pedersen 1991). Compared to untrained young people, a reduced number of lymphocytes and T cells can be observed in immunologically highly trained athletes.

From an immunological point of view, the granulocytes are not very intelligent. They seem to be activated mostly for the unspecific mechanism of removal of structures which have been changed through work. The reduced number of T lymphocytes and their subsets is a positive training adaptation. The reduction correlates with the aerobic metabolic capacity measured in $m \cdot s^{-1}$ at $4 \, mmol \cdot l^{-1}$ lactic acid (anaerobic threshold) in a field step test. The untrained subject showed an aerobic capacity of $3.35 \, m \cdot s^{-1}$ and the national football team (May 1990) of $3.95 \, m \cdot s^{-1}$.

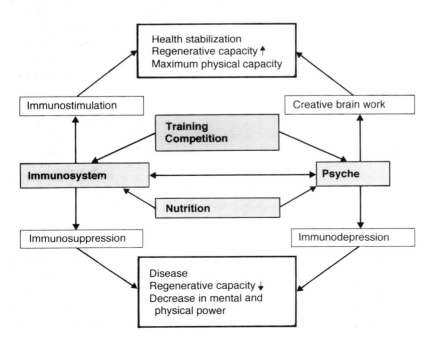

Fig. 12.1 The interaction between training/competition and psyche/immune system for health stabilization and fitness or disease.

There is a close correlation between the reduction of the T-cell subsets, the frequency, and amount of regenerative training practised during and at the end of each training phase and/or as separate training, e.g. on the day after a game or an intensive training phase.

In order to illustrate that the reduction of cell counts is also a sign of immunosuppression and the development of susceptibility to infections, the example of the preparatory training of the German Olympic field hockey team for the Olympic Games in 1988 (Fig. 12.2), although not in soccer, is presented here (Liesen *et al.* 1989a). The initial values were measured at the end of a regenerative training phase. The number of cells was only half as high as in healthy subjects of the same age. The players, however, did not show any signs of susceptibility to infections or injuries. Their immune system had a high functioning capacity.

Five weeks of an extensive and intensive general fitness training with aerobic basic training, speed training sessions, and daily regenerative work-loads, 12–14 training sessions per week, led to no significant reduction of the cell counts. The functioning of the immune sytem was also not reduced. During the next 10 days following this examination three games against "easy teams" were played, hockey-specific exercises and games demanding high concentration and difficult technical–tactical exercises were carried out twice a day. In addition, the psychological pressure was increased 4 weeks before the opening of the Olympic tournament in Seoul due to very high expectations from the public, the Olympic officials, and the players themselves. All this led to a dramatic decrease of the cell counts and a susceptibility to infections in seven players. Five developed stomach infections, one an infection in the urogenital tract, and one an acute gastritis. This suppression of the cell counts was also detected in the other T-cell subsets, B cells, and natural killer cells. The hockey-specific training and the games led to a high level of stress hormones, especially those which have a catabolic effect on the metabolism such as ACTH. However, according to our examinations this is not sufficient enough to cause such immuno-suppression. Any intellectual work, especially highly concentrative and/or creative work, affects the immune system (Fig. 12.3). The authors' experiments of the last couple of years show that the combination of psychological and concentrated work with intensive and extensive physical exercises can suppress a high-functioning immune system in top athletes within a few days.

Six weeks before the Football World Cup (1990) the German national team players showed a low aerobic regenerative capacity and a low functioning of the immune system. Therefore, the team coach (F. Beckenbauer) and his assistants (H. Osiek and B. Vogts) concentrated mainly on regenerative training work-loads during the preparation period. Intensive, football-specific technical–tactical elements were only carried out for 2–3 min with only a few repetitions, with 3–5 min active regenerative phases in between. The goal of this training was to increase the regenerative capacity and a psychological, neuro-logical, endocrinological, and immunological stabilization for the World Cup tournament. To compensate for the immunosuppressive distress reaction of a game

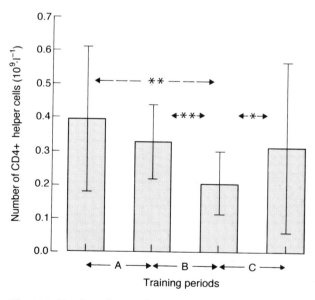

Fig. 12.2 Number of CD4+ helper cells during the period of preparation for the 1988 Olympic Games of the German field hockey players (silver medal winners) ($n = 11$). Time A: 5 weeks of training, 12–14 sessions·week^{-1}. Time B: 2 weeks of hockey-specific training with a high concentration on technical–tactical tasks and creativity. Time C: comparable training to B; three matches against international top teams and psychological stress, and under immunomodulation by a phytopharmacum (Esberitox®). *, $P < 0.05$; **, $P < 0.01$.

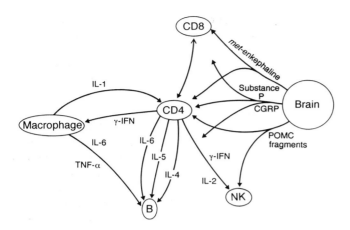

Fig. 12.3 Central stimulation by cognitive or concentrated brain work and the stress for the immunocytes. B, B cells; CD, cluster differentiation; CGRP, calcitonin gene-related peptide; IFN, interferon; IL, interleukin; POMC, pro-opiomelanocortin; TNF, tumor necrosis factor.

the players were advised to practise only regenerative elements during their free time and in their training sessions during the tournament. Considerable support for this regeneration is gained by the additional treatment with a phyto-based immunomodulant (Esberitox®) combined with vitamin C and B_{12}, (Liesen et al. 1989c, Liesen & Uhlenbruck 1992).

Nutrition and substitution of vitamins, minerals, and trace elements

Football is a game with a high level of intensity and a lot of mental stress. High physical and psychological strain causes a high demand of glycogen, which has to be taken in with the food (Karlsson 1969, Saltin 1973, Jacobs et al. 1982). Therefore, nutrition for football players should include 60–65% carbohydrates, not more than 15% fat, and about 20–25% proteins.

The analysis of the nutrition of German professional football players shows that these recommendations are not obeyed. The amount of carbohydrates eaten is considerably lower, and the amount of fat and, in particular, the amount of protein is much too high.

Moreover, the carbohydrates consumed do not contain enough vitamin B, minerals, and trace elements necessary for energy metabolism. Such malnutrition leads to limitations of performance and to health problems. Analysis and control of performance development shows that it is necessary to consume vitamins B_1 and B_2 at 15 mg·day^{-1} for about 2–3 weeks before an extensive and intensive training or competition period.

A deficiency of minerals and trace elements has been diagnosed for nearly every second German football player ($n = 750$) (Haralambie 1969, 1982; Keul et al. 1988; McDonald & Keen 1988; Beuker & Helbig 1989; Liesen et al. 1989c; Berg & Keul 1990, 1991; Tiedt et al. 1990, 1991). The main reason is that the food German players normally eat does not contain the necessary amount of these substances (Table 12.1), and that considerable amounts of these substances get lost because of a high excretion of sweat, urine (due to the level of distress during a football game), and micro-hemorraghia through the intestinal tract.

An insufficiency of magnesium hinders the development of training adaptation (Fig. 12.4). Players of a professional football team who showed on more than one occasion a low serum concentration for magnesium showed no increase of endurance capacity (measured by the 4 mmol·l^{-1} lactic acid anaerobic threshold) after a 5-week preparatory training for the new season.

Only the players with normal magnesium levels showed an increase in performance due to a multiplication of magnesium-dependent enzymes in the glycolysis and citric acid cycle.

In football players who show a decrease of magnesium concentration below 0.72 mmol·l^{-1} and an increase of the uric acid serum concentration up to a level which is either within or even above the clinical norm, high risk for muscular overloads or even injury exists. In nearly all cases a continuation of training and competition leads to myogelosis, to muscle strains, or even to ruptures of muscle fibers. Intensive treatment aimed at increasing magnesium levels and decreasing the uric acid level, in combination with physiotherapy, can reduce the danger within 3–5 days.

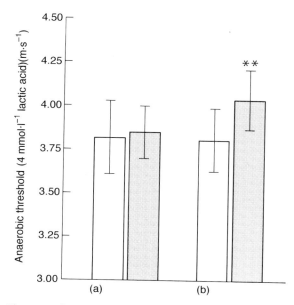

Fig. 12.4 The influence of magnesium (Mg) on metabolic aerobic adaptions by a 5-week preparatory training of professional football players. The players with Mg serum levels > 0.76 mmol·l^{-1} only got an increase in their aerobic capacity. (a) Levels of Mg < 0.74 mmol·l^{-1} ($n = 9$); (b) levels of Mg > 0.76 mmol·l^{-1} ($n = 7$). □, before training; ▨, after training. **, $P < 0.01$.

During training or competition periods football players need an additional intake of magnesium of about 300 mg·day^{-1}. Choosing the right beverages, this additional need can be covered by mineral water which has a high content of magnesium. Mineral water should contain a magnesium level of 100–200 mg·l^{-1}; the calcium concentration should not be more than twice the magnesium concentration, otherwise the magnesium resorption can be disturbed. The sodium concentration should be lower than that found in sweat (i.e. < 1000 mg·l^{-1}), otherwise additional potassium efflux is possible; the chloride level should not be higher than 600 mg·l^{-1} and the sulphate concentration not higher than 400 mg otherwise diarrhea may result.

Mineral water contains almost no trace elements. Their importance for the health preservation of the skeletal system, the muscular system, the tendinous and ligamentous apparatus, for a stable immune system, and a high regenerative psychological and physical performance capacity, is uncontested. Due to these reasons and because of hardly any or very little storage capacity (except for copper and iron) in the body for minerals and trace elements regular substitution in low doses is recommended for football players.

Mineral drinks on the national and international market are not suitable to cover the additional needs for minerals and trace elements of top athletes. In fact,

Table 12.1 The estimated need, mean intake (in Germany), absorption, uptake, and loss by perspiration for some minerals and trace elements

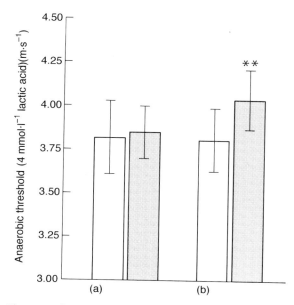

	Need (mg·day^{-1})	Intake (mg·day^{-1})	Absorption (%)	Uptake (mg·day^{-1})	Sweat (mg·l^{-1})
Sodium	500–1000	4100	100	4100	1000
Potassium	1000	3200	90	2880	300
Calcium	800	860	30	258	160
Magnesium	300	350	35	122.5	36
Iron	10–15	15	10	1.5	1.2
Copper	1.7	2	30	0.6	0.06
Zinc	10	10	20	2	1.2
Iodine	50–100 (µg·day^{-1})	40 (µg·day^{-1})	95	38 (µg·day^{-1})	10 (µg·l^{-1})

their high sugar concentration $(25-50\,g\cdot l^{-1})$ hinders the evacuation of the stomach and the resorption during and after physical work-loads. Low doses of glucose polymer (Jacobs 1989) or maltodextrin can reduce glycogen depletion.

During the preparatory training of the German national football team for the World Cup or the European Cup, the players had to learn to drink larger amounts than their bodies demanded during and after training sessions. Therefore, the training was interrupted about every 5 min and mineral water enriched with a low-dose trace element preparation (Basica, Protina-Klopfer), fresh orange juice for a better taste, and about 1 g of vitamin C per liter was offered. This organization of training can minimize the loss of fluids which reduces performance and regenerative capacity (for example it is possible to lose 2% of body weight through perspiration). During meals, after training sessions, or after a competition, 150 mg of magnesium in combination with a trace element preparation in 0.2 l mineral water or fruit juice (ratio of 1 : 2) is offered to the players. Such careful substitution can prevent a subclinical deficiency of minerals and trace elements. Functional disturbances and a susceptibility to injury and infections and a psychological instability can be prevented. Finally, the regenerative capacity of the player from extreme physical and psychological loads is accelerated.

References

Berg A. & Keul J. (1990) Spurenelementversorgung beim Sportler. In Wolfram G. & Kirchgessner M. (eds). *Spurenelemente und Ernährung*, pp. 175–185. Wissenschaftliche Verlagsgesellschaft, Stuttgart.

Berg A. & Keul J. (1991) Ernährungserfordernisse aus sportmedizinischer Sicht. Zum Nährstoffbedarf des Sportaktiven. *Akt. Ernähr. Med.* **16**, 61–67.

Beuker F. & Helbig J. (1989) Vergleichende Untersuchungen zur Wirkung einer Magnesiumsubstitution bei Läufern und Kraftsportlern (Doppelblindversuch). *Magnesium-Bul.* **11**, 34–36.

Ekblom B. (1986) Applied physiology of soccer. *Sports Med.* **3**, 50–60.

Haralambie G. (1969) Serum glycoproteins and physical exercise. *Clin. Chim. Acta* **26**, 287–291.

Haralambie G. (1982) Serum zinc in athletes in training. *Int. J. Sports Med.* **2**, 135–138.

Haralambie G. & Flaherty D.K. (1970) Serum glycoprotein levels in athletes in training. *Experientia* **26**, 959–960.

Haralambie G. & van Dam B. (1977) Untersuchung über den Vitamin-Elektrolyt-Status bei Spitzenfechterinnen. *Leistungssport* **7**, 214–219.

Hillmann W., Liesen H., Budinger H. & Hollmann W. (1982) Untersuchungen zur anaerob-laktaziden Belastung im Hallenhockeytraining und -spiel. In Heck H., Hollmann W., Liesen H. & Rost R. (eds) *Sport: Leistung und Gesundheit*, pp. 583–590. Deutsch Ärzte Verlag, Köln.

Jacobs I. (1989) Effect of glycose polymer ingestion on glycogen depletion during a soccer match. *Can. Int. Sports Sci.* **14**(2), 112–116.

Jacobs I., Westlin N., Karlsson J., Rasmusson M. & Houghton B. (1982) Muscle glycogen and diet in élite soccer players. *Eur. J. Appl. Physiol.* **48**, 297–302.

Karlsson H.G. (1969) *Kohldratomsättning under en fotbollsmatch*. Report Department of Physiologiy III, reference 6, Karolinska Institute, Stockholm.

Keul J., Jacob E., Berg A., Dickhut H.H. & Lehmann M. (1988) Zur Wirkung von Vitaminen und Eisen auf die Leistungs- und Erholungsfähigkeit des Menschen und die Sportanämie. *Leichtathletik* **27**, 1082–1086, 1115–1118.

Liesen H. (1983) Schnelligkeitsausdauertraining in Fussball aus sportmedizinischer Sicht. *Fussballtraining* **1**(5) 27–31.

Liesen H. & Hollmann W. (1981) *Ausdauer und Stoffwechsel*, pp. 103–132. Hofmann Verlag, Schorndorf.

Liesen H., Kleiter K., Mücke S., Order U., Widenmayer W. & Riedel H. (1989a) Leucocytes and lymphocyte subpopulations in players of the German Olympic field hockey team during the preparatory training period for the Olympic Games in 1988. *Deut. Zeitschr. Sportmed.* **40** (special issue), 41–52.

Liesen H., Riedel H., Order U., Mücke S. & Widenmayer W. (1989b) Reference values of leucocytes and lymphocyte subsets in male top athletes during a controlled moderate training period. *Deut. Zeitschr. Sportmed.* **40** (special issue), 4–14.

Liesen H., Riedel H., Widenmayer W., Order U., Mücke S. & Geist S. (1989c) Substitution and preventive treatment in top athletes. In Böning D., Braumann K.M., Busse M.W., Maassen N. & Schmidt W. (eds) *Sport — Rettung oder Risiko für die Gesundheit?*, pp. 531–538.

Liesen H. & Uhlenbruck G. (1992) Sports immunology. *Sport Sci. Rev.* **1**, 94–116.

McDonald R. & Keen C.L. (1988) Iron, zinc and magnesium nutrition and athletic performance. *Sports Med.* **5**, 171–184.

Mackinnon L.T. & Tomasi T.B. (1986) Immunology of exercise. *Ann. Sports Med.* **3**, 1–4.

Northoff H. & Berg A. (1991) Immunologic mediators as parameters of the reaction to strenuous exercise. *Int. J. Sports Med.* **12**, Suppl. 1, 9–15.

Öberg B., Ekstrand J., Möller M. & Gillquist J. (1984) Muscle strength and flexibility in different positions of soccer players. *Int. J. Sports Med.* **5**, 213–216.

Order U., Riedel H., Liesen H., Widenmayer W., Hellwig T. & Geist S. (1989) Leucocytes and lymphocyte subsets. *Deut. Zeitschr. Sportmed.* **40** (special issue), 22–29.

Pedersen B.K. (1991) Influence of physical on the cellular immune system; Mechanisms of action. *Int. J. Sports Med.* **12**, Suppl. 1, 23–29.

Pedersen B.K., Tvede N., Christensen L.D., Klarlund K., Kragbak S. & Halkjaer-Kristensen J. (1989) Natural killer cell activity in peripheral blood of highly trained and untrained persons. *Int. J. Sports Med.* **10**, 129–131.

Pohl A.P., O'Halloran M.W. & Pannel P.R. (1981) Biochemical and physiological changes in football players. *Med. J. Aust.* **1**, 467–470.

Reilly T. & Vaughan T. (1976) A motion analysis of work-rate in different positional roles in professional football match-play. *J. Hum. Movement Studies* **2**, 87–97.

Saltin B. (1973) Metabolic fundamentals in exercise. *Med. Sci. Sports* **5**, 137–146.

Tiedt H.J., Grimm M. & Unger K.D. (1991) Verlaufsuntersuchung von Eisen, Kupfer, Zink, Calcium, Magnesium, Ferritin und Transferrin im Serum sowie Hämoglobin und Hämatokrit im Blut bei Leistungssportlern. Teil 2. *Med. Sport* **31**, 161–165.

Tiedt H.J., Grimm M., Zerbes H. & Kühne K. (1990) Der Einfluss Alter, Geschlecht und Sportart auf den Serumspiegel von Eisen, Kupfer, Zink, Calcium und Magnesium bei Leistungssportlern. *Med. Sport* **30**, 244–247.

Weicker H. & Werle E. (1991) Interaction between hormones and the immune system. *Int. J. Sports Med.* **12**, 30–37.

Chapter 13

The team physician

Proper medical care has an important function in any sporting endeavor and football is not an exception. All teams should have access to medical attention. The delivery of this medical care will differ according to the organization and the interest of the local medical staff. The team physician, as the co-ordinator of the medical staff, is responsible for the ultimate decisions on medical management or policies involving the care of the team. A close liaison must be maintained between the medical staff and the coaching staff. Contact should be frequent to keep the coaching staff appraised of the diagnoses, progress, and prognoses of medical problems involving the team. The availability of the team physician should not be limited to coverage of games. Illnesses are more common than injuries in athletes while injury exposure is more frequent in practice because of the greater number of hours spent preparing for competition. A dedicated team physician will ensure that a well-organized coverage system is in place and functional.

One of the primary responsibilities of a team physician is to be available to the athlete who is requesting attention. A broad base of knowledge in sports medicine is required of the physician who wishes to provide optimal care to a team. He or she should not only have a profound knowledge of orthopedics, nutrition, exercise physiology, cardiology, and other related medical areas but should also know football tactics and other aspects of the sport. This is important since a wide variety of illnesses and injuries can be incurred by an active athlete.

Ultimate responsibility for the medical management of an athlete rests on the team physician but input from other qualified professionals can provide invaluable aid. When possible, the physician should organize a group approach to medical care to encompass the broad range of needs that a player may require to successfully complete a season. The team physician will see a wide variety of maladies and should be able to manage the vast majority of them. On occasion, however, additional advice concerning management will be needed. Referral to the appropriate specialist may be required for more elusive diagnoses. A football team will most often require the services of an orthopedic consultant to assist in operative management and fracture care.

Another cornerstone of the sports medicine team is the athletic trainer or the physical therapist. Most musculoskeletal problems encountered on a team will be successfully treated by this person, who also will be responsible for rehabilitation. A close alliance of the team physician and the rehabilitation specialist will be mutually beneficial to all involved with the group. Advice from a nutritionist can be a welcome addition in promoting dietary changes that will enhance the health, endurance, and performance of the team.

Responsibilities of a team physician

The responsibilities of the team physician start with the pre-participation physical examination. The examination prior to the start of the training season should be aimed at identifying potential problems that could surface with participation in football. A general medical examination should be conducted and particular attention must be paid to the musculoskeletal examination to ensure adequate treatment of any previous injuries. If a problem is identified, steps should be taken to rectify the situation to allow full participation. The purpose of the pre-participation examination should be to allow safe participation and not to disqualify athletes from play. The pre-participation examination is also an excellent avenue for the team physician to educate the team members on appropriate health-care issues to promote and maintain health outside the realm of athletics.

The duties of a team physician continue with medical supervision of the team. This will include evaluation of both the illnesses and injuries experienced by the members of the team. The team physician must, therefore, be well grounded in the principles of outpatient medicine as well as knowledgeable in the treatment of musculoskeletal problems. A broad base of knowledge will be required of a physician attempting to provide care to a large group of individuals such as a football team. Questions in exercise science as well as pharmacology and psychology will arise at some point during a tenure as team physician. A team physician must be able to address the physical and emotional needs of the team members. Physicians in the primary care fields such as family practice, pediatrics, and internal medicine are particularly suited to functioning as team physicians because of their wide exposure of training. Specialists can also be successful team physicians, provided a core of basic medical knowledge is maintained along with the particular body of information unique to their specialty.

An example of problems arising in a football team of non-professional status can be drawn from a university team in the USA with 20 males aged 18–22 years followed through a 4-month season. There were 90 visits to the team physician during that time. Fifty-seven of the visits (63%) were due to a medical problem while the remaining 33 consultations were the result of a musculoskeletal injury. Twenty-five of the consultations (27%) involved an infectious etiology with 14 (15%) of the visits being upper respiratory infections. There were three dental injuries and two concussions. There were 10 contusions with three strains, one diagnosis of tendinitis, and 13 sprains, mostly of the ankle. Two upper extremity fractures were sustained during the season.

Athletes are also subject to the same diseases as the general public and will often become ill during the season. Management of an illness will not differ significantly in content but timing may be altered in order to allow safe competition. The aim should be to allow the player to compete as symptom-free as is reasonably possible. Upper respiratory infections will be the most frequent malady requiring attention. Symptoms may include fever, chills, nasal congestion, fatigue, and a cough. Viruses are the usual inciting factor and treatment is directed at easing symptoms. Numerous medications are effective in reducing the various symptoms but attention must be given to banned medication lists at the higher levels of competition (see Chapter 18). Bacterial infections, such as streptococcal pharyngitis (step throat) or otitis media (middle ear infection), will be treated in the same manner, with the addition of an antibiotic.

Gastrointestinal disturbances can be particularly problematic when a competition is approaching. These illnesses are usually viral in nature and self-limited to 2 or 3 days. The so-called "traveler's diarrhea" may be bacterial or protozoan in nature, however, and requires antimicrobial medications. Treatment for the gastrointestinal diseases centers on fluid replacement. Prevention of dehydration through administration of fluids is the cornerstone of treatment and requires liter-for-liter replacement of the lost fluid. Antimotility drugs may be used to reduce abdominal cramping but sedation can be a problem and administration of these drugs may prolong the carrier state of the illness. The athlete and the team physician should be aware of the possibility that some drugs may not be allowed according to the doping rules (see Chapter 18).

The presence of a fever (temperature over 38°C or 100.4°F) in any of these illnesses complicates the decision to return to activity. A fever will cause decreased strength and endurance and can increase the chance of dehydration. Antipyretic medications should be administered to control the elevated temperature. The decision to play will be affected by the ability of the antipyretic medications to reduce the temperature to a normal range and the symptomatology of the athlete. Younger players should be held to stricter guidelines when deciding on the timing of a return to activity.

The use of medications will require additional considerations during competition. Side-effects from medicines can be particularly disabling in a match apart from the doping aspects. The risk of medication administration should be weighed against the potential benefit of reducing the symptoms of the disease. The team physician must be aware of any banned medications that might apply to the level of play in which the team is involved.

Game coverage is one of the many rewards for being a team physician. The intensity and excitement of a match are pleasurable for the fans and the staff alike. The team physician's responsibilities continue during the match, however, and attention must be constant. Duties on the day of a match may range from treating the new onset of an illness in a player or the gastric distress of the coaching staff, to providing emergency care for an injured player during the match (Fig. 13.1). Various and sundry supplies may be needed by the medical staff during a match. A well-equipped medical bag is essential for the proper administration of care. The bag itself should be constructed of a durable

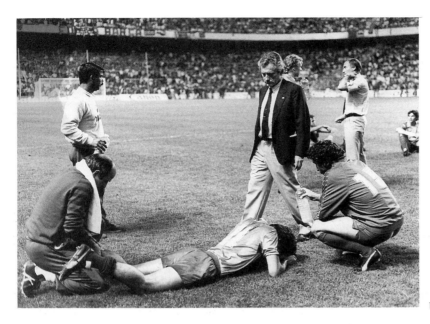

Fig. 13.1 The team physician on duty.

material. Compartments within the bag will aid in easy retrieval of the needed supplies. Kits for various purposes will often speed access and the delivery of care. Medications may be needed on a frequent basis. Medications for viral and bacterial infections will be useful. Anti-inflammatory and pain medications will also be required for treatment of some injuries. A supply of dressings for wounds and a suture kit for lacerations will be required on a regular basis. A dental kit and an eye kit may also be helpful on occasion. Supplies for emergency situations may rarely be needed but should be available at all times (Table 13.1).

Injuries in football

Several studies have investigated the incidence of injuries in the football leagues of Europe. An analysis was conducted during the Norway Cup, an annual international youth tournament in which 1459 teams with 25 000 players participated in 2987 matches (Nielsen & Yde 1989). Fifty-six per cent of the 1534 consultations by the medical staff were for injuries sustained during tournament play. Thirty-two per cent were the result of accidents while 12% involved ill-nesses. Of the injuries, 25% were contusions while 20% were sprains and strains. Fractures accounted for

Table 13.1 Physician's medical bag

Supplies	Medications
Eye kit	Antihistamines
Suture kit	Cough suppressants
Dental kit	Antacids
Oral airway	Asthma inhaler
Stethoscope	Antibiotics
Sphygmomanometer	Antimotility agents
Ophthalmoscope	Nasal spray
Otoscope	Otic solution
Scissors	Anti-emetics
Thermometer	Anti-inflammatories
Tourniquet	Local anesthetic
Malleable splints	Sunscreen
Reflex hammer	Alcohol pads

3.5% of the injuries. Two-thirds of the injuries occurred in the lower extremity with contusions dominating the picture. Sixteen per cent of all injuries involved the ankle. The injury rate was found to be $14 \cdot 1000$ match h^{-1} in the boys and $32 \cdot 1000$ match h^{-1} in the girls. Nine of 10 injured athletes were allowed to play the next day.

A similar study was undertaken during two Danish international youth tournaments in 1984 (Schmidt-Olsen *et al.* 1985). The 6600 participants, aged 9—19 years, played 945 matches in 5 days. Of the 392 medical consultations, 346 (88%) were due to injuries sustained during the tournament. Of the remaining 12% of consultations, 54% were the result of accidents and 46% resulted from an illness. Injuries to the lower extremity accounted for 80% of the injuries in this report. Contusions were reported in 33% of cases while blisters and abrasions accounted for 20%. Thirteen per cent of injuries involved the foot and ankle. Boys were injured at a rate of 16.1·match h^{-1} while the rate for girls was 29.2·match h^{-1}. The oldest girls had the highest incidence overall at 47.2·match h^{-1} while the young girls had the lowest. The oldest boys had an incidence of 20.6·match h^{-1}. The relative frequency of injury was thought to be 5% in these large youth tournaments. Only 3.7% of these injuries were considered severe.

Two prospective studies were done in Denmark. The first registered injuries for a 1-year period involving 496 boys (Schmidt-Olsen *et al.* 1991). These players recorded 312 injuries. Injury incidence increased with the age of players. Seventy per cent of the injuries occurred in the lower extremities, with 10% involving the upper extremities. Fourteen per cent had back pain, 4% of the injuries were fractures with two-thirds involving the upper extremity. The mean incidence of injury for the year was 3.7·1000 h^{-1} of football. The older boys (16—17 years) had an incidence rate of 4·1000 h^{-1}. No differences were found between injury rates in the autumn and spring seasons.

The second group was 123 male players in a Danish football club (Nielsen & Yde 1989). There were 93 adult males (over 18 years) and 30 boys (16—18 years). An injury was defined as an incident occurring in a game or practise that resulted in missing at least one game or practice session. Eighty-nine players sustained 109 injuries: 43 occurred during practice and 66 occurred during games. Eighty-four per cent of the injuries were located in the lower extremity. Ankle injuries were the most common (36%) and were found equally at all levels. There were 20 knee injuries. Overuse injuries comprised 37% of all injuries. Ankle injuries and strains had the highest rate of re-injury. Players in the youth and recreational leagues were most frequently injured during tackling (48 and 44%) while 54% of the competitive league injuries occurred during running. Thirty-eight of the injuries required treatment at a hospital. Fifty per cent of injuries were treated by the players themselves. Thirty-five per cent of the injuries caused an absence for more than 1 month. Twenty-eight per cent of the injured players still had complaints at 1 year of follow-up. The injury incidence during games was highest with the competitive players while injury during practise was more prevalent with the recreational players. The youth players had a high incidence of injury in this study.

A questionnaire survey, performed in a Danish emergency room on all football injuries seen over a 1-year period, evaluated 715 injuries in 646 males and 69 females (Hoy *et al.* 1992). Eighty-six per cent of the players were injured during matches while 9% involved insufficient warm-up and 5% occurred during training. The most common mechanism of injury was contact with another player. Earlier injuries influenced the current episode in 6% of cases. Forty-six per cent of the injuries were considered moderate and 44% were classified as minor in severity. Forty-nine per cent of the injuries involved the joints while 30% were abrasions and lacerations. Ankle sprains were the most common injury. Fractures accounted for 18% of injuries with an equal distribution between upper and lower extremities. Twenty per cent needed further care in the out-patient clinic and 7% were hospitalized. The yearly incidence of injury was 5.5% in players less than 18 years old, 17% in players aged 18—25, and 18% in players over 25 years. The severity of the injuries was also found to be less in the younger players.

A French study undertook the analysis of insurance claims submitted as a result of football injuries (Berger-Vachon *et al.* 1986) The number of accidents recorded was 6153 for 123 175 registered amateur players who played approximately 70 000 matches, 70 000 practise games, and participated in approximately 150 000 training sessions. Risk of injury was increased in the higher skill levels. Females and males over 35 had the same injury rate as the juniors. Joint injuries were the most frequent with the ankle involved 20.3% and the knee 13.8% of the time. Fractures accounted for 16.6% (5.4% upper extremity and 6.2% lower extremity) and contusions were reported at 21% (11.9% lower extremity). Fractures were the most common injury in players less than 14 years old. Sprains accounted for over half of the injuries reported in females.

An emergency room study conducted in Saudi Arabia evaluated 848 sports-related injuries (8.4% of emergency visits); 542 (64%) were the result of football play (Sadat-Ali & Sankaran-Kutty 1987). Soft-tissue injuries numbered 358 (66%). Contusions and lacerations numbered 125 (23%). Ruptured tendons occurred in 11 (2%) patients. Sprains were found in 141 (26%) patients with half involving the ankle. Strains accounted for 40 injuries (7.5%), chiefly involving the gastrocnemius and quadriceps. Ligamentous disruptions were noted in 32 (6%), mostly in the ankle and knee. There were 184 bone and joint injuries (34%). Subluxations and dislocations of the digits were seen in 16 (3%). Eleven patients had dislocations of shoulders or elbow. Fractures numbered 157 (29%). Of all injuries, 21% were considered severe with 44% classified as moderate. The lower extremity was involved in 320 (59%) of the injuries.

A Swedish study followed a senior male football division prospectively for 1 year (Ekstrand & Gillquist 1983). The 180 players were examined prior to the season. In 124 players, 256 injuries were sustained during the year. The yearly incidence of injury per player was 0.88 for a minor, 0.38 for a moderate, and 0.16 for a major injury. Eighty-eight per cent of the injuries were localized to the lower extremity. Of these, 177 (69%) were the result of trauma and 79 (31%) were due to overuse. Sprains accounted for 29% of all injuries with 59% involving the ankle and 34% occurring in the knee. Strains accounted for 45 injuries (18%), 80% of which were localized to the lower extremity. Fifty-one knee injuries were seen. Thirty-five (69%) were caused by trauma and 16 (31%) through overuse. Forty-four ankle injuries (17%) occurred with 43 sprains and one lateral malleolar fracture. The lateral ligamentous complex was injured in 39 (91%) of the 43 cases. Seventeen (47%) of the ankles had been previously sprained. Two-thirds of the traumatic injuries occurred in games, 59% of which occurred during contact with another player. Seventy-nine (31%) injuries were over-use, of which 84% occurred during practice.

Football is becoming increasingly popular on the North American continent. A study of youth football in the USA included 4018 players (age 8–18 years). Injuries reported numbered 176 (McCarroll *et al.* 1984). The overall injury rate was 4.38% with the under-19 age group having the highest incidence at 8.74%. Injury rates lessened as age decreased. Competitive teams had higher injury rates than recreational teams. The most common injury was a sprain (26.7%) with contusions comprising 25%. The ankle was the most commonly injured joint, followed by the knee.

A telephone study conducted in the USA contacted the coaches of 80 teams on a weekly basis to request injury information (Sullivan *et al.* 1980). There were 931 boys and 341 girls ranging in age from 7 to 18 years, with one-half being under the age of 10 years. Twenty-nine players sustained 34 injuries, five of which were recurrences. Sixteen boys had 19 injuries while 13 girls incurred 15 injuries. Each player amassed approximately 40 h of participation, yielding an injury rate of $0.51 \cdot 1000\,h^{-1}$ for boys and $1.1 \cdot 1000\,h^{-1}$ for the girls. Seventeen injuries prevented participation for more than 7 days. The injury rate was $7.7 \cdot 100\,h^{-1}$ in the older age groups compared to $0.8 \cdot 100\,h^{-1}$ in the younger age groups. Contusions were the most common injury with 13 episodes followed closely by 12 sprains. The upper extremity was involved in six injuries, the head and neck on five occasions and the trunk in one. The lower extremity accounted for 22 injuries.

A review of insurance claims related to football was performed through the largest insurer of secondary school students in the western USA (Pritchett 1981). There were 436 claims among 10 634 players. Minor injuries such as contusions and sprains accounted for 76% of the injuries but involved only 49% of the total cost. The lower extremity involved 58% of the injuries and costs. An ankle sprain was the most common injury site (19%). Knee injuries comprised 11.7% of the total and 28% of the costs. Contusions occurred in 30.7% of the injuries and sprains and strains accounted for 38.1%. The incidence of fracture was 18.8%.

Another report from the USA compared injuries in youth outdoor to youth indoor football (Hoff & Martin 1986). Responses were obtained on 455 players (62.9%) in the outdoor league. The indoor league had a response rate of 60.6% (366 players). Forty players sustained 46 injuries in the outdoor league while 63 players incurred 74 injuries during the indoor league. The majority of the injuries were minor — only two outdoor and six indoor injuries caused an absence of more than 7 days. During game play, the incidence rate of injury per 100 h was 4.5 times higher in the indoor league as compared to the outdoor league. Injury rates were lowest in the younger age groups. Physical contact between two players resulted in 66.6% of the injuries (60.9%) in the outdoor league and 70.3% indoor. Medical assistance was required in 6.5% of the injuries among respondents in the outdoor league while 24.3% of injuries sustained during indoor play needed medical services.

Injury management

The majority of injuries sustained through participation in football do not require hospital attention. Most injuries are to the lower extremities and involve damage to the soft tissue. Any approach to injury rehabilitation must attempt to restore normal function to the extremity in question. The major considerations in the treatment of injuries must be to regain proper range of motion, endurance, and strength. Initial management is aimed at controlling the swelling and pain associated with acute injuries. Ice should be applied to the injured area as soon as possible. Frequent application of the ice throughout the next several days will reduce swelling and allow earlier mobilization of the body part. Compression and elevation during the initial stages of the injury will also reduce the associated swelling.

Relative rest should be instituted as an integral part of the rehabilitation program. Relative rest implies refraining from the offending activity while starting an exercise program that will allow strengthening of the musculature surrounding the injured area. As flexibility of the affected area begins to return to normal, strengthening exercises should be initiated. The initial approach emphasizes endurance through low-resistance high-repetition exercises. Non-weight-bearing exercises (open kinetic chain) may need to be utilized at the onset but, as improvement is seen, weight-bearing exercises (closed kinetic chain) should be added to simulate functional movement. As improvement continues, advancement to sport-specific activity is in order. Jogging with slow changes in direction can be started with a progression to sharp turns. Individual work with a ball can then be instituted. As fluidity and ease of movement return, advancement to drills and then to play can be accomplished. The rehabilitation program should be continued beyond the complete return to play to reduce the chance of recurrence.

Two-thirds of major injuries in football are preceded by a minor injury in the previous 3 months.

Serving the professional club

The team physician's job starts as soon as a new player is recruited by the club. The first task is to give the green light to the signing of the player or advise the club's administrators against the recruitment. This is obviously done via the appropriate medical examination, including clinical and orthopedic exploration, sample analysis, radiology tests, and intensive exercise ratings. This should allow the team physician to draw a medical picture of the new arrival and to decide whether the signing is appropriate or not.

Internal medicine very rarely reveals motives to advise against a signing, but some pathologic conditions do crop up from time to time. They are usually, to use an understatement, bad news for the player and the physician, and mainly concern congenital cardiomyopathy and coronary artery malformations.

However, osteo-articular anomalies are relatively frequent, usually as a consequence of prior injuries or previous surgery. Spondylolysis, spondylolysthesis, chronic instability of the knee or ankle, osteochondritis, and other conditions are by no means uncommon among players who are transferred from one club to another. It is here that the team physician faces a responsibility within the organization as a whole.

Among the players who have already been admitted to the dressing-room, the physician's priorities begin with measures to prevent injuries and illnesses which can make players unavailable for selection and thus possibly affect the team's performance. The players must receive clear guidance on correct hygiene and anti-infectious precautions. It is also essential to stress with the coach the elementary ground rules — a thorough warm-up before training sessions and games; stretching exercises; and a training regimen administered in the right sort of doses to avoid the build-up of fatigue, especially since many professional players have little knowledge of these matters.

If working conditions allow it, the presence of the team physician in the dressing-room every day is not only desirable but important. The daily presence of the physician helps to detect and diagnose illnesses or, for example, overuse injuries in their initial stages when remedies are easy to find and when recovery times can be minimized. In this respect the collaboration of the physical therapist, who has maximum daily contact with the players, has a very special importance. Good team-work, in the sense of passing on information to the physician, is of prime importance in "preventive medicine." Once a pathological process — whatever the origin — has been established, the diagnosis and treatment of injuries or other problems should always be carried out with a view to solving the problem in the shortest possible time, mainly because a player represents a high value from the point of view of the club, the team-mates, and the fans.

If the team physician decides that the player is unable to conclude the diagnosis or treatment, this is the moment to turn to the specialists who co-operate with the club. It is important to be able to depend upon a good support team of surgeons and traumatologists. If possible, the complexity of modern traumatology and orthopedics presents a valid argument for working with a pool of specialists. Recently, the trend toward super-specialization has produced generations of professionals specifically dedicated to knees, feet, shoulders, arthroscopy, and so on, and this generally guarantees better results. Having access to a rehabilitation center is also fundamental — and preferably one which has been well set-up and well-run! Perfectly good surgical techniques can lead to ultimate failure if the rehabilitation process is incorrect.

In fact, this is a point which requires special attention. In an ideal world, the rehabilitation of injured players would always be carried out using the facilities at the stadium or the training ground and under the supervision of the club's physician and physical therapists.

It is also worth pointing out that, in all cases, physical rehabilitation work by injured players or post-surgical cases, begins as soon as the patient can physically get himself or herself to the gymnasium. Once there, systematic work-outs should begin, aimed at toning up the whole body while, at the same time, showing maximum respect for the injury zone. Speeding up the return to physical activity gives positive results on two fronts. On the one hand, the work-outs lay the foundation for an accelerated return to general fitness once normal training can be resumed. And on the other hand, they also generate benefits from a psychological viewpoint, as the injured player immediately feels that he or she is working toward reappearance in the team.

Preparation for a professional match

We could define the preparation period as the whole time-span between one match and the next. In other words, the preparation begins with the treatment of knocks and injuries produced in the previous match, continues through recovery and rehabilitation exercises, and then to a training schedule. This schedule should firstly ensure full recuperation from the previous efforts, and secondly provide technical exercises aimed at thorough preparation for the following game.

The intensive pre-match preparation period could be defined as the 24 h prior to kick-off. As from the day before the match, each player must put aside any interests which are not specifically related to the job in hand. This is the fundamental reason for favoring pre-match "concentrations" where the group can undertake a conscientious preparation for the game. This prevents the players from worrying about business interests, studies, family problems, and anything which could be a drain on psychic resources. In the hotel or residence, the player is usually insulated from crying children, telephone calls, untimely visits, and other potential distractions. This gives the team coach the chance to talk to the players, to discuss the peculiarities of the opposition and mentalize the players for the match.

The team physician can help by being present with a barrage of therapeutic weapons for the players who need them. It is important that meals and drinks are planned and supervised to a high degree. Generally, the evening meal on the day before the match could consist of a rice dish, a main course of fish, and then pastries. On match day, the program is built from the basis of kick-off time. If the match is to begin at 5 p.m., the normal procedure would start with a light breakfast of fruit juice, tea or coffee, and toast and jam. The midday meal would typically be scheduled for between 4 and 4.5 h before kick-off. The usual menu consists of spaghetti, rice, or other carbohydrate-rich meal. If it is an evening kick-off at 7 or 8 p.m., lunch is delayed until 1.30 p.m. and, in that case, a light tea will be made available at around 5 p.m., consisting of coffee or tea with biscuits, teacakes, or something similar.

At the same time, it has to be borne in mind that a

professional football team with players of varying origins is, logically, going to present a variety of culinary preferences and types of diet. For this reason, the usual "design" of the menu for team meals is decided in a committee where the players are represented. This way, the club ensures not only that a correct dietary preparation is carried out, but also satisfies the gastronomical wishes of the players. This is especially necessary when the team is away for several days due to pre-season training camps, summer tournaments, or fixtures in international tournaments.

The match-day program is also designed to allow the team to arrive at the ground 1.5 h before kick-off time. This gives the athletic trainer enough time to complete pre-match duties. It also allows the players to perform some proper warming-up exercises. At the same time, the atmosphere in the dressing-room should be as quiet and isolated as possible, so that the players can work on their concentration and get into the right frame of mind for the match. This is why the dressing-room door should remain shut to reporters, supporters, club directors, and others. The basic idea is to encourage a quiet atmosphere, a positive approach and a mood of optimism and this is much more easily obtained if access is restricted to the coach, the physician, the physical therapist, and the team's delegate.

Additional basic points arise from the obvious fact that approximately half of the season's matches and training are carried out away from home. In other words the players, the coaches, the directors, and the rest of "the team" have to be prepared for frequent journeys within their own country or abroad. The fundamental rule for all these journeys is trying to make traveling time as short and as comfortable as possible. If an away trip involves crossing time zones, then the effects of jet lag must be taken into account. This presents a need for a series of measures to be taken as soon as the party has boarded the plane, for example, it is better to stay awake during daytime travelling. Players should be encouraged to move around the aisles while they are on planes and to do some stretching and isometric exercises while sitting.

On arrival at the destination, it is important that the accommodation is in a quiet area and that the food should be recognizably similar to the players' usual diet at home. Clubs that can afford to do so often travel with their own chef and, occasionally, with their own food. This has also become routine for national teams who travel to compete in international matches. The acclimatization programs conducted by most professional teams before taking part in these competitions are well planned and include both medical, nutritional, physiological and other factors. If away games involve long-distance traveling, it is advisable to conduct a light training session as soon as possible after arrival at the destination, although the day and time of arrival may have an influence on this aspect of programing. If possible, the session should be at the ground where the match is to be played. These sessions should be relatively short but conducted at a lively pace and moderate intensity, the object here being to put the player into the right neuropsychological frame of mind.

For the physician, one of the very important tasks during travels of this type is to contact as soon as possible the medical staff of the home team with a view to starting the game well informed on subjects such as the stadium's capacity, measures for the evacuation of injured people in case of emergency, and other contingency plans which are invaluable should anything untoward happen.

The team physician — heard but not seen

The physician's day-to-day participation in the life of a football team is a peculiar role in that, apart from the purely professional capacity, it requires more than a fair degree of diplomacy.

As a general rule, the physician is taken onto the staff and employed by the club's president and/or the board of directors. In contractual terms, he or she is therefore in their employ, responsible to them and usually has the prime obligation of keeping them up to date on the state of health of the players. When it comes to signing new players or extending players' contracts, most professional clubs consult the team physician before proceeding.

At the same time, the team physician almost automatically establishes a very close working relationship with the team's coach, who also has to be given exhaustive information about the state of health of the members of the squad, so as to be able to program training sessions, select the team, and so on.

The physician's position in the middle of this "eternal triangle" requires him or her to seek and find an ethical balance which clears the field for the physician to work in favor of the patient, i.e. the player. There are obviously pathologies which can be openly discussed with the team coach or with the board of directors if need be. At the same time, however, there can sometimes be types of illness (e.g. sexually transmitted diseases) which entail moral and social implications and which demand from the physician the most strict observation of professional discretion and secrecy.

Given the peculiar working conditions, it is understandable that the team physician is very often regarded by the coaching staff as a "mole" planted in the dressing-room by the board of directors with a license to spy. It is equally understandable that the board of directors often feels that the physician has become a fully integrated member of the coaching staff.

Maintaining a balanced posture evidently depends to a very large extent on the individual skills and astuteness of the physician. To a certain extent the job can be said to be relatively easy if the physician always keeps at the front of his or her mind the basic perception that the most important element in this game is the player and that the physician must place all his or her professional skills and attention at the disposition of the patient.

A secret is a secret

Having made a passing reference to the Hippocratic oath, it is worth mentioning that one of the most delicate moments for the team physician comes when one of the players is being transferred to another club. The position of the physician, though, is quite clear. In these cases the team physician is not authorized to pass on information about current or previous pathology contained in the case history without the express permission of the individual player concerned.

The media

At many clubs, especially those with a large following and intensive media coverage, the physician is often in the position of being questioned by reporters about the fitness or state of health of injured players. At certain clubs, this has even become part of the daily routine. It is usually argued that the player is a VIP of great interest to the general public and that the fans,

therefore, have a right to be informed, as long as the information cannot be considered an intrusion into the player's private life. So, in practical terms, the physician is often obliged to keep the media informed about the injuries, possible recovery times, parameters for the player's absence, and chances of being fit to play in certain matches. In this situation, the physician must evidently be able to communicate in simple terms which offer no scope for confusion and which, at the same time, restrict to a minimum the precise details of the pathology suffered by the player. In practise, it is unquestionably better if the team physician keeps as low a profile as possible in the media and only makes "public appearance" when they are strictly necessary and with the consent of the player concerned.

References

Berger-Vachon C., Gabard G. & Moyen B. (1986) Soccer accidents in the French Rhone-Alpes soccer association. *Sports Med.* **3**, 69–77.

Ekstrand J. & Gillquist J. (1983) Soccer injuries and their mechanisms: a prospective study. *Med. Sci. Sport Exerc.* **15**, 267–270.

Hoff G.L. & Martin T.A. (1986) Outdoor and indoor soccer: injuries among youth players. *Am. J. Sports Med.* **14**, 231–233.

Hoy K., Lindblad B.E., Terkelsen C.J. & Helleland H.E. (1992) European soccer injuries: a prospective epidemiologic and socioeconomic study. *Am. J. Sports Med.* **20**, 318–322.

McCarroll J.R., Meaney C. & Sieber J.M. (1984) Profile of youth soccer injuries. *Phys. Sportsmed.* **12**(2), 113–117.

Nielsen A.B. & Yde J. (1989) Epidemiology and traumatology of injuries in soccer. *Am. J. Sports Med.* **17**, 803–807.

Nilsson S. (1978) Soccer injuries in adolescents. *Am. J. Sports Med.* **6**, 358–361.

Pritchett J.W. (1981) Cost of high school soccer injuries. *Am. J. Sports Med.* **9**, 64–66.

Sadat-Ali M. & Sankaran-Kutty M. (1987) Soccer injuries in Saudi-Arabia. *Am. J. Sports Med.* **15**, 500–502.

Schmidt-Olsen S., Bunemann K.H., Lade V. & Brassoe J.O.K. (1985) Soccer injuries of youth. *Br. J. Sports Med.* **19**, 161–164.

Schmidt-Olsen S., Jörgensen U., Kaalund S. & Sorensen J. (1991) Injuries among young soccer players. *Am. J. Sports Med.* **19**, 273–275.

Sullivan J.A., Gross R.H., Grana W.A. & Garcia-Moral C.A. (1980) Evaluation of injuries in youth soccer. *Am. J. Sports Med.* **8**, 325–327.

Chapter 14

Injuries

Table 14.1 Type of injury (%)

	Total	Minor	Moderate	Major
Sprain	29	16	7	5
Overuse	23	17	5	2
Contusion	20	15	5	0
Strain	18	9	7	2
Fracture	4	1	1	2
Dislocation	2	0	2	0
Others	4	4	0	0
Total	100	62	27	11

Minor injury, absence from practise for less than 1 week; moderate injury, absence from practise for more than 1 week but less than 1 month; major injury, absence from practise for more than 1 month.

Football is the most popular sport in the world, with approximately 40 million organized players (and *c.* 100—150 million participants in total). As the popularity of football has grown, football injuries have become the object of increasing medical interest. It is estimated that in Europe 50—60% of all sports injuries and 3.5—10% of all hospital-treated injuries are due to football (Franke 1977, Ekstrand 1982, Keller *et al.* 1987).

Type, localization, and incidence of injuries

A fundamental problem associated with an epidemiologic assessment of data on sports injuries is the inconsistent manner in which injury is defined and information collected and recorded. Current literature on football injury epidemiology relies upon a variety of definitions of injury. The meaningful comparison of data collected in future football studies and comparison of football injury data with those reported for other sports requires a universal definition of athletic injury. It has been suggested that only those injuries resulting in lost time from practise or play should be included in the statistics. The duration of restricted athletic performance should also be reported in future studies since this represents a useful measure of the severity of injury.

Ekstrand and Gillquist (1983), Brynhildsen *et al.* (1991), Jörgensen (1984), and others have all used a common definition of injury as an event occurring during scheduled games or practise and causing the player to miss the next game or practise session. Injuries were classified into three categories according to severity (Table 14.1). The type and localization of injuries from the studies by Ekstrand are shown in Tables 14.1 and 14.2.

Expressed as a percentage of total injuries, lower

Table 14.2 Localization of injury (%)

	Total	Minor	Moderate	Major
Foot	12	10	2	0
Ankle	17	11	5	2
Leg	12	6	4	2
Knee	20	11	5	4
Thigh	14	6	5	2
Groin	13	9	3	1
Back	5	4	1	0
Others	7	5	2	0
Total	100	62	27	11

See Table 14.1 for definitions.

extremity injuries represent 82—88% for senior male amateur players (Ekstrand 1982, Jörgensen 1984), 73% for male professional players (Albert 1983), 80% for senior female players (Brynhildsen *et al.* 1991), and 65—68% for youth players (Nilsson & Roaas 1978, Sullivan *et al.* 1980).

To evaluate the real risk for football injuries, the exposure factor, i.e. the time the player is at risk, has to be taken into account (Table 14.3).

This section refers to a selection of common sport-

Table 14.3 Football injury exposure rate

Athlete	No. injuries· 1000 h^{-1}	Reference
Youth		Sullivan *et al.* (1980)
Male	0.5	
Female	1.1	
Youth		Nilsson & Roaas (1978)
Male	1.4	
Female	3.2	
Senior		
Male		Ekstrand (1982)
Practice	7.6	
Game	16.9	
Female		Brynhildsen *et al.* (1991)
Practice	2.1	
Game	6.5	
Senior		Jörgensen (1987)
Male	4.1	

specific injuries occurring in football players. Since injuries to the lower extremity are dominant in football, the next is limited to such injuries. Concerning injuries not included in this section, like fractures, luxations, etc., the reader is referred to general textbooks in orthopedics and sports medicine traumatology.

Foot and ankle

Turf toe syndrome

Turf toe syndrome is a sprain of the plantar capsule of the base joint of the big toe (metatarsophalangeal joint). It is common in playing football on an artificial surface and is caused by a forceful dorsiflexion of the big toe due to increased friction between the shoe and the surface.

Symptoms and diagnosis

The symptoms are pain, tenderness, and swelling in the base joint of the big toe. It is particularly painful during push-off in running and passive dorsiflexion of the joint causes pain.

Treatment

Initial treatment includes rest, ice, compression, and elevation (RICE) treatment, anti-inflammatory agents, and relief of weight-bearing. After 2–4 days, weight-bearing can be resumed, but 2–4 weeks of rest is recommended before return to football. During the rehabilitation phase, the great toe can be taped to limit dorsiflexion.

Hallux rigidus

Hallux rigidus is a chronic injury resulting from repeated minor injuries to the base joint of the great toe.

Symptoms and diagnosis

The dorsiflexion of the great toe is limited and this is detrimental to the performance of football players, who need 90° of dorsiflexion of the base joint of the great toe at push-off.

Treatment

A stiff-soled shoe might reduce pain and occasionally surgery is indicated.

Football toe (subungual hematoma)

Subungual hematoma is often called "football toe" because it is more common in football than in other sports. The injury is usually caused either by jamming of the longest toe against the toe-box or on an opponent's stepping on the shoe.

Symptoms, diagnosis, and treatment

Subungual hematoma produces severe pain which can be eliminated by making a hole through the nail with a red-hot needle or straightened paper clip.

Morton's syndrome

Morton's syndrome is a local swelling of a plantar digital nerve, caused by compression of the nerve between the metatarsal heads (Fig. 14.1). A player with hypermobile foot with excessive pronation or a depressed anterior arch is predisposed to this entity.

Symptoms and diagnosis

The most common symptom is pain on the plantar aspect of the foot. The pain may radiate into the adjacent toes and is relieved by rest.

Treatment

Conservative treatment consists of wide-fitting shoes and arch support with a pad which can spread the metatarsal bones. Surgical excision through a dorsal incision is very effective.

Plantar fasciitis

Plantar fasciitis is an insertion tendinitis of the plantar aponeurosis (fascia) at the origin at calcaneus. It is considered as an overuse injury and excessive pronation is a predisposing factor (Fig. 14.2). A calcaneal spur seen on X-ray is the result and not the cause of traction, chronic inflammation, and subsequent calcification.

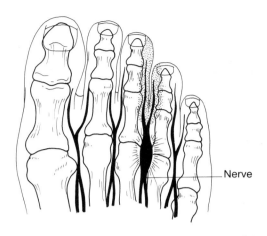

Fig. 14.1 Morton's syndrome. When the front arch is weak, a nerve can get trapped between the metatarsal bones. The nerve then swells, increasing pressure which in turn may cause radiating pain and numbness in the toes (shaded areas). (From Peterson & Renström 1988.)

Symptoms and diagnosis

An intensive palpation tenderness over the medial insertion of the plantar fascia onto the calcaneus gives the diagnosis. Differential diagnoses are tarsal tunnel syndrome and calcaneal nerve entrapment.

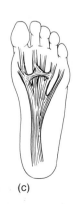

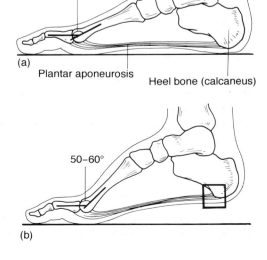

Fig. 14.2 Plantar fasciitis. (a) The foot and plantar aponeurosis (fascia) when the whole foot is loaded against the surface. (b) The plantar aponeurosis stretched during take-off. The boxed area indicates the seat of inflammation at the origin of the plantar aponeurosis from the heel bone. (c) The plantar aponeurosis seen from underneath. (From Peterson & Renström 1988.)

Treatment

Treatment consists of rest and unloading of the longitudinal foot arch by the use of arch support (orthotics) or arch taping. Local steroid injections can be of help but are painful. Plantar fasciitis may take 2—3 months to resolve and sometimes surgical intervention is necessary.

Footballer's ankle

Acute or repeated overstretching of the ankle joint causes traction in the attachment of the joint capsule and can lead to the development of osteophytes in the anterior edge of the tibia and/or on the neck of the talus (Fig. 14.3). The condition is frequently seen in professional football players.

Symptoms and diagnosis

The symptoms are pain across the ankle joint which is aggravated at kicking. On physical examination there is tenderness and slight swelling in the anterior aspect of the ankle joint and sometimes the osteophytes can

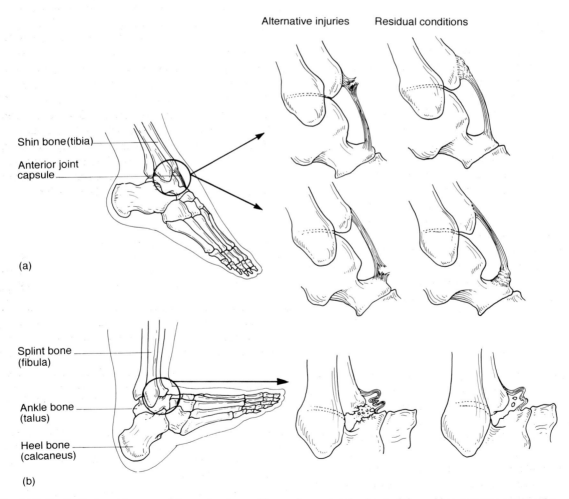

Fig. 14.3 Footballer's ankle — possible mechanisms of bone changes at the front of the ankle joint: (a) overstretching in passive plantar flexion; (b) overstretching in passive dorsiflexion. (From Peterson & Renström 1988.)

be palpated. The mobility of the ankle joint is usually impaired. The diagnosis is verified by X-rays showing osteophytes.

Treatment

Conservative treatment consists of anti-inflammatory drugs or steroid injections. Surgery can be necessary and consists of excision of osteophytes. The excision can be done arthroscopically or by a small arthrotomy. The post-operative administration of non-steroidal anti-inflammatory drugs (NSAIDs) is sometimes recommended to reduce the risk of recurrent osteophyte formation.

Ankle sprain

Ankle sprains are the most common injuries in football. They constitute about 20% of all football injuries and the incidence in senior players is reported to be between 1.7 and $2 \cdot 1000\,h^{-1}$ of exposure to football.

Most ankle sprains affect the lateral ligamentous complex and these injuries are caused by inversion and plantar flexion of the ankle. The anterior talofibular ligament (TFA) is injured first (70%). In about 20% of cases, there is a combination injury with tear of the TFA as well as the calcaneofibular ligament. In young growing athletes with strong ligaments and in elderly patients with brittle bones, an inversion/plantarflexion trauma could cause a bony avulsion at the tip of the lateral malleolus, whilst the ligaments remain intact. Injuries to the deltoid ligament on the medial side are uncommon, accounting for less than 10% of all ankle sprains. The mechanism behind these injuries is pronation and outward rotation of the foot.

Symptoms and diagnosis

The diagnosis of an ankle sprain is made by the presence of swelling and tenderness over the injured ligament. The clinical anterior drawer test is positive in case of rupture of the TFA, but this test can be difficult to evaluate in acute injuries with pain and swelling. An X-ray examination is suggested to exclude fractures and bony avulsions and X-ray with an anterior drawer test confirms the diagnosis of lateral ligament injury.

Concerning differential diagnosis, a syndesmosis injury should be suspected in cases with tenderness over the junction of the tibia and fibula and a widening of the ankle mortise at X-ray. If left untreated, a syndesmosis injury could later cause lateral subluxation of the talus which impairs performance in football.

Treatment

The initial treatment of ankle sprains consists of limiting bleeding and swelling by the use of RICE therapy (Table 14.4). The treatment should be immediate and intensive. A compression bandage suitable for ankle sprains is a horseshoe-shaped pad around the lateral malleolus (over the three ligaments) combined with overlaying elastic bandage (Fig. 14.4). The compression bandage should be used for 3–7 days or until the swelling has disappeared. The bandage should be kept on over night. The use of crutches is recommended during this period to minimize loading. As soon as pain subsides, mobility training including flexion and extension of the ankle joint is started.

When swelling subsides, the elastic bandage should be replaced by a supportive tape bandage. The ankle joint should be taped continuously for 5–6 weeks. To avoid skin problems and loosening of the tape, retaping each week is recommended. Healing of the ligament takes 6–8 weeks, but with proper taping and rehabilitation, return to football can take place earlier.

Table 14.4 Rest, ice, compression, and elevation (RICE) therapy. The immediate treatment is the same for almost all acute traumatic football injuries of the lower extremity

Rest is necessary because continued exercise or other activity could extend the injury. Crutches should be used in a non-weight-bearing toe-touch or partial weight-bearing manner

Ice decreases the bleeding from injured vessels and causes them to contract. The more blood that collects in a wound, the longer it takes to heal. Ice has also a local pain-relieving effect

Compression limits swelling which, if uncontrolled, could retard healing. A compression bandage usually consists of a pad placed over the injured part and an elastic bandage applied with some degree of tension over that

Elevation of the injured part to above the level of the heart uses the force of gravity to help drain excess fluid

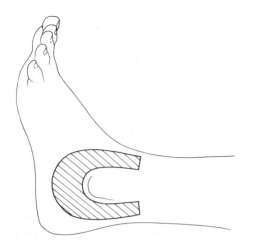

Fig. 14.4 Acute treatment of ankle sprains: a horseshoe-shaped pad around the lateral malleolus for compression.

During the healing phase, intensive rehabilitation is recommended. The principles of intensive and football-specific rehabilitation after an ankle sprain and other injuries to the lower extremity are described in Fig. 14.5. The basic principle is a stepwise increase of the stress on the injured ligament with avoidance of pain and swelling. When the player is able to walk without limping, jogging can begin, followed by running in a figure of eight, zig-zag running, and running with turns. When the player is able to run and turn around 360° without pain, individual ball exercises are introduced, followed by kicking, jumping, and sprinting.

When the player can do all football-specific exercises without pain, participation in team training can begin, where tackling situations are included. Full, pain-free participation in team training is mandatory before matches. If a step in the rehabilitation ladder creates pain or swelling, the player should return to the previous step for a couple of days and then try the higher step again. The ankle joint should be taped during the rehabilitation period and then during practise sessions and matches for the first 6 months after the injury.

For rehabilitation of proprioceptive control, balance training on an ankle disk is recommended.

As a rule, the results of conservative treatment are so favorable that surgical treatment is only indicated to a limited extent. If a ligament injury still causes instability problems 4–6 months after conservative treatment, surgery is indicated. The results after suture or reconstruction of a ligament injury are favorable. An ankle sprain may also cause cartilage injuries or osteochondral fractures on the talus. The symptoms are pain and tenderness (common on the medial side),

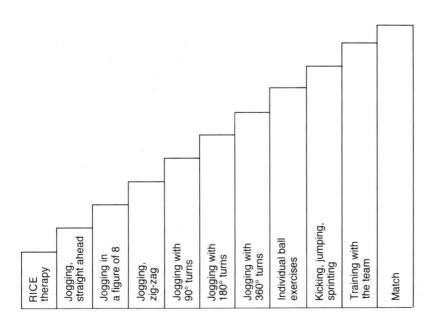

Fig. 14.5 Rehabilitation after injury to the lower extremity. Stepwise increase of the stress on the injured structure with avoidance of pain and swelling.

swelling and locking. Arthroscopy or arthrotomy are valuable for diagnosis and treatment.

Achilles tendon injuries

Injuries to the Achilles tendon could be caused by trauma (total or partial rupture of the tendon) or by overuse (Achilles tendinitis or Achilles bursitis). Two factors predispose to Achilles tendon injuries: (a) the great load that is put on the tendon in athletic activities; and (b) the poor circulation of the tendon. Concerning the load, the critical limit for tendons is estimated to be about $5000\,N\cdot cm^{-2}$. The cross-section area of the Achilles tendon is about $2\,cm^2$ and since the forces put on the tendon is about $5000-10\,000\,N$ in sprinting activities, it is clear that many activities in football put a stress on the Achilles tendon which is close to its critical limit.

Injuries of the Achilles tendon usually occur at the zone of poor circulation, which is located $2-6\,cm$ above it's insertion at calcaneus.

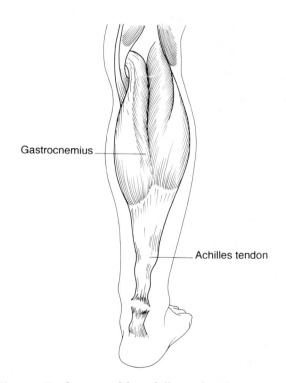

Gastrocnemius

Achilles tendon

Fig. 14.6 Total rupture of the Achilles tendon (from Peterson & Renström 1988).

Total rupture of the Achilles tendon

Total ruptures usually occur in degenerated tendons and are therefore more common in elderly players or in players previously affected by Achilles tendinitis (Fig. 14.6).

Symptoms and diagnosis

Typically, the player feels like he has been kicked on the tendon. The player can usually walk normally, but is unable to stand on tiptoe. There is a distinct tenderness over the ruptured area and a gap in the tendon can be felt. Definite diagnosis is made with the Thompson test. In this test, the calf is squeezed, and if the ankle fails to flex, the Achilles tendon is ruptured.

Treatment

Treatment of a complete rupture of the Achilles tendon in an active football player should be surgical.

Partial rupture of the Achilles tendon

Partial ruptures of the Achilles tendon are common in football players and they often become chronic and cause prolonged problems (Fig. 14.7).

Symptoms and diagnosis

Usually the player experiences a sharp pain in the tendon on jumping, sprinting, and other explosive movements. A nodule is palpable in the tendon, usually $2-6\,cm$ above the os calcis.

Treatment

Conservative treatment consists of rest, a heel lift, and anti-inflammatory medication. If conservative treatment fails, the nodules should be exposed and degenerative areas of the tendon resected. The rehabilitation period after surgery is usually $4-6$ months before football can be resumed.

Achilles tendinitis

Achilles tendinitis is the most common tendinitis seen in football players. It is an overuse injury resulting

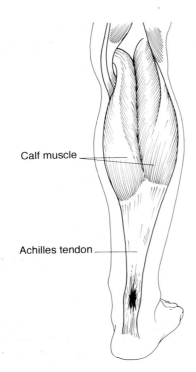

Calf muscle

Achilles tendon

Fig. 14.7 Partial rupture of the Achilles tendon (from Peterson & Renström 1988).

from prolonged repeated loading. Anatomical malalignments such as flat feet, pes cavus, or muscle tightness of the calf muscles predispose to this injury.

Symptoms and diagnosis

The major symptom is pain, which is aggravated by activity and relieved by rest. The player usually complains of stiffness in the morning and before and after activity.

Treatment

The treatment consists of rest, heel lift, ice massage, and anti-inflammatory medication for a couple of weeks. If the player does not rest, the acute inflammation may turn into a chronic condition where the pseudosheath of the Achilles tendon becomes fibrotic and stenotic and may require surgical decompression consisting of removal of the entire pseudosheath.

Achilles bursitis

The retrocalcaneal bursa is located between the Achilles tendon and os calcaneus. Inflammation and hypertrophy of this bursa is common in football players due to either kicking in the area or pressure from the football shoes (Fig. 14.8). A prominent posterior tubercle of the os calcis may be an additional cause of the bursitis.

Symptoms and diagnosis

The pain and tenderness at palpation are located at the insertion of the tendon, more distal than the location of an Achilles tendinitis or a partial rupture.

Treatment

Conservative treatment with ice or injection of cortisone in the bursa is usually favorable. In chronic cases, surgery is indicated. During the exploration, the bursa and the bony prominence are removed.

Medial lower leg pain

Pain on the medial side of the lower leg can arise from the periost (periostitis), from the posterior deep muscle compartment (compartment syndrome), or from the tibia (stress fracture).

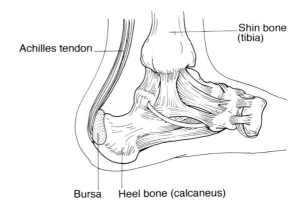

Achilles tendon

Shin bone (tibia)

Bursa   Heel bone (calcaneus)

Fig. 14.8 Achilles bursitis, where there is inflammation of the bursa át the attachment of the Achilles tendon to the calcaneus (from Peterson & Renström 1988).

Periostitis (shin splints)

Periostitis of the medial margin of the tibia is a musculo-tendinous inflammation. It is an overuse injury, which often afflicts football players when they change surfaces or shoes or when they increase the intensity of training and matches.

Symptoms and diagnosis

The symptoms are pain and tenderness over the distal margin of the tibia. The periostitis is often bilateral. Typically, the pain is intensive at the beginning of an activity and diminished after warm-up.

Treatment

The primary treatment is rest from the causative factor(s), until the tenderness over the tibia has disappeared. Surgery, in the form of fasciotomy, may be necessary in chronic cases.

Posterior deep compartment syndrome

The muscles of the lower leg are enclosed in four compartments of connective tissue which are anchored to the tibia and fibula. Compartment syndromes are caused by increased pressure inside the compartments. Acute compartment syndrome can be the result from a blow or a kick to the calf and chronic compartment syndrome is a result of the increase of muscle bulk following training (Fig. 14.9). The deep posterior compartment contains the flexor digitorum, flexor hallucis longus, and tibialis posterior muscles.

Symptoms and diagnosis

The major symptom of a posterior deep compartment syndrome is a gradually increasing pain at the medial margin of the tibia, sometimes associated with weakness and numbness of the foot.

Treatment

The treatment consists of rest, ice massage, anti-inflammatory medication, and, in chronic cases, fasciotomy.

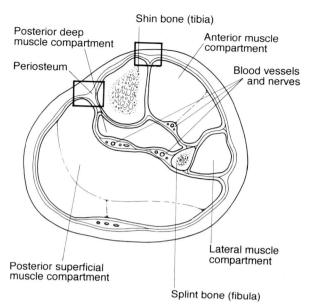

Fig. 14.9 Compartment syndrome. Cross-section of the lower leg; the muscles are enclosed in four well-defined muscle compartments. The squares indicate common sites of tenderness at the anchor points of muscle compartments to the periosteum of the shin bone. (From Peterson & Renström 1988.)

Stress fractures

Stress fractures are common overuse injuries in football players. The most common localizations are at the tibia and the fibula, but stress fractures are also commonly seen in the metatarsal bones, in the femur, and in the pelvic ring.

Symptoms and diagnosis

There is usually a sharp pain and a localized tenderness over the area of a stress fracture. A fresh stress fracture is usually not visible on plain X-ray, but may be visible as a subperiostal bone formation on a repeat X-ray 2–3 weeks after the onset of symptoms. A bone scan gives the definite diagnosis, but the clinical examination with a very localized, strong palpation tenderness, is usually enough for diagnosis.

Treatment

Tibial stress fractures usually do not require immobilization with plaster, but they do require complete cessation of running and other football activities for 6–8 weeks. Other activities, such as bicycling, swimming, and water-jogging, are recommended to maintain fitness and muscle strength.

Knee

Disorders of the knee (Fig. 14.10) may be mechanical (traumatic injuries) or inflammatory (overuse injuries), intra-articular or extra-articular. In order to evaluate the knee properly, a comprehensive history and physical examination must be performed, supported by radiography and, when appropriate, laboratory studies. At times, arthroscopy is useful as a diagnostic tool and also for treatment.

This section will briefly describe some overuse injuries (iliotibial band friction syndrome, patellar tendinitis, and tibial epiphysitis) and some traumatic injuries (ruptures of the meniscii, the medial collateral ligament (MCL), and the cruciate ligaments).

Iliotibial band friction syndrome

Iliotibial band friction syndrome is an overuse injury primarily caused by running. The mechanism behind it is friction of the iliotibial band when it moves over the lateral femoral condyle (Fig. 14.11). A tightness of the hip abductors predispose to the injury.

Symptoms and diagnosis

The player complains of pain on the lateral aspect of the knee and at examination there is localized tenderness at palpation of the lateral femoral condyle. Examination of the knee does not show any symptoms of lateral meniscus rupture or other intra-articular injury.

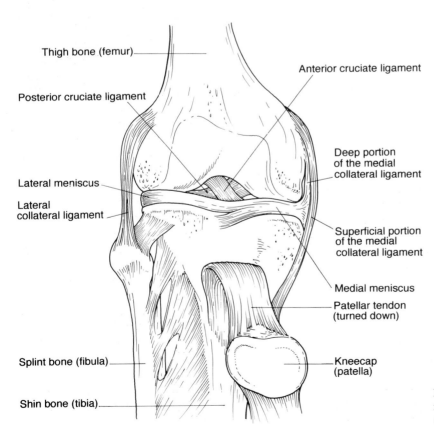

Thigh bone (femur)

Posterior cruciate ligament

Lateral meniscus

Lateral collateral ligament

Splint bone (fibula)

Shin bone (tibia)

Anterior cruciate ligament

Deep portion of the medial collateral ligament

Superficial portion of the medial collateral ligament

Medial meniscus

Patellar tendon (turned down)

Kneecap (patella)

Fig. 14.10 Anatomical diagram of the right knee joint seen from the front (from Peterson & Renström 1988).

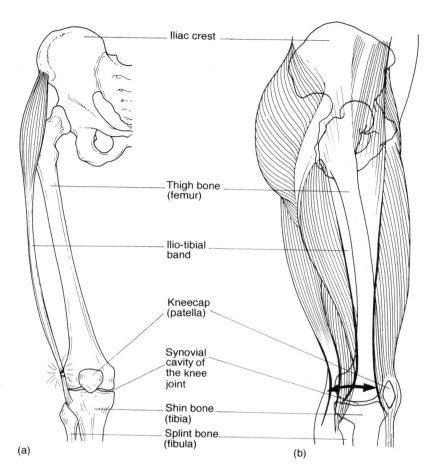

Iliac crest

Thigh bone
(femur)

Ilio-tibial
band

Kneecap
(patella)

Synovial
cavity of
the knee
joint

Shin bone
(tibia)

Splint bone
(fibula)

(a) (b)

Fig. 14.11 Iliotibial band friction syndrome. (a) Diagram showing how the ilio-tibial band slips backwards and forwards over the lower, lateral part of the femur when bending and straightening the knee joint. (b) Lateral view of the thigh muscles. (From Peterson & Renström 1988.)

Treatment

Treatment consist of rest, ice, anti-inflammatory medication, and stretching of the iliotibial band. Local injections of steroids are usually very helpful. In chronic cases, surgery is indicated. The surgical procedure consists of an X-incision or similar incisions to release the tight iliotibial fibers from the femoral condyle.

Patellar tendinitis

Jumper's knee is a clinical syndrome with tendinitis, degeneration and sometimes partial rupture of the patellar tendon. The symptoms generally appear after kicking and jumping and is more common in goalkeepers (Fig. 14.12). Usually the injury is located at apex patella but a localization near the tuberositas

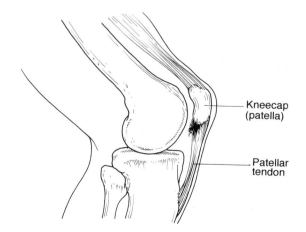

Kneecap
(patella)

Patellar
tendon

Fig. 14.12 Patellar tendinitis — a partial rupture of the top posterior portion of the patellar tendon (from Peterson & Renström 1988).

tibiae or above patella (quadriceps tendinitis) is not uncommon.

Symptoms and diagnosis

The symptoms are anterior knee pain and distinctly located tenderness over the affected part of the tendon. The pain is aggravated by contraction of the quadriceps.

Treatment

Treatment consists of adequate warm-up and ice massage after activity, anti-inflammatory medication, ultrasound, stretching of the quadriceps and hamstrings muscles, and activity modification to avoid jumping and other movements that trigger the pain. Local steroid injections are not recommended. Surgery is indicated in chronic cases and consists of incision of the tendon and removal of the degenerative areas.

Resection or drilling of the inferior pole of the patella is sometimes recommended. It is also important to consider the patellar alignment and sometimes a lateral release, a vastus medialis advancement, or an excision of osteophytes or calcified fragments are needed.

The rehabilitation period after surgery is long, usually 4–6 months before the player can return to football. Since the patellar tendon has a poor blood supply, it is important that the post-operative rehabilitation is slow, usually an immobilization period of 4–6 weeks is recommended.

Tibial epiphysitis (Osgood–Schlatter disease)

Osgood–Schlatter disease is a common injury in the adolescent football player. It used to be found mostly in boys in their growth spurt, but has recently been seen in girls aged 10–12 years. The etiology is somewhat unclear, but is usually considered as an inflammation or a minor avulsion fracture of the developing ossification center of the tibial tubercle (Fig. 14.13). In jumping and kicking movements in football, the extensor mechanism applies great tensile stress on the apophysis.

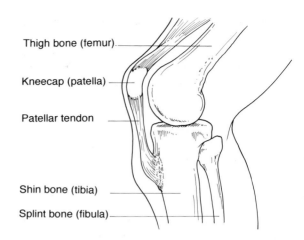

Fig. 14.13 Tibial epiphysitis. The bone is inflamed and broken up at the attachment of the patellar tendon to the shin bone. (From Peterson & Renström 1988.)

Symptoms and diagnosis

The pain is located over the tibial tubercle and aggravated by jumping and kicking. Usually, there is swelling and tenderness over the insertion of the patellar tendon to the tibia. An X-ray examination may show fragmentation of the tibial tubercle.

Treatment

Concerning treatment, it is important to stress that the disease heals spontaneously. To reduce symptoms, jumping and other pain-inducing activities should be avoided. Cortisone injections are not recommended and immobilization or surgery are generally not necessary. The enlargement of the tibial tubercle will usually remain in the adult player.

Meniscal injuries

Meniscal injuries are common in football, according to some studies, football causes the highest incidence of meniscal injuries in all sports. The mechanism of injury is usually a rotation of the femur relative to the tibia. Such rotational forces can be produced in contact situations, like in tackling, or in non-contact situations such as when a player's foot is fixed to the ground or in various cutting maneuvers. Meniscus injuries can also occur as a result of hyperflexion or hyperextension of the knee (Fig. 14.14).

Injury to the medial meniscus is more common than injury to the lateral meniscus. This is partly because the medial meniscus is attached to the medial collateral ligament and partly because tackles in football are more often directed toward the lateral side of the knee, causing increased forces on the medial meniscus. Meniscus injuries often occur in combination with other knee ligament injuries.

Symptoms and diagnosis

The symptoms of a meniscus injury is pain, swelling, giving way, and locking. The pain is located at the injured side (medial or lateral). The typical swelling in an isolated meniscus injury develops gradually over 1–3 days. Locking, with a lack of full extension, indicates a displaced meniscus tear such as a bucket-handle rupture. The diagnosis is fairly certain if two or more of the following examination findings are present:

1 Palpation tenderness over the affected meniscus.
2 Pain over the meniscus at hyperextension of the knee.
3 Pain over the meniscus at hyperflexion of the knee.
4 Positive McMurray test.

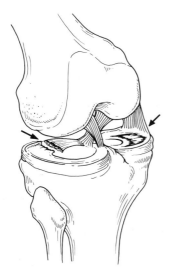

Fig. 14.14 Medial and lateral meniscus injuries (right knee). *Right*: a longitudinal rupture; *left*: a transverse rupture. (From Peterson & Renström 1988.)

The diagnosis is verified by arthroscopy, which provides a diagnosis with 98% accuracy and with low morbidity. The arthroscopic technique permits precise classification of type, extent, and location of the meniscus tear.

Treatment

Arthroscopic surgery techniques permit partial meniscectomy to be carried out in order to remove the damaged part of the meniscus and to retain maximum functional meniscal tissue. Arthroscopy also permits recognition of candidates for spontaneous healing or meniscal repairs of lesions within the vascular zone. A player who has been operated for a meniscus injury transarthroscopically, can usually start jogging 7–10 days after surgery or as soon as swelling has disappeared, and return to football 2–4 weeks post-operatively.

MCL injuries

The mechanism of injury to the MCL is most commonly an impact to the lateral side of the knee, which forces the joint into valgus (Fig. 14.15). There are three types of sprains: grade I, II, and III. In grade I injuries, there is stretching but not disruption of the MCL. There is tenderness at the site of injury and pain but no laxity at valgus stress testing. Treatment is conservative and football can be resumed when pain has disappeared, usually within a few weeks. In grade II injuries, there is a partial rupture of the MCL. In valgus stress testing there is a mild or moderate laxity (up to 5 mm of excess, compared to the non-injured leg) with a firm end-point. The treatment is conservative, and rehabilitation usually takes 3–6 weeks. In grade III injuries, there is a complete rupture of the MCL. Valgus stress testing shows more than 5 mm laxity without a distinct end-point.

If the medial joint opens up more than 10 mm, a cruciate ligament is usually also injured.

The treatment of grade III sprains is debatable, but the recent trend has been to also treat grade III injuries conservatively. An arthroscopy is recommended to rule out concomitant injuries. A grade III sprain to the MCL combined with an anterior cruciate ligament (ACL) injury should be treated surgically in a football player.

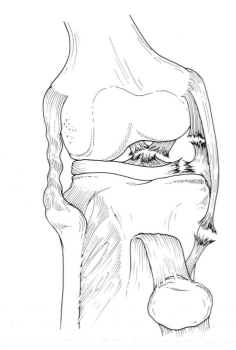

Fig. 14.15 Collateral and cruciate ligament injuries (right knee). In an extremely violent impact, the posterior cruciate ligament can also rupture, resulting in damage to the medial meniscus and the medial collateral ligament as well as the anterior and posterior cruciate ligaments. (From Peterson & Renström 1988.)

ACL injuries

Injuries to the ACL are fairly common in football (see Fig. 14.15). The yearly incidence has been estimated to be $1 \cdot 100$ players^{-1} in senior players. ACL injuries can occur in contact (60%) as well as in non-contact (40%) situations. The mechanism in a contact injury is either hyperextension of the knee or a valgus-outward rotation. The non-contact injuries usually occur in dribbling, cutting, or quick changes of direction.

It has been shown that knee injuries occurring in non-contact situations often occur to players with previous knee injury and persistent instability. Another important factor is the shoe–surface interface. The relationship between knee injuries and the fixation of the foot to the ground is not yet fully evaluated in football. In American football, the severity and incidence of knee and ankle injuries were reported to be significantly lower when using shoes with lower fric-

tion properties. However, severe injuries typically occur in collision situations independent of the surface. Football is characterized by sprinting, cutting, and pivoting situations, where shoe–surface relations are essential and frictional forces must be within an optimal range. High friction between shoe and surface may produce excessive forces on the knees with a risk of ACL injuries. However, too little friction may be the reason for slipping, which affects performance negatively, and may cause other injuries. Future research should address this compromise between performance and protection.

Symptoms and diagnosis

The symptoms of an acute ACL injury are sudden pain, a sense of giving way, and severe swelling of the knee within 1–2 h. The severe swelling is pathognomonic of hemarthrosis. It has been shown that more than 70% of all athletes with hemarthrosis following acute knee trauma have a torn ACL.

A football player with an adequate trauma and swelling of the knee within 6 h should be considered to have an ACL injury and the diagnosis should be confirmed by an arthroscopy and a stability test under anesthesia. During arthroscopy it is important to diagnose associated joint pathology such as meniscus tears and chondral lesions.

Treatment

The treatment of an ACL injury in a football player should as a rule be surgical. The ACL is the key ligament of the knee and tears of the ACL with resulting instability are a major cause of disability and are not readily tolerated by football players. Several studies have pointed out that football players with untreated ACL injuries who try to continue playing football show a high incidence of re-injury, loss of function, and as a rule had to discontinue the sport.

The acute ACL tear should have a primary repair and an augmentation of the repair. Suture of the ACL alone, leads to re-elongation in 50% of cases. The satisfactory surgical reconstruction of the chronic ACL-insufficient knee is a challenge. Replacement of the injured ACL using autologous tissues surrounding the knee joint, as well as a variety of synthetic material has been described (Fig. 14.16). A successful result

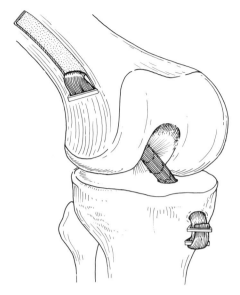

Fig. 14.16 Intra-articular reconstruction of the anterior cruciate ligament by employment of a fascia lata strip.

after ACL reconstruction depends however on several factors such as selection of patient, selection of graft, operative technique, and rehabilitation.

Optimal rehabilitation is without doubt a prominent factor in surgical success and it has been stressed that post-operative rehabilitation is just as important as the details of the surgery. Rehabilitation after ACL reconstruction begins immediately after the operation. Continous passive motion (CPM) seems to be advantageous in that it maintains nutrition to and the physical characteristics of cartilage, ligament, and muscle, as well as avoiding contracture problems. Immediate movement under very strict protective conditions is beneficial for the joint. The graft needs to be stressed if it is to remodel along the lines of functional demands. According to Wolff's law the early healing period is governed by the principle requiring absolute control of forces to prevent disruption or elongation of the graft. Walking is initiated at a later stage since this creates large ACL forces. Restriction of quadriceps exercises and symphysis of hamstring muscles have also been described as appropriate in order to avoid stress on the ACL. Stationary cycling seems to be advantageous in that it increases the range of movements as well as providing exercise for the thigh muscles without putting stress on the ACL. A football-specific rehabilitation phase is

equally important since the goal for the football player is to return to pre-injury activity level. This period is designed to achieve maximum strength and restore neuromuscular co-ordination and endurance. In optimal cases the player can return to football participation within 5–6 months after ACL surgery.

Posterior cruciate ligament (PCL) injuries

Injuries to the PCL are relatively uncommon in football and their treatment is controversial (see Fig. 14.15). The PCL is a 38-mm long, strong ligament, which is responsible for 90% of the resistance to posterior displacement of the tibia. Hyperflexion of the knee, with or without pretibial trauma, is the most common mechanism of PCL injury in football.

Symptoms and diagnosis

Diagnosis should be based on the history of injury, the presence of a posterior sag, and a posterior drawer test. X-rays should be performed to rule out bony avulsions from the tibia, and arthroscopy is recommended to confirm the diagnosis and to rule out other pathology.

Treatment

Football players with an isolated PCL injury generally function well without surgery. As a rule, they can return to football and other contact sports without any significant functional problems. At clinical examination they often show a significant posterior drawer but they show good results in functional tests. In order to maintain the high degree of knee function required in football, a player with PCL deficiency must strive to attain and maintain at least 100% quadriceps strength equality. Acute injuries should be treated with a program consisting of early motion within the limits of pain, and intensive quadriceps and hamstrings progressive resistance exercises. Similar to the rehabilitation of ACL injuries, stationary biking, water jogging, and co-ordination exercises are important in the rehabilitation program.

Long-term follow-up of conservatively treated PCL injuries have not shown any deterioration with time. Indication for surgery exists is selected cases: in isolated PCL injuries with a bony avulsion from the tibia, in acute PCL injuries with associated pathology, and in chronic PCL injuries with combined instability.

Thigh

Muscle ruptures

Musculotendinous injuries or strains (Fig. 14.17) are some of the most common injury types in football, but also some of the easiest to prevent. In a Swedish study in 1980 (Ekstrand 1982), the incidence of musculo-tendinous injuries in male senior football players was found to be 18%. After introduction of preventive measures such as stretching, proper warm-up, and cool-down, the incidence was found to be lower than 5% in a similar study in 1990 (J. Ekstrand unpublished data).

Most muscle injuries affect the lower extremity especially the quadriceps, hamstrings, adductors, and gastrocnemius. Muscle ruptures can be total or partial. Total ruptures can be palpated as a defect in the muscle under contraction. Surgery should be considered for total ruptures of thigh muscles. Partial ruptures are more common and they are as a rule treated conserva-tively. There are two major causes of muscle ruptures in football players: (a) compression, as a result of direct impact; or (b) distraction as a result of over-stretching or overload.

Symptoms and diagnosis

The diagnosis is usually clinical with pain, tenderness, and spasm in the affected muscle. The clinical diag-nosis of an acute muscle injury can however sometimes be unreliable. Real ruptures of muscle fibers and hema-tomas due to bleeding from connective tissue vessels can both create the same pain and tenderness, but the prognosis is quite different. While hematomas due to

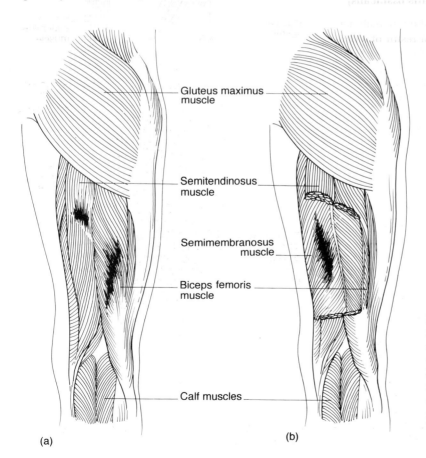

Gluteus maximus
muscle

Semitendinosus
muscle

Semimembranosus
muscle

Biceps femoris
muscle

Calf muscles

(a)

(b)

Fig. 14.17 Muscle ruptures. (a) *Left*: a rupture of the semitendinosus muscle at the back of the thigh; *right*: a rupture of the biceps femoris muscle. (b) Rupture of the semimembranosus muscle at the back of the thigh. The middle parts of the semitendinosus muscle and the biceps femoris have been removed to show the rupture. (From Peterson & Renström 1988.)

bleeding from connective tissue vessels disappear in a few days, real ruptures take 2–12 weeks to heal. Therefore it is valuable to complement the clinical diagnosis with other diagnostic measures such as sonography, computerized tomography (CT), or creatinine kinase (CK) measurements.

Treatment

The treatment of muscle injuries should be intensive RICE therapy (see Table 14.4). The rehabilitation should be gradual according to the principles outlined in Fig. 14.5. Re-injuries are known to be common. However, re-injuries could be minimized by exact diagnosis, intensive immediate treatment, guided rehabilitation, and prophylactic measures such as stretching.

Heterotopic bone formation (myositis ossificans)

Heterotopic bone formation may follow hematoma formation in an injured muscle as a result of a contusion or strain. The most common location in football players is the quadriceps femoris and lateral hamstrings muscles. By the use of stretching for prevention and RICE therapy for acute treatment of muscle injuries, the development of myositis ossificans is rarely seen. The size of the heterotopic bone formation may cause functional impairment.

Symptoms and diagnosis

The diagnosis is verified on X-ray examination. Osteogenic sarcoma should thought of in the differential diagnosis.

Treatment

Surgical excision of the ossification should be considered if there is functional impairment.

Groin

Groin pain is becoming increasingly recognized as a common condition in football players. Renström and Peterson (1980) reported that 5% of all football injuries were located in the groin region, and others have reported that up to 28% of football players have a history of groin pain. The etiology of pain may be difficult to determine and the results of treatment can be frustrating. The symptoms of groin injuries are often vague and non-specific and it is important to consider a variety of diagnostic possibilities.

Rupture of the adductor longus, rectus abdominis, iliopsoas, and rectus femoris muscles

The most common etiology of groin pain is a strain injury to the muscles of the groin region, including the adductor longus, rectus abdominis, iliopsoas, and rectus femoris muscles (Fig. 14.18). The ruptures are usually partial.

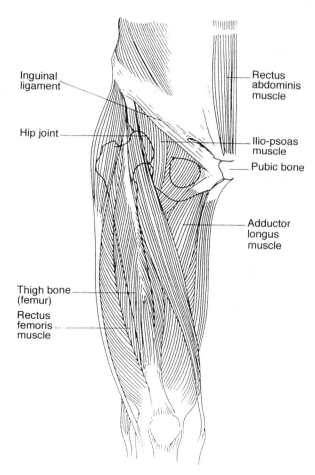

Fig. 14.18 Muscles of the groin region (from Peterson & Renström 1988).

Symptoms and diagnosis

The major symptom is a momentary pain in the groin region. A clinical examination should be performed when the muscle is relaxed as well as contracted. All four muscles should be analyzed and maximal pain and tenderness at contraction points out the affected muscle.

Treatment

The treatment is conservative with immediate RICE therapy and then a gradual rehabilitation to the pain limit. Surgery is seldom indicated.

Tendinitis of the adductor longus, rectus abdominis, iliopsoas, and rectus femoris muscles

Tendinitis of these muscles are to be considered as overuse injuries. They are often the result of overload, for example after increased intensity of training and matches, after training on hard surfaces, or after frequent change of playing surfaces.

Symptoms and diagnosis

The pain is commonly located in the muscle origin of the affected muscle and may radiate down the leg or upward toward the lower abdomen. The pain typically decreases after warm-up but returns after activity. Sprinting, jumping, and shooting aggravate the pain. In chronic cases, the pain may be constant and functional impairment is common.

Treatment

Conservative treatment is recommended for at least 6 months before consideration of surgery. Conservative treatment consists of rest, physiotherapy, anti-inflammatory medication, and in selected cases local cortisone injections.

Trochanter bursitis

The greater trochanteric bursa may be affected by contusion (hemobursa) or by overuse (bursitis). Hemobursa is especially common in goalkeepers and it is caused by falls or blows. Minor bleeding resolves

spontaneously. Major bleeds sometimes need aspiration and drainage of the bursa (Fig. 14.19). Protection of the trochanter region by padding is sometimes needed in goalkeepers, especially when playing on hard surfaces.

Symptoms and diagnosis

The major symptoms are pain and tenderness over the greater trochanter region.

Treatment

Treatment consists of anti-inflammatory medication and local steroid injections. Surgery might be necessary in prolonged cases.

Hernia

An incompetent abdominal wall in the groin, with or

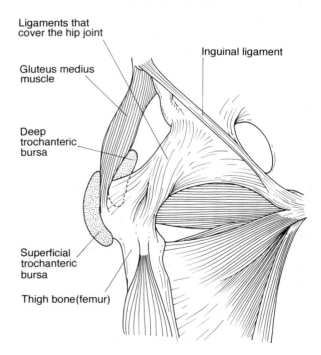

Ligaments that cover the hip joint

Inguinal ligament

Gluteus medius muscle

Deep trochanteric bursa

Superficial trochanteric bursa

Thigh bone (femur)

Fig. 14.19 Trochanter bursitis — inflammation of the superficial and deep bursae of the greater trochanter (from Peterson & Renström 1988).

without a detective inguinal hernia may be the cause of groin pain.

Symptoms and diagnosis

The pain is aggravated by exertion and sometimes by coughing and sneezing. Only about 8% have obvious hernias that are revealed by physical examination. The majority have incipient hernias where physical examination is normal but diagnosis can be verified by herniography, which involves injection of contrast intraperitoneally.

Treatment

The treatment is surgical, usually a herniorraphy, as for example a modified Bassiniplasty, is recommended.

Ilioinguinal nerve entrapment

Ilioinguinal nerve entrapment is known to be a consequence of herniorraphies, appendectomies, or other low abdominal incisions. This gives rise to pain, most often in connection with the operation, but sometimes delayed until months after surgery. Less well known is the "spontaneous" ilioinguinal nerve entrapment which is not uncommon in football players. The entrapment is probably due to the special anatomy of this nerve. It penetrates the abdominal muscle layers in a stepwise way.

Symptoms and diagnosis

The pain is usually sudden, intense, or stabbing. It is triggered by exercise and relieved by rest. Usually there is tenderness over the affected ilioinguinal nerve where it penetrates the abdominal muscle layers in the lower abdominal region. Diagnosis is verified by pain relief after injection of local anesthetics at the point of maximum tenderness.

Treatment

The treatment is surgical resection of the nerve.

Hip joint pathology

Pain in the groin may be referred from the hip joint. Perthe's disease and epiphyseolysis should be considered in children and adolescents as well as osteoarthritis in the adult player.

Diagnosis

The diagnosis should be suspected when hip movements, especially rotation, is impaired and the diagnosis is verified by an X-ray examination.

Genitourinary afflictions

Prostatitis, epididimitis, urethritis, hydrocele, gynecological disorders, and other genitourinary afflictions can cause pain which radiates out toward the groin.

References

Albert M. (1983) Descriptive three year data study of outdoor and indoor professional soccer injuries. *Athl. Train.* **18**, 218–220.

Brynhildsen J., Ekstrand J., Jeppsson A. & Tropp H. (1990) Previous injuries and persisting symptoms in female soccer players. *Int. J. Sports Med.* **11**, 489–492.

Brynhildsen J., Tropp H. & Ekstrand J. (1993) Injuries in women's soccer — a prospective study. In press.

Ekstrand J. (1982) *Soccer injuries and their prevention.* Medical dissertation No. 130, Linköping University, Sweden.

Ekstrand J. & Gillquist J. (1983) Soccer injuries and their mechanisms: A prospective study. *Med. Sci. Sports Exerc.* **15**, 267–270.

Franke K. (1977) *Traumatologie des Sports* (Traumatology in Sports). VEB Verlag, Volk und Gesundheit, Berlin.

Jörgensen U. (1984) Epidemiology of injuries in typical Scandinavian team sports. *Br. J. Sports Med.* **18**, 59–63.

Keller C.S., Noyes F.R. & Buncher C.R. (1987) The medical aspects of soccer injury epidemiology. *Am. J. Sports Med.* **15**, 105–112.

Nilsson S. & Roaas A. (1978) Soccer injuries in adolescents. *Am. J. Sports Med.* **6**, 358–361.

Pardon E.T. (1977) Lower extremities are the site of most soccer injuries. *Phys. Sports Med.* **6**, 43–48.

Peterson L. & Renström P. (1988) *Sports Injuries, their Prevention and Treatment.* Martin Dunitz, London.

Renström P. & Peterson L. (1980) Groin injuries in athletes. *Br. J. Sports Med.* **14**, 30–36.

Sullivan J.A., Gross R.H. & Grana W.A. (1980) Evaluation of injuries in youth soccer. *Am. J. Sports Med.* **8**, 325–327.

Further reading

Blyth C.S. & Mueller F.D. (1974) Soccer injury survey. *Phys. Sports Med.* **9**, 45–52.

Ekstrand J. (1989) Reconstruction of the anterior cruciate ligament in soccer players. *J. Sci. Football* **2**, 19–27.

Ekstrand J. & Nigg B. (1989) Surface-related injuries in soccer. *Sports Med.* **8**(1), 56–62.

Kraus J.F. & Burg F.D. (1970) Injury reporting and recording. *J. Am. Med. Assoc.* **213**(3), 438–444.

Nicholas J.A. & Hershman E.B. (1986) *The Lower Extremity and Spine in Sports Medicine*. CV Mosby, St Louis.

Vinger P.F. & Hoerner E.F. (1986) *Sports Injuries*. PSG Publishing, Littleton, Massachusetts.

Chapter 15

Locomotor injuries
in young players

Football is probably the most popular organized sport in the world with about 120 million registered players, approximately 3% of the population of the world. According to recent studies, football remains the fastest growing team sport. In consequence of this popularity, the number of young players is significantly increased.

Nevertheless, in association with this growth, football injuries have become the object of increasing medical interest. It is estimated that in Europe 50–60% of all sports injuries and 3.5% of all hospital-treated injuries are due to football. This is mostly due to an increased number of participants, but questions have been raised about the relative safety of football, particularly among young players.

Epidemiology

Epidemiology studies of the rates of occurrence of football injuries in youth players are relatively rare and difficult to compare. Firstly, there is presently no common operational definition of athletic injury. The present football injury epidemiology literature therefore relies upon a variety of definitions. Secondly, there is a difference between investigations based on injuries occurring during an entire season, instead of a tournament. The total exposition is greater.

In general, it is more useful to compare the injury rates when they are expressed as incidence per unit exposure time, e.g. per 1000 h of practise or games. Nevertheless, in reviewing the present epidemiology literature, certain similarities and conclusions still can be made. It has been suggested that there is a general decrease in the incidence of injuries in younger age groups when compared to senior players. In fact, senior athletes still sustain 15–30 times more injuries than youth athletes. This lesser incidence of injury in young people can perhaps be due to smaller mass and lesser velocity with resultant lesser force. Also other factors such as a more compliant use of protective equipment and less incidence of illegal play or tactics include this discrepancy.

Although not subjected to statistical analysis, female players appear to sustain twice the number of injuries as male players. Probably, this is due to the lack of tradition for girls' football. An additional observation which appears to be consistent is the vast majority of football injuries occurring in the lower extremity. Injuries about the foot, ankle, and knee are at the highest level of occurrence. Remarkably, there is a relatively higher proportion of head and upper extremity injuries among young players compared to senior players. This may be due to more frequent falls on an outstretched hand or the increased fragility of growing upper extremity epiphyses. The increased incidence of head injuries may result from insufficient technical expertise in heading the ball, or the increased ball–head weight ratio for young players. It is well known that leather balls gain extra weight when they are wet which may result in head injury. Therefore, it is recommended that a lighter weight ball be used which is made from synthetic, non-absorbing material.

Sites of injury

In general, the mechanism of injury in football as found in young players can be divided into direct extrinsic lesions (59%), muscular intrinsic lesions (13%), and capsuloligamental lesions (26%). The first group consists of muscular and bone contusions (54%), with fractures (5%). In addition it is important to be aware that the special factors to be concerned about in children's sports injuries include the presence of growth tissue and the fact that the child is still subject to growth processes.

According to the sites of injury, the majority occur, as already mentioned, in the lower extremity (± 66%).

Hip and pelvis

Injuries occurring about the hip and pelvis consist mostly of acute traumatic injuries, the most dramatic of which is frank dislocation of the hip. Every effort must be made to obtain an immediate reduction in a safe fashion of a dislocated of the hip.

The other class of acute traumatic injuries of the hip and pelvis is that of avulsion of the apophyseal attachments about the hip and pelvis. The most important localizations are the apophyseal insertion of the sartorius and tensor fasciae latae (anterior superior iliac spine), the rectus femoris (anterior inferior iliac spine), the hamstrings (ischial tuberosity), and the iliopsoas (lesser trochanter). Also the abdominal muscles (iliac crest) and the adductor brevis and longus (pubic tubercle) can be involved.

During the process of endochondral ossification, the cartilage of the apophyseal attachments will be replaced by bone, because of the rich vascularization of the area. This takes place at the age of 13–17 years. During that period, the cartilage is very sensitive to traumatic injuries. In most cases, an acute avulsion occurs because of a brutal action. A young player of 14 years will feel a violent pain, compared to a muscular lesion, presenting with an antalgic attitude, flexing the hip and knee, and limping. Active mobilization is difficult, specific isometric evaluation is impossible, and direct pressure at the place of avulsion is very painful. Frequently, a reactionary muscular contracture can be palpated and sometimes we can observe a subcutaneous ecchymosis. The radiographic evaluation is important.

In almost every instance, these can be treated conservatively with relative rest during the period of healing, followed by proper rehabilitation.

Leg and thigh

Acute injuries to the upper leg and thigh are relatively common among young players. Thigh contusions can be a cause of significant disability. These are treated by immediate rest, and ice massage, if necessary followed by conservative rehabilitation. The complication of myositis ossificans formation must be part of the differential diagnosis.

Hamstring strains are another debilitating injury of the football player, that mostly occurs at the musculotendinous junction. Acute care involves rest, ice, and compression. Complete rehabilitation must include not only restoration of the normal range of motion of the hamstrings but also restoration of strength. The role of stretching is very important in the prevention of injury. This appears to have statistical support among young players.

Knee

Younger players participating in football present frequently with knee injuries (20%). These must be evaluated very carefully. The classification of extensor mechanism injuries, internal derangements, and ligamentous injuries must be supplemented by a fourth category, that of apophysitis of the knee.

Two pathologies are frequently described: (a) apophysitis of the patella, noted as Sinding–Larsen–Johansson disease; and (b) apophysitis of the tuberosity of tibia, noted as Osgood–Schlatter disease. Sinding–Larsen–Johansson disease is an apophysitis of growth, concerning the distal part of the patella. It is due to minimal traumas (like repetitive shots at the anterior part of the knees), and successive micro-traumas. The young player is mostly about 10–13 years. Frequently, the complaint is located at one side only.

Isometric extension of the knee and direct pressure at the distal point of the patella is very painful. Normally, some tumefaction around the patella can be seen. The whole rehabilitation process can take 1 year.

Younger players, 11–15 years, are candidates for Osgood–Schlatter disease, especially when they are complaining of pain at the tuberosity of the tibia. This happens often at both sides (25%). Normally, it is the result of repetitive trauma, due to very intensive training. The player is able to localize the origin of pain exactly, namely at the tuberosity. The action of playing is very painful.

At the tuberosity of tibia, some tumefaction and peritendinous oedema will be found. Isometric extension and passive flexion of the knee is painful, as is palpation of the tuberosity. Also important is the radiologic evaluation, that shows a fragmentation of an irregular bone nucleus at the tuberosity. Both diseases are treated by immediate rest (> 1 month), relative immobilization, and cryotherapy. If the evolution is favorable, then training can proceed slowly.

Lower leg

Injuries of the lower leg are also often encountered in football players. In assessing lower leg injuries, the differential diagnosis must include that of stress fracture, compartment syndrome, tendinitis, and fasciitis as a training-related injury, all known as a non-specific diagnosis of "shin splints." The prevention of lower leg injuries with the use of shin protectors among young players is particularly important.

Foot and ankle

At the foot and ankle, ligament sprains account for one-third of injuries regardless of age. Recent studies prove that ankle sprains occur more frequently in football players with previous injury to the lateral ankle ligaments. There is no evidence to suggest that physiologic laxity is associated with any increase in injury rate. New ankle injuries often occur at previous injury sites, and are mostly due to an incomplete rehabilitation. Especially with younger players participating football, heel pain is very often found to be apophysitis of the calcaneus — Sever's disease. This appears to be an avulsion injury or apophysitis of the calcaneus, due to repetitive trauma. The evolution takes about 18 months, and appears mostly between the age of 8 and 15 years. The treatment consists of rest from sport, and the use of a shock-absorbent heel pads.

Injury prevention

The great majority of football injuries occur among young players, therefore prevention appears to be a high priority, and must be promoted in youth football programs. It is very important to perform proper pre-participation screening of the candidates to ensure not only the absence of eliminating conditions, but also the physical capacity to participate in football. For example, children who are undergoing periods of relatively rapid growth may be unaware of their true physical capabilities, and therefore might be more susceptible to injury. An additional factor is the presence of proper training and playing instruction.

Environmental factors contributing to the occurrence of football injuries includes field conditions and the use of protective equipment, in particular the use of taping and shin protectors.

Chapter 16

Goalkeeper injuries

Every football team has 11 players on the team, but only one goalkeeper. The challenges and requirements on how to play in this position differ essentially from what is required of the other positions of the team. The goalkeeper needs not only to have a specific athletic agility and quick reaction time, but also a different psyche. Goalkeepers should have a certain height to reach the ball, not only because of the size of the goal, but also to be able to dominate the air in the penalty area in, for example, heading situations. Goalkeepers are, in general, taller than the average field player.

A goalkeeper must, of course, be a football player and be ready to play the ball with his or her feet as any of the other players. This is especially true with the new rule stipulating that when passing the ball with the feet back to the goalkeeper it is no longer permissible for the player to take the ball with the hands. The goalkeeper must also be able both to kick the ball far out into the field and to throw the ball with some precision to the different players who are in a free position and so speed up the game.

The goalkeeper needs not only to be well conditioned, but must also be quick and have very fast reactions. The goalkeeper must be agile and be able to move quickly in all different directions. On corner kicks, the goalkeeper must jump high and compete for the ball and be accurately positioned to grip or box the ball. His or her sense of timing must, therefore, be very good. The goalkeeper must, in other words, be a well-rounded athlete with a well-developed sense for the play of football (Fig. 16.1).

From a psychological point of view, being a goalkeeper is especially demanding, as it requires an ability to concentrate continuously on the game. A goalkeeper can be outside the playing situations for 10 min, and then suddenly be in the center of the action. One single error can result in a goal and lead to major criticism even if the goalkeeper might have made 15 outstanding saves prior to the one visible mistake. The goalkeeper must be able to withstand criticism from the other players, coaches, spectators, the press, etc. In the next match, the goalkeeper may be the main focus of attention.

With all of this in mind, it seems relevant to say that

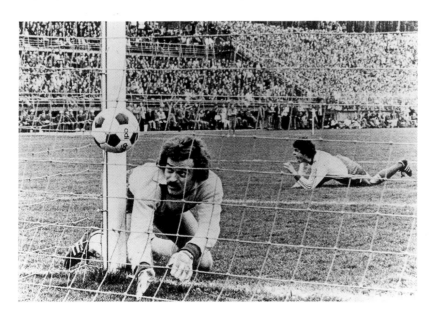

Fig. 16.1 The goalkeeper as the last line of defense cannot be successful all of the time. © IOC archives.

being a goalkeeper is a challenge, and requires a specific talent and an unusual athletic ability with a special psyche.

Injury aetiology

A number of factors affect the goalkeeper's risk for injury such as athletic ability, the team's capacity, the position in the field, equipment, artificial light, the environment, and especially the turf (Peterson & Renström 1980b).

Football is becoming increasingly intense, which results in more intensive body contact, tougher tackles, etc. The playing season is long with varying climatic conditions, which affects the different turfs. These factors may account for an increased risk for injury.

The goalkeeper is often involved in risk situations for an injury and therefore has a specific injury pattern somewhat different from the other players on the team (Tables 16.1–16.3).

Trauma situations

As mentioned above, the goalkeeper needs special qualifications and talent to be a good goalkeeper. Reaction patterns must be well developed so that the goalkeeper can quickly and adequately react when shot at with the ball. There is an intense body contact with other players on the ground, in the air during collisions, when running for the ball against the opponents, and so on. Especially in crowded situations such as corners, the goalkeeper has to act in the air, which is filled with players fighting for the ball. The goalkeeper must be able to jump high to grip the ball on corner situations and similar occasions. He or she often has to grip the ball in the air and might then

Table 16.1 Injury frequency in relation to player's position in men assuming 1−4−3−3 team formation

Field position	Injury frequency			
	Renström *et al.* (1977)		Hunt & Fulford (1990)	
Goalkeeper	17	(8.5)*	28	(14)
Back	87	(43.1)	45	(22.5)
Midfielder	54	(27)	120	(60)
Forward	50	(25)	6	(3)
Referee	0	(0)	1	(0.5)
Total	178	(100)	200	(100)

* Figures in parentheses express results as a percentage.

Table 16.2 Percentage of total injuries sustained by each position (males) assuming a 1−3−3−4 team formation

Athlete	Striker (%)	Midfielder (%)	Back (%)	Goalkeeper (%)	Reference
Professional	38	30	18	10	McMaster & Walter (1978)
Youth	32	17	32	18	Sullivan *et al.* (1980)
Senior	36	27	27	9	Ekstrand & Gillquist (1983)

Table 16.3 Injury rate by player position in female football (Engström et al. 1991) assuming a 1−4−4−2 team formation

Player position	No. players on team	No. injuries	%	Incidence of injury (%)
Goalkeeper	1	6	8	9
Back	4	24	31	36
Midfielder	4	32	41	36
Forward	2	16	20	18

Table 16.4 Location of injuries in retired goalkeepers in football, team handball, ice hockey, and bandy (field hockey on ice) (Björnum et al. 1980)

	Football (n = 11)	Team handball (n = 7)	Ice hockey (n = 6)	Bandy (n = 9)
Knee	6	2	2	2
Hip		2		2
Ankle	3	1	1	1
Shoulder		1		2
Elbow		2		2
Wrist	3	2	1	1
Hand−fingers	3	7	3	5
Head	3			
Back	1	1	1	2
Kidneys	2			

land on the ground without the protection of the hands and arms. This means that the goalkeeper is often subjected to direct trauma against the body, which increases the risk for contusions, abrasions, and other injuries produced by direct trauma. The goalkeeper can also land on another player's feet and, thereby, twist an ankle or a knee joint. Ankle and knee injuries are common in goalkeepers. The goalkeeper may also be injured by ground contact, which frequently occurs in the saving of goals and also in collisions with the goal-posts. Goalkeepers must sometimes throw themselves in front of the players that are attacking. The player can then kick the goalkeeper, and contusion injuries, such as muscle hematomas can be the result. Occasionally, the goalkeeper can also hit the goalposts with the head, as well as the rest of the body and, thereby, be subjected to head contusions and so on.

The goalkeeper must often turn quickly and throw the body in another direction. As football shoes have cleats, the shoes might stick to the ground, and a rotation trauma may occur with ligamentous and joint injuries in the knee and ankle as a result.

When the ball is shot directly at the goalkeeper, the ball can hit the fingers and the hands. Distortions, dislocations, and fractures of the fingers and the hands are not uncommon in goalkeepers. The ball, as well as the opponents fingers, hands, elbows, etc., can also hit the face and the goalkeeper can sustain eye injuries. Table 16.4 shows the location of injuries that retired goalkeepers have sustained in different sports in a study by Björnum et al. (1980). These male goalkeepers

had been active on average for 25 years and were between 34 and 55 years old.

Playing level of the team

Investigations report that the risk for injury is greater in the higher top-level divisions (Nilsson & Roaas 1978, Peterson & Renström 1980b). In higher divisions, the playing intensity is higher, and the players are more prone to take chances for goals. On the other hand, during recreational play and in lower divisions, the players are not as experienced, and might therefore constitute a risk for injury for the goalkeepers because of careless and less skillful players. There are, however, no figures available on exactly what this means for the goalkeepers.

Of injuries in football, 73% occurred during games in more than 70% of cases (Peterson & Renström 1980b). The players trained 2.5 times as often as they played games, which means that the risk for injury was much higher during games. This is especially true for goalkeepers, as they usually are not tackled or severely challenged during practise.

Most injuries occur in the beginning of the first period and toward the end of the second period of a match (Peterson & Renström 1980b). They occur in the beginning because of lack of warm-up, and initial increased intensity of a match. Toward the end of the match, muscle fatigue results in decreased co-ordination, judgment, risk taking, etc. There are no figures available on when goalkeepers are mostly injured.

Shoes

The most important equipment in football is the shoe. Ligament injuries in knee joints and ankles are often caused by a rotation trauma with fixation of the foot to the ground during body contact or changing direction. The design of the shoe and its relation to the playing surface is a most important factor for the cause, incidence, and severity of knee injuries.

The goalkeeper must often change directions quickly and it depends, therefore, on a very good grip between the shoe and the turf. On natural grass, this is given by cleats. These cleats can, on the other hand, also be stuck in the ground, as the cleats have dug themselves into the grass when the body is turned. A twisting trauma to the ankle and knee joints occurs thus causing injuries.

Cleats should not be used on artificial turf, as they will increase the incidence for injury. In Peterson and Renström's study (1980b) 73% of the players who were injured on artificial turf used cleated shoes compared to a total number of 43%. These results indicate that cleats are an important factor in the injury mechanism on artificial turfs.

Equipment

Shin guards are the most important equipment for protection and prevention of injuries for goalkeepers, as they are for the other players. La Federation Internationale de Football Associations (FIFA) has decided on mandatory use of shin guards for all players. Unfortunately, there are no international standard norms or test procedures available for shin guards in football. Nationally, the Swedish Football Federation has approved standard norms and test procedures for shin guards for football (Andreasson & Peterson 1992). Shin guards should cover the lower leg, and if possible the malleoli and the head of the fibula and unload the tibia from direct impact, thus reducing the risk of penetration and wounds, as well as reducing the risk for fractures and muscular contusions and hematomas.

Genital protectors, e.g. boxes (cups), should be used. They should enclose the penis and the testes to protect from direct blows.

The goalkeeper is at risk for sustaining not only contusion injuries, but also abrasions and friction burn injuries when throwing the body on the ground. The contusion injuries should be prevented by trousers with padding, as well as padding for knees, especially knee caps and for elbows (Fig. 16.2).

Abrasions and friction burn injuries are best prevented by wearing complete equipment. On artificial turf, the goalkeeper should wear long trousers in order to avoid contact between the turf and the skin. In the study by Renström et al. (1977) on the first artificial turf used for football in Europe (in Göteborg, Sweden), it was found that during the first few months of use some friction burn injuries were reported, but these decreased after the initial period with education. With adequate prevention, careful cleaning, and bandages, these friction burn injuries may be regarded as a minor problem.

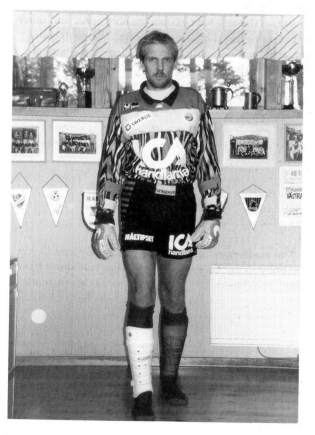

Fig. 16.2 Goalkeeper's equipment includes pants with protection for the hips, and shirts with protection for the elbows.

The injury causing mechanisms on grass and gravel are very similar, but artificial turf shows a different picture. Grass and gravel injuries are caused by kicking without the ball much more commonly than tripping, while the reverse is the case for artificial turfs (Renström *et al.* 1977, Peterson & Renström 1980b). The reason for this was considered to be a difference in playing techniques.

The turfs

The conditions of the turfs are important. On very dry natural grass or gravel, the ground is hard and uneven and may increase the risk especially for contusions and abrasions for goalkeepers. When natural grass is soft and in good condition, it is probably the best turf to play on for a goalkeeper.

When the artificial turf is dry, there is increased friction, and thereby also increased risk for injuries for goalkeepers. Ligament and muscle injuries occurred as often on dry as on wet surfaces while fractures occurred more on dry turfs (Renström *et al.* 1977, Peterson & Renström 1980b).

Specific injuries

The types of injury sustained by goalkeepers are presented in Table 16.5.

Table 16.5 Type of injury in goalkeepers

Type of injury	Renström *et al.* (1977)	Hunt & Fulford (1990)
Sprain (ankle)	4	8
Fracture	4	9
Bruise	3	6
Laceration	2	1
Dislocation	—	2
Head injury	2	—
Other	2	2
Total	17/178 (10%)	28/200 (14%)

Abrasions and friction burns

Goalkeepers throw themselves quite daringly to the ground, or land on the ground after gripping or trying to grip the ball. The goalkeeper then often lands directly on the body without the protection of the hands and arms. The goalkeeper may land directly on the uncovered skin, and abrasions may be the result on grass and gravel and friction burn injuries on artificial turf.

These injuries should, as soon as possible, be cleaned out, as there is always a risk for infection. These injuries can be aggravated if not properly taken care of, especially if they occur on the artificial turfs and result in suffering for several days. Immediate care is, therefore, important. Prevention with clothing, especially when playing on the artificial turfs, is recommended.

Head

Head injuries are common in goalkeepers. They occur in collision with the opponents, or can also be caused by a kick or blow from other players. Serious injuries also occur when the goalkeeper collides with the goalpost. Head contusions and fractures of the skull are not uncommon and this injury is considered potentially serious if the player becomes unconscious. If the goalkeeper has had a head contusion with unconsciousness, he or she should not be allowed to continue to play and should be examined by a doctor and observed for the acute period. Serious brain hemorrhage can occur due to head contusions, which may be life threatening. Sometimes there is bleeding from the ear which is a serious sign of a fracture of the skull base. This player should immediately be transported to a hospital for treatment. In summary it is important to stress that the goalkeeper with a major trauma to the head, should be taken off the field. If there is a persistent headache or nausea, the player should be kept under observation.

Facial injuries are common among goalkeepers. They include wounds to the face, which should be taken care of by stopping the bleeding and securing healing by taping or suturing as soon as possible. Facial fractures are common in body contact with the players and the goal-posts and includes serious injuries such as fractures of the maxillary bone with depression of the maxillary bone, which can cause double vision. The goalkeeper should be checked for double vision when there is any sign of maxillary bone fracture. When there is a displacement of the fragment, surgical treatment is often required.

Fractures of the zygomatic bone are also common and there is a tenderness on the zygomatic bone in front of the ear and there is pain on chewing. Sometimes surgical treatment is needed when the bone is dislocated.

Fractures of the mandibular bone can occur in collision with other players, the ground or the goal-post. There is tenderness in front of the ear below the zygomatic bone, and pain occurs when the patient clenches the teeth. Usually the teeth are out of alignment when pressed together with the upper jaw. When there is a displacement, surgery is needed. Dental injuries can also occur.

Fractures of the nasal bone is the most common fracture in goalkeepers and occur in body contact and falling to the ground or against the poles. Usually there is bleeding from the nose, and tenderness on palpation. Sometimes visible displacement is present.

When there is dislocation of the nasal bone, surgery is indicated.

Eye injuries may occur when the goalkeeper receives a blow from an opponent or the ball in the eye. There may be bleeding in the anterior chamber of the eye. The blood can then form fluid localized between the iris and the cornea at the bottom of the anterior chamber of the eye. The vision is severed and the goalkeeper should not continue to play, but should receive treatment from an eye specialist as soon as possible. Detachment of the retina can also occur on a contusion to the eye and this may give a reduced vision in a specific area.

Shoulder

Shoulder dislocations are not uncommon in goalkeepers and occur when they land on the arm or elbow, after throwing themselves after the ball (Fig. 16.3). They can also be pushed in the air by a nodding player and land straight on their arm, forcing an anterior dislocation. A goalkeeper with an anterior dislocation has major pain, and should of course be taken off the

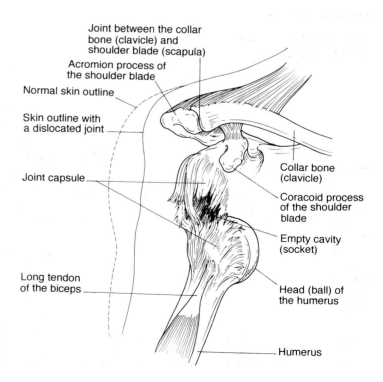

Joint between the collar bone (clavicle) and shoulder blade (scapula)

Acromion process of the shoulder blade

Normal skin outline

Skin outline with a dislocated joint

Joint capsule

Long tendon of the biceps

Collar bone (clavicle)

Coracoid process of the shoulder blade

Empty cavity (socket)

Head (ball) of the humerus

Humerus

Fig. 16.3 Anterior dislocation of the right shoulder joint, as a result of extensive injuries to the surrounding soft tissues (from Peterson & Renström 1988).

field in order to secure as rapid a reduction as possible. A goalkeeper with a shoulder dislocation can usually not return to goalkeeping until 2 months after the incident. Too early a return to football, or an incomplete rehabilitation, may cause recurrent dislocation and instability, which may require reconstructive surgery later for restoring the function.

Acromioclavicular joint separations are rather common injuries when the goalkeeper falls straight onto the shoulder with the ball gripped by the hands (Fig. 16.4). These injuries can be classified according to their severity. The treatment is mostly conservative and return to goalkeeping is usually possible within 1−2 months.

Fracture of the clavicle (Fig. 16.5) may occur when the goalkeeper falls on the shoulder as an alternative injury to acromioclavicular joint separations. There is tenderness over the clavicle and crepitation can be present on motion. X-rays will confirm the diagnosis and the treatment is conservative as a rule.

Rotator cuff tears can occur when the goalkeeper falls straight onto the shoulder or arm. These injuries often take a long time to heal because of poor vascularization and tendon degeneration. It is important to treat them well with rest and careful mobilization. Return to goalkeeping is not recommended before there is a full range of motion without pain. Sometimes surgery is required.

The goalkeeper often throws the ball as far out on

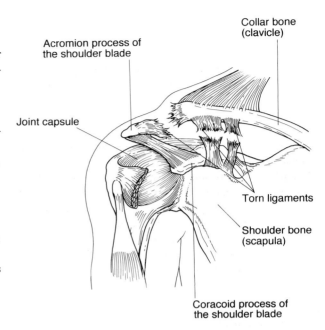

Fig. 16.4 Dislocation of the joint between the clavicle and the acromion process of the scapula (right shoulder) (from Peterson & Renström 1988).

the field as is possible, thus typical throwing injuries such as labrum tears in the joint, rotator cuff tears, or other muscle tendon strains in any of the muscles around the shoulder may occur.

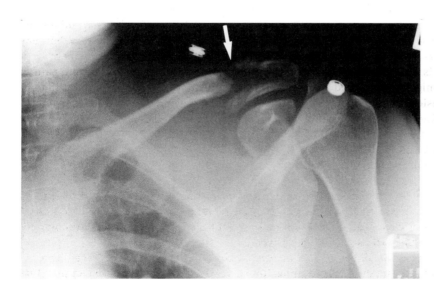

Fig. 16.5 Radiogram of a fractured clavicle (left shoulder) (arrow). Courtesy of Dr R.E. Leach.

Elbow

Hemorrhagic bursitis can occur over the olecranon bursa when the goalkeeper throws the body to the ground, especially if not wearing a preventive pad. At the time of trauma, a hemorrhage will occur in the bursa. If this hemorrhage is not evacuated, the bursa will react with calcification and adhesions. Loose bodies can also be formed. If this is not treated well, chronic bursitis will be the end result. A chronic bursitis will often cause secondary, recurrent swelling. Sometimes excision of the bursa in goalkeepers might be necessary. Prevention of these injuries includes a good padding over the olecranon, and this should be a mandatory equipment for all goalkeepers.

Occasionally, more severe injuries such as fractures and dislocations of the elbow can occur, but they are rare.

Hand and finger

Fractures to the wrist are not uncommon for goalkeepers, e.g. after throwing themselves onto the ground. These fractures, however, heal well, but the goalkeeper will be unable to return to sports for 2−3 months.

Fractures to the scaphoid can occur, especially if the goalkeeper lands with the wrist dorsiflexed. There is tenderness over the snuff box area, and pain during motions of the wrist. Because of poor circulation of the scaphoid bone, these injuries need immobilization for up to 10−12 weeks, and the goalkeeper will be away from competition for up to 4 months.

Fractures, dislocations, and distortions of the fingers (Fig. 16.6) are common in goalkeepers. They are usually treated conservatively, but if there is a major displacement of the fracture, surgery might be indicated.

Gamekeeper's thumb (Stener's lesion) or ulnar collateral ligament lesion can occur. These injuries are among the most common injuries that a goalkeeper can sustain. They occur not only when the goalkeepers throw themselves to the ground, but also when the ball hits the thumb from straight ahead. These injuries need surgery in 50−70% of the cases in order to secure adequate apposition and healing of the ligaments, and to secure good future functional capacity. A goalkeeper, who needs surgery for this injury, will be away from goalkeeping for 3−4 months. The gloves are not well designed from a preventive point of view.

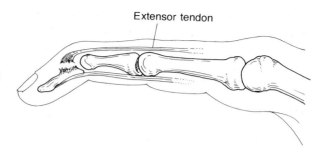

Fig. 16.6 A jammed finger from ball contact by the goalkeeper can result in joint injury and tendon damage (as in the rupture of the attachment of the long extensor tendon shown). (From Peterson & Renström 1988.)

Back

Low back pain is not more common among goalkeepers than other players. Disc herniation is not uncommon. Back injuries may, however, occur in goalkeepers due to the high speed and energy involved in collisions, both against the opponents, the ground, and the goal-posts.

Injuries to the cervical spine may be caused by flexion or extension mechanism, and also with actual compression when hitting the goal-posts. This may result in severe injuries with fractures or dislocation and instability. Any goalkeeper complaining of pain in the neck or radiating pain into the arms after a trauma to the head or neck, should be taken off the field and carefully examined.

Fractures of the vertebrae in the thoracic and lumbar spine are uncommon among football players, but may occur in goalkeepers in collision with opponent players or the goal-post. This may give severe pain in the thoracic or lumbar spine, with or without the radiating pain to the lower extremities. Players complaining of back pain after trauma should be carefully examined.

Chest

Chest injuries may be serious injuries and are common among goalkeepers, due to the intense body contact with the opponent players, and with the ground and goal-posts.

Fractures of the ribs are common and may be a serious injury, because the fractured rib can puncture a lung and cause a leak of air (pneumothorax) or bleeding (hemothorax) from the lung into the pleura. This may give rise to a life-threatening condition. Pain when breathing and pain on compression on the fractured ribs are warning symptoms and the goalkeeper should be removed from the field and examined by X-ray.

Abdominal

Abdominal injuries are not common, but occur in goalkeepers, due to their playing position and body contact.

Abdominal injuries may be serious and life-threatening injuries should be dealt with very carefully. Rupture of the spleen may occur when the goalkeeper receives a blow on the left side of the abdomen or the lumbar spine or the lower left ribs. The spleen may rupture and cause bleeding, which can sometimes begin in the closed capsule of the spleen, but more often the bleeding penetrates the ruptured capsule into the abdominal cavity, causing serious life-threatening conditions. The player may complain of pain, but it is important to recognize a fast, weak pulse, pallor, sweating, and sometimes drowsiness, and as this may lead to a loss of consciousness. The player should be taken to the hospital immediately for treatment.

Rupture of the liver may occur in goalkeepers when they receive a blow to the right side of the upper abdomen. The rupture will cause bleeding into the abdominal cavity, along with bile leakage which will cause peritonitis and may prove fatal. A major rupture of the liver shows symptoms of pain and shock, and the patient should be taken to the hospital immediately.

The kidney may be injured on the left or right side due to a blow to the abdomen, or lumbar back. Rupture of the kidney may result in bleeding in the urine. The bleeding can also spread to the extra-abdominal space and give rise to a life-threatening condition. The patient should be sent to hospital and kept under observation.

A direct contusion from a knee into the abdomen may result in an injury to the intestine, especially the duodenum which may be injured when being compressed against the vertebral spine (Saartok *et al.* 1992). This may lead to penetration into the abdominal cavity or the retroperitoneal cavity, and may give rise

to peritonitis. This should be suspected when there is pain in the upper abdomen or back along with nausea, vomiting, and pain. Shock symptoms should call for immediate hospital care.

A contusion to the lower abdomen can cause an injury to the bladder and, thereby, blood in the urine. The patient should be observed in hospital. A contusion to the testis, or to the penis can cause painful bleeding and swelling and should be treated immediately with ice and rest to avoid further hematoma. These injuries could be prevented by boxes (cups).

Hip

A hip pointer can occur when goalkeepers land on their hip region after throwing themselves to the ground. They then can have a contusion against the bony parts of the pelvis with major bleeding as a result. Goalkeepers should wear protective pants with padding. The hip pointers are uncommon in top-level goalkeepers because of this protection, but recreational goalkeepers can still injure themselves this way. The treatment is rest and a gradual return to football.

A direct trauma to the lateral aspect of the greater trochanteric region, may cause trochanteric bursitis. A direct trauma causes a hemorrhagic bursitis with bleeding in the bursa. If this hemorrhage is not evacuated, a chronic condition with calcification, adhesions, and loose bodies may occur, and thereby a chronic bursitis. These injuries should be prevented by good padding. If they occur, the bleeding should be evacuated.

Thigh

Thigh muscle hematomas can occur when the goalkeeper, as well as the other players, sustain contusions against their thighs. Collision with other players is common. A knee can often be pressed into the lateral thigh muscles, and intra- or intermuscular hematomas can be the result. Immediate rest, ice, compression, and elevation should be started. If these injuries are not treated well initially, a so-called "Charlie's horse" may result with myositis ossificans as a severe complication. The initial treatment is, in other words, essential, and the goalkeeper should not return to sports until the full range of motion to the knee joints is restored without pain.

Knee

Meniscus injuries are some of the most common injuries in football, and occasionally goalkeepers also are injured. Goalkeepers wear shoes with cleats, which may be caught in the ground. A change of direction will result in a twisting motion of the knee, and, thereby, the meniscus can rupture. A meniscus tear in an athlete usually requires arthroscopic surgery. Return to sports varies depending on the size and location of the injury, but usually it is possible to return to play after 1−2 months. If the meniscus is repaired, the healing time is often around 4 months.

Anterior cruciate ligament (ACL) and posterior cruciate ligament (PCL) injuries, as well as medial collateral ligament (MCL) injuries, are not as common in goalkeepers as in other players, but may occur. ACL injuries are potentially severe and usually require surgical intervention. PCL are not uncommon in goalkeepers when the lower extremity can be pressed posteriorly in a collision where the impact hits the tibia below the knee, and thereby forces a traumatic, posterior drawer. These injuries are most commonly treated surgically, but sometimes conservatively. If they are isolated then the return to sports is variable, but the rehabilitation time often takes 4−6 months.

MCL injuries are common, but more benign. They are usually treated non-surgically with early range of motion and muscle strength exercises. Return to football is possible after 2−3 months, if not earlier.

Prepatellar bursitis may occur after landing on the patella. The contusion may cause bleeding — resulting in a chronic bursitis when not treated adequately. When there is bleeding in the bursa, it should be evacuated. Surgical removal may be necessary in chronic bursitis that gives long-lasting problems.

Lower leg

Tibia and fibula fractures are not uncommon in goalkeepers when they collide with opponents. They are treated with immobilization for a variable period of time.

Ankle

Ankle sprains are the most common injuries in goalkeepers, as well as in other players. They may occur when the goalkeeper is up in the air and comes down with the foot on another player's foot, and twisting occurs such as supination−internal rotation, or pronation−external rotation. These injuries most commonly involve the anterior talofibular (ATF) ligaments and are in 20% combined with the calcaneofibular (CF) ligaments. Ankle sprains usually heal well with functional treatment. The return to sports varies between 1 week for a mild sprain to a couple of months for a very severe sprain. After having ankle sprains, the goalkeeper should wear protective ankle bracing or taping in order to prevent recurrent injuries.

Residual problems after ankle sprains are not uncommon, and can cause ligament instability with recurrent sprains, which may require reconstruction. Osteochondral lesions, or osteochondritis dissecans on the talus can occur and should be suspected in athletes with persistent pain. These injuries can heal with rest, but if the pain persists, arthroscopic surgery is the treatment of choice. Return to sports depends on the size and location of the injury.

Achilles tendon

Achilles tendon injuries can occur as overuse injuries, as the goalkeeper is in constant motion and often uses eccentric action of the calf muscles. Overuse syndrome problems increase if the goalkeeper is practising much on hard or uneven turf. The risk for injury increases if cleated shoes are used on hard turf.

Achilles tendon ruptures may occur if the goalkeeper is jumping and lands in a bad position. For complete tears, the treatment is most commonly surgery. Return to goalkeeping is possible after 6 months.

Foot

Plantar fasciitis does occur in goalkeepers. The goalkeeper is often standing on their toes with the toes dorsiflexed, and, thereby, increasing the tension on the plantar fascia, especially when jumping or sprinting. This is especially the case if the goalkeeper has foot malalignments such as cavus feet or increased pronation. Plantar fasciitis should be treated with great care, as this injury has a tendency to be chronic. Orthosis in the football shoes is often required, as well as stretching of the plantar fascia and the calf muscles.

Various foot deformities such as hallux valgus, hallux rigidus, and hammer toes may occur. They are treated with orthosis, often complemented with a metatarsal bar, or by having good shoes. Surgery is sometimes indicated.

Turf toe syndrome may occur when the foot and toes are jammed into an unyielding ground with high friction such as an artificial turf that is glued to the ground. The plantar fascia of the metatarsal phalangeal joints may then be ruptured and stretched; the result is a stiff big toe with pain at push-off. These injuries can take a long time to heal and should be treated as soon as possible with rest, ice, and protection.

Injury prevention

Goalkeepers need to protect certain areas that are prone to injuries. Goalkeepers are prone to receive injuries over unprotected elbows and patella. They need, therefore, to have specific pads over the elbow to protect the olecranon, and over the patella to protect that area from direct trauma. Hemorrhagic bursitis may, as mentioned earlier, be the result. These protective pads should be mandatory for goalkeepers.

Goalkeepers need also to have pants that are well padded on the sides to prevent hip pointers and trochanteric bursitis. Genital protectors should be worn.

As well as for other players, it is mandatory for goalkeepers to have shin guards. The goalkeeper can be kicked on the shin and they are very sensitive to pain and injury. Fractures may occur in the lower leg, and shin guards may protect to some extent from this.

For general prevention, the goalkeeper needs to do lots of special training such as general agility training. The goalkeeper faces specific demands and should, therefore, train individually, as well as with the team. The goalkeeper should exercise with more stretching than the other players, and also train specific movements and reaction speeds. Special training on concentration would be valuable.

Conclusion

A successful football team depends on an outstanding goalkeeper. Such a goalkeeper must be agile and have quick reaction speeds. A successful goalkeeper must also have the ability to concentrate on the match movements, and be consistent in his or her actions.

The goalkeeper is prone to injury because of the increased risks of the position. He or she must not only be alert and stop the ball when the opponent shoots at the goalkeeper, but must also be able to throw themselves and grip the ball, and be able to land without the hands as protection. This requires very good techniques, and the use of protective equipment over areas such as the elbow, knee, hip, and genitals. The goalkeeper must also train individually, as well as with the team. The special demands on the goalkeeper must be well known and respected by the team and the coaches.

References

Andreasson G. & Peterson L. (1992) *European Congress on Football*. Stockholm, Sweden.

Björnum S., Peterson L. & Renström P. (1980) *Injuries in Goalkeepers*. Proceedings of the Swedish Society of Sports Medicine, Halmstad, Sweden.

Ekstrand J. & Gillquist J. (1983) Soccer injuries and their mechanisms. A prospective study. *Med. Sci. Sports Exerc.* **15**, 267–270.

Engström B., Johansson C. & Törnkvist H. (1991) Soccer injuries among élite female players. *Am. J. Sports Med.* **19**(4), 372–375.

Hunt M. & Fulford S. (1990) Amateur soccer: injuries in relation to field position. *Br. J. Sports Med.* **24**(4), 265.

Keller C.S., Noyes F.R. & Buncher C.R. (1987) The medical aspects of soccer injury epidemiology. *Am. J. Sports Med.* **15**(3), 230–237.

McMaster W.C. & Walter M. (1978) Injuries in soccer. *Am. J. Sports Med.* **6**, 354–357.

Nilsson S. & Roaas A. (1978) Soccer injuries in adolescents. *Am. J. Sports Med.* **6**, 358–361.

Peterson L. & Renström P. (1980a) Fotbollsskador-frevens och art (Soccer injuries — frequency and type). *Läkartidningen* **77**(41), 3621–3623.

Peterson L. & Renström P. (1980b) Några faktorer av betydelse för skador i fotboll (Some factors of importance for injuries in soccer). *Läkartidningen* **77**(41), 3623–3625.

Peterson L. & Renström P. (1988) *Sports Injuries, their Prevention and Treatment*. Martin Dunitz, London.

Renström P., Peterson L., Edberg B., Svenneng J. & Olofson B. (1977) Fotbollsplan med konstgräs (Soccer field with artificial turf). *Naturvårdsverket Sweden* **846**, 1–128.

Saartok T., Peterson L., Karlbom A. & Karlsson L. (1992) Blunt abdominal trauma in soccer causing duodenal rupture: Case report and review. *Scand. J. Med. Sci. Sports* **2**(1), 40–43.

Sullivan J.A., Gross R.H., Grana W.A. *et al.* (1980) Evaluation of injuries in youth soccer. *Am. J. Sports Med.* **8**, 325–327.

Chapter 17

Injury prevention

The essence of sports medicine is the prevention of injuries. To prevent injuries occurring in a certain sport, it is necessary to be sport specific, i.e. to analyze the incidence, type, and localization of injuries as well as the mechanisms behind the injuries in just that sport. The purpose of this section is to summarize briefly some mechanisms involved in football injuries and then discuss various methods of prevention.

Injury aetiology

The assessment of etiological factors responsible for football injuries is a necessity for injury prevention. The cause of a football injury is often multifactorial. Ekstrand *et al.* (1983a) analyzed possible injury mechanisms and the avoidability of football injuries by compiling information from a pre-season examination and test, a prospective study of injuries, and a training analysis in a Swedish football league. The results are summarized in Table 17.1.

Injury prevention

Pre-season examination

Pre-season examination and testing of football players are valuable in preventing injury. Incorrect training and individual player factors such as muscle tightness, malalignment, muscle weakness, and joint instability are related to many football injuries. A pre-season examination provides the opportunity to analyze and correct individual factors predisposing to injury. It is suggested that a pre-season examination should include a physical examination as well as measurements of flexibility and muscle strength.

Table 17.1 Etiology of injuries (%). Combinations of factors were fairly common

Player factors		
	Joint instability	12
	Muscle tightness	11
	Inadequate rehabilitation	17
	Non-training	2
	Total	42
Equipment		
	Shoes	13
	Shin guards	4
	Total	17
Playing surface		24
Rules		12
Other factors		29

Physical examination

It is recommended that a pre-season examination begins with an enquiry about past injuries and an examination to evaluate persistent symptoms from past injuries. Since leg injuries dominate in football, the musculoskeletal profile of the lower extremity should be analyzed to evaluate persistent symptoms after past injuries. Such examination includes the following.

Ankle tests

Mechanical instability can be evaluated by the drawer test. If there is mechanical instability, ankle taping is recommended, see below.

Functional instability, i.e. a feeling of "giving way" and recurrent sprains can be evaluated by stabilometry. Stabilometry is an objective method for the study of postural control where the body sway is measured on a force plate. However, a modified Romberg test can also be used to evaluate functional instability. The player stands on one leg with the other leg raised and flexed at the knee, the arms folded across the chest and the eyes closed (Fig. 17.1). The player should be able to stand for 60 s without putting the raised foot to

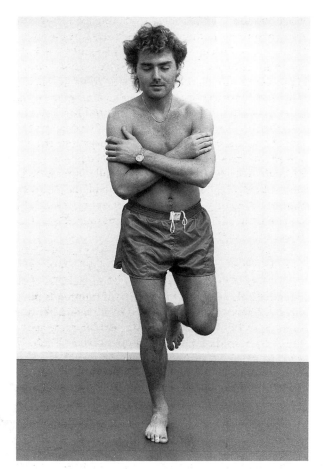

Fig. 17.1 Analysis of functional instability of the ankle joints (modified Romberg test). The player stands on one leg with the other leg raised and flexed at the knee, the arms folded across the chest and the eyes closed.

the ground. Correction movements of the standing leg are allowed. If the player fails to stand for 60 s (three attempts are allowed), he or she is considered to have functional instability and should be recommended ankle disk training (see below).

Test of the knee joint

Measurement of range of movement (ROM) and clinical instability, such as the anterior drawer test or Lachmann test, are used for the evaluation of sagittal stability. They can be complemented by objective measurement by using a laxity tester. A player with an insufficient

anterior cruciate ligament (ACL) knee is usually unable to continue football and should be recommended a reconstruction of the ACL (Ekstrand 1989a,b).

Test of the hip joint

Coxarthrosis should be excluded by clinical examination, i.e. analysis of rotation.

Malalignment test

Screening for malalignments or other possible biomechanical risk factors for overuse injuries, should be included in the physical examination. Examples of malalignments include: pes cavus, pes planus, Q-angle over 20°, limb length discrepancy, soft heel pads, etc. The use of a mirror-box facilitates the analysis (Fig. 17.2).

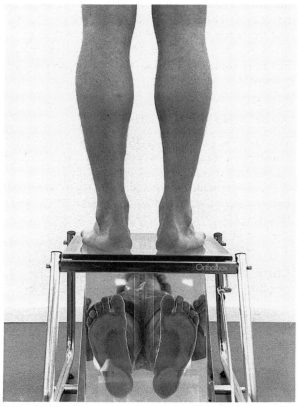

Fig. 17.2 The mirror-box for the screening of malalignments of the lower extremity.

Measurement of ROM

To disclose muscular tightness of the lower extremity, a pre-season examination should include measurement of six movements of the lower extremity:

1 Hip flexion with the knee straight.
2 Hip extension.
3 Hip abduction.
4 Knee flexion lying prone.
5 Ankle dorsiflexion with the knee straight.
6 Ankle dorsiflexion with the knee bent.

In the absence of coxarthrosis, gonarthrosis, and neurologic disease, these movements are thought to be limited by muscles and ligaments, and to be restricted in the presence of muscular tightness of the hamstrings, iliopsoas, adductors, rectus femoris, gastrocnemius, and soleus.

Commonly used clinical methods for ROM measurement have a measurement error of 7–10%, and showed that the accuracy of measurement could be improved (measurement error < 2%) by the use of goniometers and by secure fixation and marking of anatomical landmarks (Ekstrand et al. 1982). Players with muscle tightness are recommended stretching exercises (see below).

Measurement of muscle strength

The maximal muscle strength of the knee extensor (quadriceps) and the knee flexor (hamstrings) muscles can be measured with great accuracy by using an isokinetic dynamometer. In the absence of such devices muscle strength can be evaluated by using functional tests such as the one-leg long-jump (Tegner 1985) or vertical jump (Gauffin 1991).

Correction of training, warming up, cooling down, and stretching techniques

Football players are in general less flexible than non-football players of the same age (Ekstrand et al. 1982). There is a correlation between muscle tightness with strains and tendinitis (Ekstrand et al. 1983a).

The muscle tightness observed in football players is probably correlated to the design of football training. In a field study it was found that the duration of warm-up was adequate but its content was not optimal (Ekstrand et al. 1983b). Since 90% of football injuries affect the lower extremities, stretching exercises for the leg muscles (adductors, hamstrings, quadriceps, iliopsoas, and triceps surae) should be included in the warm-up and cool-down exercises. A special warm-up program with contract–relax stretching for the legs combined with a cool-down program after training has been devised. Möller et al. (1985) found that this program increased ROM by 5–20%. Players with muscle tightness detected by ROM measurement at pre-season examination, should be recommended individual stretching exercises as well. Other corrections of training design are also valuable in reducing injuries. Shooting at goal before warm-up should be avoided since it increases the risk of muscle strains (Ekstrand 1982).

Planning of the football season is also of importance. Ekstrand et al. (1983b) found a correlation between team success and the amount of training which would seem logical, provided the quality of training is adequate. They also found a curved relationship between injuries and training; teams with less than average training showed an increase in the number of injuries with increased training, probably the result of prolonged exposure. It was found, however, that teams with more than average training sustain fewer injuries with increased training, probably a reflection of the well-known fact that well-trained athletes sustain fewer injuries. Another important aspect of the planning of a season is that a high practice–game ratio seems to be beneficial with a tendency toward better performance with fewer injuries.

Ankle taping, bracing, and disk training

Ankle sprains are common in football (Ekstrand 1982, Tropp 1985) mostly affecting joints with a previous history of sprain. Several methods for prevention of ankle sprains have been documented (Ekstrand 1982, Tropp et al. 1985). Based on findings at the pre-season examination it is recommended that players with mechanical instability of the ankle joints are selected for taping or bracing and players with functional instability (FI) are selected for ankle disk training.

Ankle taping

Prophylactic taping has become one of the main methods to prevent ankle sprains. The mechanism behind the effect of taping is not fully understood. It is assumed that external support increases ankle stability by re-inforcing the ligaments and restricting motions such as extreme inversion (Fumich *et al.* 1981, Tropp 1985). A neuromuscular reflex mechanism has also been proposed (Boland & Glick 1981).

Another question to be answered is, who should be taped, by whom, and by which method? Ekstrand *et al.* (1983b) showed good results by selecting players with mechanical instability for taping, letting the coach, trainer, or doctor tape the players before games using a "stirrup and horseshoe technique" followed by a figure of eight lock around the heel, and let the players tape themselves before practise sessions using only stirrups and horseshoes. The reasoning behind this procedure was the finding that match injuries are twice as common as practise injuries (Ekstrand 1982).

Ankle bracing

Since ankle taping is expensive and the technique can be difficult to learn, an alternative to ankle taping would be valuable for players with mechanical insta-bility (Tropp *et al.* 1985). Various functional semi-rigid ankle braces are available and semi-rigid supports have been found effective in restricting ankle inversion and reducing the risk of ankle sprain (Stover 1979, Tropp *et al.* 1985). Some players, however, may complain of discomfort from the use of ankle braces.

Ankle disk training

The most common residual disability after ankle sprain is FI. Tropp (1985) found impaired postural control and pronator muscle weakness to be correlated to FI. Players with FI are predisposed to recurrent ankle sprain (Tropp 1985). Impaired postural control and pronator muscle weakness as well as the subjective feeling of instability can be improved by co-ordination training on an ankle disk.

The exercises are performed on an ankle disk, which is a section of a sphere (Fig. 17.3), the supporting leg being held straight and the other leg flexed at the knee. The arms should be folded across the chest.

The recommended dose and duration of training is 5 min for each leg, 5 days a week, for 10 weeks (Tropp 1985). In players with a history of ankle problems, ankle disk training seems to be the method of choice

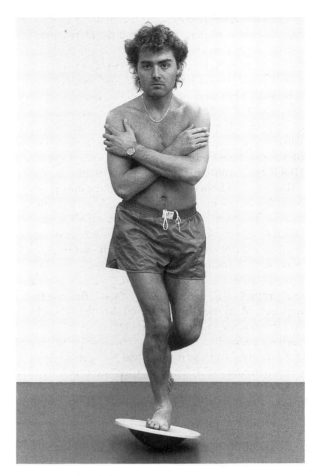

Fig. 17.3 Ankle disk training. The exercise is performed on an ankle disk which is a section of a sphere, the supporting leg being held straight and the other leg flexed at the knee. The arms should be folded across the chest.

because it diminishes FI and breaks the vicious circle of recurrent sprain and subsequent atrophy (Tropp 1985). After an initial sprain, further ankle disk train-ing is indicated even if the player is able to return to football play, because of the increased risk of re-injury. This may prevent residual disability and injury pre-disposition (Tropp 1985).

Equipment and playing surface

The value of optimum equipment in injury prevention

has been stressed (Ekstrand 1982, Hoerner & Vinger 1986, Hlobil *et al.* 1987). Shin guards, shoes, and insoles are important in football. It has been demonstrated that shock-absorbent, anatomically shaped shin guards, protecting a large area of the lower leg, can prevent injuries to the shin bone in football players (Ekstrand 1982). The variety of football shoes available is enormous. When selecting footwear it should be realized that there is interaction between the foot and the shoe and between the shoe and the playing surface (Hlobil *et al.* 1987, Ekstrand & Nigg 1989).

High friction between shoe and surface may produce excessive forces on the knees and ankles; too little friction, however, may be the reason for slipping, which affects performance negatively and may cause injuries (Ekstrand & Nigg 1989). Frictional resistance must be held within an optimum range.

Furthermore, it is generally assumed that the stiffness properties of the playing surface influence the frequency of injuries. It is assumed that "hard" surfaces are associated with more injuries than "soft" and "well-cushioned" surfaces. The stiffness properties of a surface might have an influence on some chronic overuse injuries which account for about one-third of all football injuries (Ekstrand & Nigg 1989). Overuse injuries can be avoided or reduced by adequate training, gradual adaption to a new surface, by the use of appropriate insoles and suitable football shoes (Jörgensen 1989), and by adapting the movement to the surface.

Rehabilitation

Incomplete rehabilitation following a sports injury is a causal factor in the recurrence of sports injuries. In a prospective study of football players Ekstrand (1982) found that 17% of the injuries were attributable to inadequate rehabilitation. Rehabilitation following a football injury is commonly neglected, yet few injuries sustained by football players are so trivial that no form of rehabilitation is necessary.

A rehabilitation program should be sports-specific, gradually increasing the stress on the injured leg, and step-by-step adaptation for the player before return to play. Return to games and practise should be decided by the doctor and physiotherapist, and a full, pain-free ROM, the regaining of co-ordination and more than 90% of muscle strength should be mandatory. In this way, "controlled rehabilitation" can reduce the number of football injuries (Ekstrand 1982).

Information and supervision

Many authors regard lack of information regarding the causes of sports injuries as a factor in their occurrence and the provision of information as an important factor in their prevention. In football, information should be given to coaches and players about:
1 The importance of disciplined play and the risk of serious own-foul injuries (Ekstrand 1982).
2 The increased incidence of injury at training camps and how to avoid such injury (Ekstrand 1982).
3 The importance of the use of protective equipment and other individual protective measures (Hlobil *et al.* 1987).
Furthermore, supervision by doctors and physiotherapists is an important part of the prophylactic program.

References

Blyth C.S. & Mueller F.D. (1974) Football injury survey. *Phys. Sports Med.* **9**, 45−52.

Boland A.J. & Glick J. (1981) Editorial comment. *Am. J. Sports Med.* **9**, 316−317.

Ekstrand J. (1982) *Soccer injuries and their prevention.* Medical dissertation No. 130, Linköping University, Sweden.

Ekstrand J. (1989a) Reconstruction of the anterior cruciate ligament in athletes, using a fascia lata graft: a review with preliminary results of a new concept. *Int. J. Sports Med.* **1**, 225−232.

Ekstrand J. (1989b) Reconstruction of the anterior cruciate ligament in soccer players. *J. Sci. Football* **2**, 19−27.

Ekstrand J. & Gillquist J. (1983a) The avoidability of soccer injuries. *Int. J. Sports Med.* **2**, 124−128.

Ekstrand J. & Gillquist J. (1983b) Soccer injuries and their mechanisms: a prospective study. *Med. Sci. Sports Exerc.* **15**, 267−270.

Ekstrand J., Gillquist J. & Liljedahl S.O. (1983a) Prevention of soccer injuries. Supervision by doctors and physiotherapists. *Am. J. Sports Med.* **11**, 116−120.

Ekstrand J., Gillquist J., Möller M., Öberg B. & Liljedahl S.O. (1983b) Incidence of soccer injuries and their relation to training and team success. *Am. J. Sports Med.* **11**, 63−67.

Ekstrand J. & Nigg B. (1989) Surface-related injuries in soccer. *Sports Med.* **8**, 56−62.

Ekstrand J., Wiktorsson M., Öberg B. & Gillquist J. (1982) Lower extremity goniometric measurements: a study to determine their rehability. *Arch. Phys. Med. Rehab.* **63**, 171–175.

Franke K. (1977) *Traumatologie des Sports* (Traumatology of Sports). VEB Verlag, Volk und Gesundheit, Berlin.

Fumich R.M., Ellison A.E., Guerin G.J. & Grace P.D. (1981) The measured effect of taping on combined foot and ankle motion before and after exercise. *Am. J. Sports Med.* **9**, 165–170.

Gauffin H. (1991) *Knee and ankle kinesiology and joint instability*. Medical dissertation No. 331, Linköping University, Sweden.

Hlobil H., van Mechelen W. & Kemper H.C.G. (1987) *How Can Sports Injuries be Prevented?* WISGZ Publication No. 25E, Medical Faculty, University of Amsterdam, the Netherlands.

Hoerner E.F. & Vinger P.F. (1986) Protective equipment: its value, capabilities and limitations. In Vinger P.F. & Hoerner E.F. (eds) *Sports Injuries*, 2nd edn, pp. 375–376. PSG Publishing, Littleton, Massachusetts.

Jörgensen U. (1984) Epidemiology of injuries in typical Scandinavian team sports. *Br. J. Sports Med.* **18**, 59–63.

Jörgensen U. (1989) *Implications of heel strike — an anatomical, physiological and clinical study with focus on the heel pad*. Medical dissertation No. 284, Linköping University, Sweden.

Möller M., Ekstrand J., Öberg B. & Gillquist J. (1985) Duration of stretching effect on range of motion in lower extremities. *Arch. Phys. Med. Rehab.* **66**, 171–173.

Stover G.N. (1979) A functional semi-rigid support system for ankle injuries. *Phys. Sports Med.* **7**, 71–81.

Tegner Y. (1985) *Cruciate ligament injuries in the knee. Evaluation and rehabilitation*. Medical dissertation No. 203, Linköping University, Sweden.

Tropp H. (1985) *Functional instability of the ankle joint*. Medical dissertation No. 202, Linköping University, Sweden.

Tropp H., Askling C. & Gillquist J. (1985) Prevention of ankle sprains. *Am. J. Sports Med.* **13**, 259–262.

Further reading

Albert M. (1983) Descriptive three year data stady of outdoor and indoor professional soccer injuries. *Athl. Train.* **18**, 218–220.

Brynhildsen J., Ekstrand J., Jeppsson A. & Tropp H. (1990) Previous injuries and persisting symptoms in female soccer players. *Int. J. Sports Med.* **11**, 489–492.

Brynhildsen J., Tropp H. & Ekstrand J. (1994) Injuries in women's soccer — a prospective study. *Am. J. Sports Med.* submitted.

Ekstrand J. & Gillquist J. (1982) The frequency of muscle tightness and injuries in soccer players. *Am. J. Sports Med.* **10**, 75–78.

Keller C.S., Noyes F.R. & Buncher C.R. (1987) The medical aspects of soccer injury epidemiology. *Am. J. Sports Med.* **15**, 105–112.

Kraus J.F. & Burg F.D. (1970) Injury reporting and recording. *J. Am. Med. Assoc.* **213**(3), 438–444.

Nilsson S. & Roaas A. (1978) Soccer injuries in adolescents. *Am. J. Sports Med.* **6**, 358–361.

Pardon E.T. (1977) Lower extremities are the site of most soccer injuries. *Phys. Sports Med.* **6**, 43–48.

Sullivan J.A., Gross R.H. & Grana W.A. (1980) Evaluation of injuries in youth soccer. *Am. J. Sports Med.* **8**, 325–327.

Chapter 18
Doping

Much has been said and written during the past few years about the problem of doping in sport. Indeed, no sport can consider itself immune from this scourge. The responsible bodies within the international organizations (FIFA and UEFA) have been well aware of the problem, especially since some major doping cases have filled the media since the last two Olympic Games. In 1979, UEFA set up a committee with the aim of handling the doping problem, how it could be controlled at matches as well as suggest sanctions in cases proved positive. The basic purpose should be to ensure that doping checks were carried out in order that the ban on doping, as contained in the competition regulations, was properly respected.

FIFA, for its part, had already gathered experience at three World Cups. The question of sanctions has always been a particularly difficult issue, since the first round of the European club competitions includes 64 matches in all UEFA member countries.

The problem was systematically solved by first introducing doping controls at the matches directly organized by UEFA, such as club cup finals and the finals of the European Championship along the same lines as the FIFA checks. The number of controls was thereafter subsequently expanded to cover other games too, so that at present controls at random at a certain number of matches of the European Cup competitions and the qualifying matches for the European and World Championships are carried out.

Above all, any tendency to allow a certain liberty in doping has been categorically rejected including references to the freedom of the individual. For sport has not only ethical constraints but also rules of the game part of which concern doping controls. Anybody failing to respect these rules should be punished by the Control and Disciplinary Committee.

Doping control regulations

The use of banned substances and the taking of such substances before or during a game with the intention of artificially improving a player's mental or physical condition, or the attempt by third parties to cause or have caused the use of such substances is to be considered as doping. Offenders in the presence of the necessary evidence are to be punished. The list of banned substances contains substances which are particularly dangerous or harmful for the human body and which may be detected by the prescribed analytical methods and thus kept under control. The banned substance list is brought up to date every year, in accordance with the list maintained by the International Olympic Committee (IOC) — see Appendix 18.1.

On the basis of the rules, UEFA and FIFA can principally carry out doping controls at any match of its competitions. Ninety minutes before kick-off the team physician has to give the official game delegate a physician's certificate which lists all the medications prescribed to that team's players over the past 48 h with exact details of the name of the medication and of its producers. This system makes the team doctors more aware of what they are prescribing and also guards against negligent use of medication by physiotherapists and by the players themselves.

Two players per team are always drawn by lot 15 min before the end of the game for doping control under the supervision of the doping medical doctor. More players may also be individually selected by the UEFA or FIFA delegate, the referee or the doping control medical physician. The players whose names are drawn for the checks have to report to the doping control room within 30 min after the game, bringing with them their identity cards and the red forms given to them by the doping control medical doctor. The doping controls take place according to international norms and in specially designated rooms with the necessary sanitary installations. All players are obliged to give full information about any medications taken before or during the game, or to indicate whether they have been given any medications by third parties. They must all undergo whatever medical examination the doping control medical doctor considers necessary.

Players are always obliged to give urine for test

analysis. The player must be allowed his or her own choice of vessel for urine delivery, glass flasks for sample storage and containers for sample shipment from among a number of each of these items:

1 The player must be informed that any items of equipment that may be used for receiving or holding urine samples must be properly cleaned prior to such use.

2 The player has the right to clean the vessels before delivering a sample.

3 Players delivering urine samples must comply with the provisions concerning dress and urine delivery must be monitored.

4 The player must deliver not less than 60 ml of urine into the vessel.

5 Each urine sample must be distributed between two bottles (A and B). Each bottle must be marked with an indelible number and the transfer of the sample into the flasks may be operated by the player.

6 The numbers marked on the bottles and containers must tally with the entry in the corresponding verification forms.

It must be emphasized that tests may not be conducted in the absence of the persons authorized to officiate at these tests. Tests should not be conducted unless acceptable standards or cleanliness are ensured. Seals, including lead seals, should be applied or fastened to the urine containers in such way that subsequent manipulation is ruled out. The athletes should inspect the seals. Players have rights as well as obligations. They may be accompanied by their own team physician and may check the whole doping control procedure right through to the sealing of the samples at which point the player and the team physician may sign a note of confirmation. The doping control medical physician then gives the player a form with a code number for the sample bottles and the transportation package. In principle, it is the doping control medical physician or his or her assistant who delivers the samples to the analyzing laboratory. The urine samples are personally handed over to the head of the laboratory who signs a note to confirm that the seals have not been broken. Thus any accusations are ruled out.

However, manipulation may occur during a test, say by serving refreshments or by a third party putting doping agents into the vessels used for urine delivery. Players should therefore abstain from drinking any

beverages unless they are factory-bottled and served with the bottle caps intact. They should also keep a watchful eye on the vessels holding their samples.

On completion of the test, the player and the persons accompanying them are required to acknowledge compliance with the rules by signing the test protocol. In the event that the test was not carried out in compliance with the rules, complaints if any should be entered in the test protocol. The samples must be analysed by a laboratory accredited by the IOC. These laboratories are subject to permanent monitoring by the IOC Medical Committee and are thus guaranteed to conduct the analyses properly and produce accurate results.

The cost of the analysis amounts to about 300 DM per individual, thus a total cost of about 1200 DM per game (1992 figures).

A finding is not considered to be positive unless and until the analysis of sample B has yielded results matching the results obtained from sample A. Sample B may be analyzed in the presence of the player concerned and/or any persons authorized to represent him or her (i.e. a national association or sports organization). Sample A and B may be analysed by the same laboratory, with the proviso that operatives involved in the analysis of sample A may not analyse sample B.

Sanctions

Sanctions are applied if the use of a doping agent has been established beyond reasonable doubt (if sample B is positive). Any person who invites players to use banned substances or encourages or promotes doping and any person who buys and sells banned substances for use in doping is liable to be punished. The national sports organizations, the international sports federations, and the governments have special responsibility in the struggle against doping. In order to increase the responsibility of the above-mentioned bodies, it is important to:

1 Stop the illegal trade with doping substances.

2 Limit the availability of banned drugs.

3 Enforce the athletes' motivations to renounce the use of doping.

In this field the IOC, international federations, national associations, and governmental bodies have developed many activities for improving the present situation. In this connection the working group "Antidoping" of the European Sport Conference shows special activities in applying the various groups of people as there are athletes, coaches, physicians, masseurs, physiotherapists, the parents of young athletes as well as students of medicine and physical education by means of adequate educational programs.

Physicians working in the field of sport, must always be aware of the fact they have a high responsibility in the struggle against doping.

Appendix 18.1: IOC doping list (1993)

I Doping classes

A Stimulants, e.g.

Amfepramone
Amfetaminil
Amineptine
Amiphenazole
Amphetamine
Bemigride
Benzphetamine
Caffeine*
Cathine
Chlorphentermine
Clobenzorex
Clorprenaline
Cocaine
Cropropamide ⎫
Crotethamide ⎭ (component of "micoren")
Dimetamfetamine
Ephedrine
Etafedrine
Ethamivan
Etilamfetamine
Fencamfamin
Fenetylline
Fenproporex
Furfenorex
Mefenorex
Mesocarbe
Methamphetamine
Methoxyphenamine
Methylephedrine

* Caffeine: a sample is defined as positive if the concentration in the urine exceeds $12\,\mu g \cdot ml^{-1}$.

Methylphenidate
Morazone
Nikethamide
Pemoline
Pentetrazol
Phendimetrazine
Phenmetrazine
Phentermine
Phenylpropanolamine
Pipradol
Prolintane
Propylhexedrine
Pyrovalerone
Strychnine
and related compounds

β_2 *agonists.* The use of only the following β_2 agonists is permitted in the aerosol form:
Salbutamol
Terbutaline

The following β_2 agonists are prohibited:
Bitolterol
Orciprenaline
Rimiterol

B Narcotic analgesics, e.g.

Alphaprodine
Anileridine
Buprenorphine
Dextromoramide
Dextropropoxyphene (di-antalvic)
Diamorphine (heroin)
Dihydrocodeine
Dipipanone
Ethoheptazine
Ethylmorphine
Levorphanol
Methadone
Morphine
Nalbuphine
Pentazocine
Pethidine
Phenazocine
Trimeperidine
and related compounds

Codein is permitted for therapeutic use.

C Anabolic agents

C1 Androgenic anabolic steroids

Bolasterone
Boldenone
Clostebol
Dehydrochlormethyltestosterone
Fluoxymesterone
Mesterolone
Metandienone
Metenolone
Methyltestosterone
Nandrolone
Norethandrolone
Oxandrolone
Oxymesterone
Oxymetholone
Stanozolol
Testosterone*
and related compounds

C2 Other anabolic agents, e.g.

Clenbuterol

D Diuretics, e.g.

Acetazolamide
Amiloride
Bendroflumethiazide
Benzthiazide
Bumetanide
Canrenone
Chlormerodrin
Chlortalidone
Diclofenamide
Ethacrynic acid
Furosemide
Hydrochlorothiazide
Mersalyl
Spironolactone
Triamterene
and related compounds

* Testosterone: a sample is defined as positive if the
administration of this substance, or its application by any
other means, causes the ratio of the total concentration of
testosterone to that of epitestosterone in the urine to above
six.

E Peptide hormones and related substances

Human chorionic gonadotrophin (HCG): it is well
known that the administration to males of HCG and
other compounds with related activity leads to an
increased rate of production of endogenous androgenic
steroids and is considered equivalent to the exogenous
administration of testosterone.

Corticotrophin (ACTH) has been misused to increase
the blood levels of endogenous corticosteroids notably
to obtain the euphoric effect of corticosteroids. The
application of corticotrophin is considered to be equivalent to the oral, intramuscular, or intravenous application of corticosteroids (see Section IIID on
corticosteroids).

Growth hormone (HGH, somatotrophin): the misuse
of growth hormone in sport is deemed to be unethical
and dangerous because of various adverse effects, for
example, allergic reactions, diabetogenic effects,
and acromegaly when applied in high doses. All the
respective releasing factors of the above-mentioned
substances are also banned.

Erythropoietin (EPO) is the glucoprotein hormone
produced in human kidney which regulates, apparently by a feedback mechanism, the rate of synthesis
of erythrocite.

II Methods

A Blood doping

Blood transfusion is the intravenous administration of
red blood cells or related blood products that contain
red blood cells. Such products can be obtained from
blood drawn from the same (autologous) or from a
different (non-autologous) individual. The most common indications for red blood transfusion in conventional medical practice are acute blood loss and severe
anemia.

Blood doping is the administration of blood or
related red blood products to an athlete other than for
legitimate medical treatment. This procedure may be
preceded by withdrawal of blood from the athlete who
continues to train in this blood-depleted state.

These procedures contravene the ethics of medicine
and of sport. There are also risks involved in the transfusion of blood and related blood products. These
include the development of allergic reactions (rash,

fever, etc.) and acute hemolytic reaction with kidney damage if incorrectly typed blood is used, as well as delayed transfusion reaction resulting in fever and jaundice, transmission of infectious diseases (viral hepatitis and AIDS), overload of the circulation and metabolic shock. Therefore the practise of blood doping in sport is banned by the IOC Medical Commission. The UEFA Medical Committee bans erythropoietin as method of doping (see Section IE on peptide hormones and related substances).

B Pharmacological, chemical, and physical manipulation

The UEFA Medical Committee bans the use of substances and of methods which alter the integrity and validity of urine samples used in doping controls. Examples of banned methods are catherization, urine substitution, and/or tampering, inhibition of renal excretion, e.g. by probenecid and related compounds.

III Classes of drugs subject to certain restrictions

A Alcohol

Alcohol is not prohibited. However, breath or blood alcohol levels may be determined at the request of an International Federation.

B Marijuana

Marijuana is not prohibited. However, tests may be carried out at the request of an International Federation.

C Local anesthetics

Injectable local anesthetics are permitted under the following conditions:
1 That procaine, xylocaine, carbocaine, etc. are used but not cocaine.
2 Only local or intra-articular injections may be administered.
3 Only when medically justified (i.e. the details including diagnosis; dose and route of administration must be submitted immediately in writing to the UEFA Medical Committee).

D Corticosteroids

The naturally occurring and synthetic corticosteroids are mainly used as anti-inflammatory drugs which also relieve pain. They influence circulating concentrations of natural corticosteroids in the body. They produce euphoria and side-effects such that their medical use, except when used topically, require medical control. Since 1975, the IOC Medical Commission has attempted to restrict their use during competitions by requiring a declaration by team physicians; because it is known that corticosteroids are being used non-therapeutically by the intramuscular and even the intravenous route in some sports.

However, the problem was not solved by these restrictions and therefore stronger measures designed not to interfere with the appropriate medical use of these compounds became necessary.

The use of corticosteroids is banned except for topical use (aural, ophthalmological and dermatological), inhalational therapy (asthma, allergic rhinitis) and local or intra-articular injections.

Any team physician wishing to administer corticosteroids intra-articularly or locally to a competitor must give written notification to the UEFA Medical Committee.

E β blockers, e.g.

Acebutolol
Alprenolol
Atenolol
Labetalol
Metoprolol
Nadolol
Oxprenolol
Propranolol
Sotalol
and related compounds

Prior notice must be given in the case of therapeutic use.

Index